MEDICAL
REHABILITATION

MEDICAL REHABILITATION

EDITED BY

John V. Basmajian, M.D., F.A.C.A., F.R.C.P.(C.)

McMaster University and Chedoke Rehabilitation Centre
Chedoke-McMaster Hospitals
Hamilton, Ontario, Canada

R. Lee Kirby, M.D., F.R.C.P.(C.)

Dalhousie University and Nova Scotia Rehabilitation Centre
Halifax, Nova Scotia, Canada

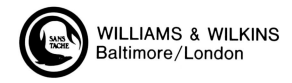

WILLIAMS & WILKINS
Baltimore/London

Editor: George Stamathis
Associate Editor: Victoria M. Vaughn
Copy Editor: Stephen Siegforth
Design: Joanne Janowiak
Illustration Planning: Lorraine Wrzosek
Production: Carol L. Eckhart

Accurate indications, adverse reactions, and dosage schedules for drugs are provided in this book, but it is possible that they may change. The reader is urged to review the package information data of the manufacturers of the medications mentioned.

Copyright © 1984
Williams & Wilkins
428 E. Preston Street
Baltimore, MD 21202, U.S.A.

Made in the United States of America

Library of Congress Cataloging in Publication Data

Main entry under title:

Medical rehabilitation.

Includes index.
1. Physical therapy. 2. Rehabilitation. I. Basmajian, John V., 1921–. II. Kirby, R. Lee. RM701.M4 1984   615.5   83-9054
ISBN 0-683-00415-8

Composed and printed at the
Waverly Press, Inc.
Mt. Royal and Guilford Aves.
Baltimore, Md 21202, U.S.A.

Preface

Medical rehabilitation has grown and changed rapidly in the past two decades. Specialized books now abound on subjects covering a spectrum from electrodiagnosis, through neurological diseases, to musculoskeletal problems, which are useful for teaching residents or for reference. Surprisingly, teachers of medical undergraduates and other health professionals with overlapping interests have not had a suitable textbook which adequately covers medical rehabilitation for nonspecialists. This book attempts to correct that situation.

We, the editors, first agreed that broad and authoritative views were necessary, combined with tight organization of the profuse materials available. To achieve breadth and authority we needed a large number of specialists with a clear idea of our aims. Outstanding leaders in rehabilitation throughout North America and abroad responded generously to our requests for contributions despite tight constraints on content and space necessitated by the intended audience. Our authors deserve all the thanks and praise that we the editors and you the readers can heap on them. The publishers have been very cooperative and equally enthusiastic; we owe them special thanks, too.

This book should be useful throughout the clinical years of undergraduate education. It is aimed at all medical students, regardless of their subsequent career plans. While we have avoided producing a book for specialists, nevertheless we expect that residents and staffs in physical medicine and rehabilitation, rheumatology, neurology, orthopedics, and plastic and neurological surgery, as well as nonmedical members of the rehabilitation team, will find much of value in these pages.

In such a condensed text, particularly in its first edition, one treads a fine line between excessive terseness and oversimplification, and also runs the risk of omitting important material. We would welcome suggestions from students, teachers, and reviewers as to how this work might be improved.

John V. Basmajian
McMaster University
R. Lee Kirby
Dalhousie University
1983

Contributors

Michael A. Alexander, M.D.
Pediatrician/Physiatrist, Children's Hospital of Pittsburgh, Pittsburgh, Pennsylvania

Thomas P. Anderson, M.D.
Professor of Physical Medicine and Rehabilitation, University of Minnesota Medical School, Minneapolis, Minnesota

Essam A. Awad, M.D., Ph.D.
Clinical Professor of Physical Medicine and Rehabilitation, University of Minnesota Medical School, Minneapolis, Minnesota; Director, Department of Physical Medicine and Rehabilitation, United Hospitals, St. Paul, Minnesota

Sikhar N. Banerjee, M.B., B.S., F.R.C.P.(C.)
Associate Professor of Medicine (Rehabilitation Medicine), McMaster University School of Medicine; Director, Amputee Program, Rehabilitation Centre, Chedoke-McMaster Hospitals, Hamilton, Ontario, Canada

John V. Basmajian, M.D., F.A.C.A., F.R.C.P.(C.)
Professor of Medicine (Rehabilitation Medicine), McMaster University School of Medicine, Director of Rehabilitation Programs, Rehabilitation Centre, Chedoke-McMaster Hospitals, Hamilton, Ontario, Canada

Leonard F. Bender, M.D., M.S.
President and Chief Executive Officer, Rehabilitation Institute; Professor and Chairman, Department of Physical Medicine and Rehabilitation, Wayne State University School of Medicine, Detroit, Michigan

Sheldon Berrol, M.D.
Associate Clinical Professor, University of California, San Francisco; Chief, Rehabilitation Medicine, San Francisco General Hospital, San Francisco, California

Duane S. Bishop, M.D., F.R.C.P.(C.)
Associate Professor of Psychiatry, Brown University; Clinical Director, Butler Hospital, Providence, Rhode Island

Murray E. Brandstater, M.D., Ph.D., F.R.C.P.(C.)
Professor of Medicine (Rehabilitation Medicine), McMaster University School of Medicine; Director, Stroke Program, Rehabilitation Centre, Chedoke-McMaster Hospitals, Hamilton, Ontario, Canada

René Cailliet, M.D.
Professor and Chairman, Department of Rehabilitation Medicine, University of Southern California School of Medicine; Director, Department of Rehabilitation Medicine, Los Angeles County-U.S.C. Medical Center, Los Angeles, California

Jacqueline L. Claus-Walker, Ph.D.
Associate Professor, Department of Rehabilitation and Physiology, Baylor College of Medicine; Director, Neuroendocrine Laboratory, Institute for Rehabilitation and Research, Houston, Texas

Sam C. Colachis, Jr., M.D.
Director, Physical Medicine and Rehabilitation, St. Luke's Hospital Medical Center, Phoenix, Arizona

Sandra S. Cole, A.C.S.E., A.C.S.C.
Departments of Psychiatry and Physical Medicine and Rehabilitation, University of Michigan Medical School, Ann Arbor, Michigan

Theodore M. Cole, M.D.
Professor and Chairman, Department of Physical Medicine and Rehabilitation, University of Michigan and University Hospital, Ann Arbor, Michigan

John Darracott, M.B., B.S., Dip. Phys. Med., F.R.C.P.(C.)
Associate Professor of Medicine (Rehabilitation Medicine), McMaster University, Hamilton, Ontario, Canada

Barbara J. de Lateur
Professor, Department of Rehabilitation Medicine, University of Washington School of Medicine, Seattle, Washington

Steven V. Fisher, M.D.
Assistant Professor, University of Minnesota; Staff Physician, Department of Physical Medicine and Rehabilitation and Consulting Physician, Regional Burn Center, St. Paul-Ramsey Medical Center, St. Paul, Minnesota

Wilbert E. Fordyce, Ph.D.
Professor, Department of Rehabilitation Medicine and Pain Service, School of Medicine, University of Washington, Seattle, Washington

Charles M. Godfrey, M.D., F.R.C.P.(C.)
Professor, Department of Rehabilitation Medicine, University of Toronto Faculty of Medicine; Director of Rehabilitation Medicine, Wellesley Hospital, Toronto, Ontario, Canada

Lauro S. Halstead, M.D.
Associate Professor, Department of Rehabilitation, Community, and Physical Medicine, Baylor College of Medicine; Attending Physician, Institute for Rehabilitation and Research, Houston, Texas

Thomas G. Kantor, M.D.
Professor of Clinical Medicine, New York University School of Medicine, New York, New York

Terence Kavanagh, M.D., Dip. Phys. Med., F.C.C.P., F.R.C.P.(C.)
Medical Director, Toronto Rehabilitation Centre; Associate Professor, Department of Rehabilitation Medicine, University of Toronto Faculty of Medicine, Toronto, Ontario, Canada

Ali A. Khalili, M.D.
Director of Physical Medicine and Rehabilitation, Grant Hospital, Chicago, Illinois

R. Lee Kirby, M.D., F.R.C.P.(C.)
Associate Professor of Medicine (Physical Medicine and Rehabilitation), Dalhousie University, Halifax, Nova Scotia, Canada

George H. Kraft, M.D.
Professor, Department of Rehabilitation Medicine, University of Washington School of Medicine, Seattle, Washington

Janice C. Ledebur, L.P.T.
Department Head of Physical Therapy and Rehabilitation, Geriatrics Center, Philadelphia, Pennsylvania

John Leszczynski, M.B., Ch.B., F.R.C.P.(C.)
Professor and Head, Department of Rehabilitation Medicine, University of Saskatchewan, Saskatoon, Saskatchewan, Canada

D. Duncan Murray, M.D., F.R.C.P.(C.)
Associate Professor and Head, Division of Rehabilitation Medicine, University of British Columbia; Head, Department of Rehabilitation Medicine, Shaughnessy Hospital, Vancouver, British Columbia, Canada

Francis Naso, M.D., F.A.C.P.
Professor of Rehabilitation Medicine and Assistant Professor of Medicine, Thomas Jefferson University; Physiatrist, Department of Rehabilitation Medicine, Thomas Jefferson University Hospital, Philadelphia, Pennsylvania

Farhad Nowroozi, M.D.
Assistant Professor, Physical Medicine and Rehabilitation, University of California, Irvine Medical Center, Orange, California

Don A. Olson, Ph.D.
Director of Education and Training, Rehabilitation Institute of Chicago; Associate Professor, Departments of Neurology and Rehabilitation Medicine, Northwestern University Medical School, Chicago, Illinois

Bernard Posner
Executive Director, President's Committee on Employment of the Handicapped, Washington, D.C.

John B. Redford, M.D.
Professor and Chairman, Department of Rehabilitation Medicine, College of Health Sciences and Hospital, University of Kansas, Kansas City, Kansas

Mary D. Romano, M.S.W.
Assistant Director, Department of Social Work Services, Presbyterian Hospital, New York, New York

Bhagwan T. Shahani, M.D., D. Phil. (Oxon)
Associate Professor, Department of Neurology, Harvard Medical School and Massachusetts General Hospital, Boston, Massachusetts

David G. Simons, M.D.
Clinical Professor, Department of Physical Medicine, University of California, Irvine; Chief, EMG and Electrodiagnostic Section, Veterans' Administration Center, Long Beach, California

Walter C. Stolov, M.D.
Professor, Department of Rehabilitation Medicine, University of Washington School of Medicine, Seattle, Washington

Samuel L. Stover, M.D.
Professor and Chairman, Department of Rehabilitation Medicine, University of Alabama in Birmingham School of Medicine, Birmingham, Alabama

Thomas E. Strax, M.D.
Assistant Medical Director, Moss Rehabilitation Hospital; Associate Professor, Rehabilitation Medicine, Temple University School of Medicine; Consultant, Geriatrics Center, Philadelphia, Pennsylvania

Robert L. Swezey, M.D.
Medical Director, Arthritis and Back Pain Center Inc., Santa Monica, California; Clinical Professor of Medicine, UCLA School of Medicine, Los Angeles, California

Perry S. Tepperman, B.Sc., M.D., F.R.C.P.(C.)
Assistant Professor, Department of Rehabilitation Medicine, Faculty of Medicine, University of Toronto; Staff Physician, Mt. Sinai and Baycrest Hospitals, Toronto, Ontario, Canada

Michael S. Weiss, M.D.
Assistant Professor, Department of Physical Medicine and Rehabilitation, University of Wisconsin, Madison, Wisconsin

David O. Wiechers, M.D.
Assistant Professor, Department of Physical Medicine, Ohio State University, Columbus, Ohio

Philip H. N. Wood, F.R.C.P., F.F.C.M.
Director, Arthritis and Rheumatism, Epidemiology Research Unit, Honorary Reader in Community Medicine, University of Manchester Medical School, Honorary Regional Specialist in Community Medicine, North West Regional Health Authority, Manchester, Great Britain

Konstantinos Yiannikas, M.B., B.S., M.D., F.R.A.C.P.
Fellow in Neurophysiology, Sydney University, Sydney, Australia

Contents

PART ONE / EVALUATION

PART TWO / **THERAPEUTIC TOOLS**

PART THREE / **REHABILITATION PROBLEMS**

PART ONE

Evaluation

CHAPTER ONE

Introduction

Medical Rehabilitation and the Student

J. V. BASMAJIAN

This introductory chapter is derived to a great extent from the recommendations on undergraduate medical education of the Association of Academic Physiatrists and the American Academy of Physical Medicine and Rehabilitation. Nevertheless, we believe that *all* medical school graduates should be able to assess the problems facing a patient disabled by neuromuscular and musculoskeletal conditions and should be able to provide advice and continuing management in most cases. Some severe conditions may require a complex rehabilitation management team and special facility such as a rehabilitation center. Thus the undergraduate and graduate physician should recognize when the special skills of other members of the rehabilitation team are required and should be prepared to work with such a team to achieve the optimal comfort and independence of patients when they are returned to the home and society. In general, the book illustrates what we believe to be the level of achievement expected of medical graduates at the time of graduation from medical school

insofar as rehabilitation of musculoskeletal and neuromuscular conditions are concerned.

The purpose of this book is to provide an introduction, for all medical students who are either entering or are in the clinical years, to the broad field of medical rehabilitation. It presents, all in one place, the information needed by practitioners to make appropriate decisions in helping patients to deal with neuromuscular, articular, skeletal, and psychosocial needs.

Rehabilitation Medicine (also known as Physical Medicine and Rehabilitation) is a specialty, and its practitioners are called physiatrists (*PHYS*-i-a-trists). Yet, this is not a "how-to" book for becoming a specialist in Rehabilitation Medicine. Rather, it presents the elements that physicians in Family Medicine and other clinical specialties must clearly understand and appreciate. This should make possible the optimal care that they and all members of the health professions must provide for the recovery of patients from chronic conditions and from the postacute stages of acute illnesses and accidents.

Recent surveys have identified Rehabilitation Medicine as one of a small number of specialties in which manpower shortages still exist, with career opportunities in community, office, or hospital-based clinical practice, teaching, and research. Every medical student should acquire a clear idea as to what this specialty entails and should be able to state the scope of its clinical practice, research activities, and the nature and degree of overlap of the specialty with other medical and nonmedical disciplines. This book will help to define these boundaries and interactions. We hope that, as a by-product of this work, a few students go on to become rehabilitation specialists.

KNOWLEDGE

Basic Sciences

The basic sciences of anatomy, physiology, pathology, kinesiology, and ergonomics must form a significant part of the student's intellectual armory. This implies an understanding of both normal and deranged structure and function of the neuromuscular and the musculoskeletal systems and their related functional integration. This includes the functional anatomy of the central nervous and peripheral nervous systems, a reasonable understanding of muscle anatomy and physiology, and the function of the muscles in an integrated fashion. All are important acquisitions in medical school before one can do a satisfactory evaluation and management of physically handicapped patients.

One does not need a detailed knowledge of all of the muscles with their origins and insertions, but one must have a clear understanding of the interplay of muscles in groups as they act across the various joints. In the same way, the detailed knowledge of all of the ligaments around all of the joints can hardly be expected to linger in the memory of most physicians. However, the principles of these structures and a well-planned methodology for seeking specific information whenever needed are requirements. The more anatomy, physiology, and pathology that a student retains at graduation, the more likely that the result will be better evaluations and better management of patients suffering neuromuscular and musculoskeletal disturbances.

Specific Conditions

Medical students should not graduate without developing a clear understanding of specific neuromuscular and musculoskeletal conditions that are encompassed in the area of medical rehabilitation. These include spinal cord injury, cerebrovascular disease of various types, cerebral palsy, multiple sclerosis, entrapment neuropathies, muscular dystrophy, polymyositis, the various types of arthritis, soft tissue injury, overuse syndromes, scoliosis, peripheral vascular disease, amputations, cardiac diseases, chronic pulmonary diseases, and neurogenic bladder. Related secondary disorders also must be understood, particularly aerobic deconditioning, disuse muscular atrophy, contractures, pressure ulcers, and various types of behavioral and psychological disorders such as grief reactions and depression. The distinctions between impairment resulting from pathology and the consequent disability and handicap should be understood.

Diagnosis and Investigation

The student should acquire a practical ability to approach the neuromuscular disorders through their signs and symptoms (e.g., pain, weakness, paresthesias) and should understand the various techniques that are available for further investigative studies. The physician should be able to select, requisition, or arrange for the various types of laboratory, electrical, or procedural investigations now available, including serum calcium, muscle enzymes, myelography, arthrography, arthroscopy, computerized tomography, bone scan, electromyography, nerve conduction studies, stress testing of locomotor or cardiopulmonary function, psychometric tests by psychologists, or the results of urodynamic testing by urologists. Before graduation, a student should be able to discuss the indications for, limitations, and methodologies of these investigations, even though the general physician will never actually do any of these tests.

Therapeutic Options

There are a bewildering number of techniques used in rehabilitation. Some of them are easy to understand, but some are really more appropriate for specialists, either physiatrists, surgeons, or allied health professionals (e.g., rehabilitation nurses, physical therapists, occupational therapists, social workers, psychologists, and others). Given a patient with a neuromuscular or musculoskeletal disorder, the physician should be able to select, requisition, or arrange for and monitor the responses to appropriate therapeutic options. These include patient education, special bed-care techniques, therapeutic exercise, orthoses and prostheses, functional aids and appliances, therapeutic heat and cold, anti-inflammatory and neuroactive drugs, surgical joint replacement, methods of re-education, milieu therapy, sexual counseling, and behavior modification. At a minimum, the student should become able to discuss the mode of action of the therapeutic options, their indications, contraindications, complications, and various special considerations. For example, the different considerations include the growing child, the athlete, the pregnant woman, the elderly, and patients with progressive illness.

Problem Lists

The student should acquire the ability to formulate a comprehensive problem list that is medically, functionally, and socioeconomically oriented. An appropriate plan for investigation and management of each problem should follow. The student should be able to discuss with reasonable ease the social, economic, vocational, and personal impact of chronic pain and disability on an individual, and on the family, friends, and community.

The Rehabilitation Team

While much of what the physician needs to learn will guide future ability to manage patients at home or in a clinical setting, it is still recognized that the rehabilitation team needs to be called on from time to time. Thus, the student must gain some understanding of the rehabilitation team and its various members. The formal part of the team usually includes a physiatrist, rehabilitation nurse, occupational therapist, physical therapist, speech pathologist, orthotist, prosthetist, vocational counselor, social worker, psychologist, community agencies and organizations, the family physician and, most important, the patient and the patient's family. The role of each will change from case to case, and at different points in a single patient's transition toward independence. Each profession has been trained to acquire special ability, but each also has limitations. It is the collective team approach, especially the well coordinated team, that has the most to offer.

Rehabilitation Literature

The rehabilitation literature is quite broad and sometimes confusing for students. The student should acquire some familiarity with the journals devoted to rehabilitation and should be prepared to follow the changes that occur as part of his or her continuing medical education or to find information relevant to a particular patient's problems. The references in this book have been selected on the above basis.

SKILLS

As part of medical education, the student should become skilled in those areas of human problems normally not seen in acute general hospital settings. Although students tend to be more impressed by the drama of acute illness and surgery, all around them on the wards of a teaching hospital there are many patients with chronic and subacute disorders and special disorders of the neuromuscular and musculoskeletal systems requiring rehabilitation. Much can be done and learned.

Interview and Physical Examination

Some special skills are required in performing an adequate interview and physical examination of patients with the disorders being considered here. Not the least of the problems is the need of more input from the family of the patient than is normally expected when dealing with acute illness. The interviewer must pay special attention to factors such as residual abilities, functional limitations, limiting factors (e.g., architectural barriers), aids (mechanical and electrical), appliances of various types, such as wheelchairs, and the socioeconomic impact of the problems. While any good physician deals with all of these concerns to some extent, in rehabilitation they become particularly important.

The *physical examination* requires an understanding of how to examine the neuromuscular and musculoskeletal systems and how to evaluate functional abilities. Even in the absence of specific complaints, the student should learn how to perform a screening examination for the early detection of significant remediable disorders (e.g., limb-length discrepancies, scoliosis).

Technical Skills

The student should be able to perform certain basic technical diagnostic tests (e.g., arthrocentesis, lumbar puncture). Certain basic treatment skills also should be acquired, such as the application of a plaster cast or shoulder sling, or intraarticular injections. These are skills that are taught in a variety of departments of a medical school but are of special importance in medical rehabilitation.

Communication

The student should learn how to make good use of family conferences and team conferences in a manner that optimizes the contributions of each person, including the family and the team members. This requires experience in co-ordination and can only be learned by taking part. Communication with patients, family members, allied health professionals, and physiatrists plays an important part in rehabilitation. The keeping of logical and concise medical rehabilitation records with sufficient information (e.g., range of motion of joints) is important for appropriate monitoring of the patient's progress.

ATTITUDES
Interdisciplinary Functions

Finally, by the time of graduation, the medical graduate should have acquired a special combination of problem-solving inquisitiveness and an empathy and compassion for patients with chronic illness and disability. Rehabilitation requires a patient-centered rather than a disease-oriented medical ethic. A concern for the social, cultural, and economic implications of a patient's disorder must remain paramount in the thinking of all the professional staff's concern for the rehabilitation patient. This implies a respect for and a willingness to work in harmony with other members of the rehabilitation team; again, this can be acquired only by some exposure to the activities of the team, with as much involvement as possible during the training in medical school.

Optimism in Rehabilitation

Rehabilitation is not an overnight phenomenon and requires a special degree of patience in seeking long-term solutions. The student should develop as much enthusiasm and eagerness as possible in seeking methods of optimizing residual abilities and in preventing secondary complications. This approach can be as exciting in its own way as work in the emergency room or intensive care unit.

A good principle to remember is that almost all patients with chronic disabilities and with multiple physical distur-bances can be made significantly better on the basis of the amount of effort put into the treatment by the patient, the family, and the rehabilitation team. The future physician should see the possibilities for becoming a significant member of that team, regardless of whether or not the future includes becoming a part of the specialty of Rehabilitation Medicine.

The Magnitude and Scope of the Problem

P. H. N. WOOD

An epidemiologic appraisal attempts to make a diagnosis of a particular health problem on a community scale. The **three principal components** of such an appraisal are:

(i) *Perception* of the problem, *i.e.*, recognition of its existence, to which the production of this book attests;

(ii) *Definition* of the problem and its constituent features, which calls for
  ● Specification of the nature of the problem,
  ● Identification of associated attributes that characterize the subpopulation at risk, which can serve as the basis for screening and preventive intervention,
  ● Examination of the frequency and severity of manifestations of the problem, and of any trends that may be evident,
  ● Documentation of the consequences to which the problem gives rise.
  (It is with these matters that this chapter will deal.)

(iii) *Review* of the potential for intervention, which is a function of etiology and which has to take account of primary, secondary, and tertiary levels of control, and of the effectiveness and efficiency of such measures; these aspects will be considered elsewhere in this book.

On the basis of such an appraisal it is possible to formulate objectives or strategies for control of the problem, and from these to derive policies (organizational or administrative responses) in order to attain these ends. An example of strategic guidelines for rehabilitation services has already been published (1).

Diagnosis on this scale tends to be less familiar to physicians, but they should recall Henry Ford's view that a scientific discovery is a fine thing in itself, but it doesn't help the world till its put on a business basis. Inescapably, epidemiologic appraisal is the complement of clinical diagnosis because it indicates the probability of occurrence of various phenomena of relevance, and even more because it is only as a result of such a process that resources are likely to be made available to enable the physician to call on what assistance and support he may need.

DISABLEMENT

At the most fundamental level, disablement reflects the consequences of adverse health experience. The nature of the problems will be considered at greater length in the next chapter, so that for the present purpose it should be sufficient to clarify the different planes of experience to which the data that follow relate. Drawing on work done for the World

Health Organization (2), which we have expanded elsewhere in regard both to practical application and the gathering of data (3), and to terminology (4), a sequence of experiences can be identified.

Adverse health experiences may be identified as diseases, disorders, and losses (e.g., amputation of part of the body). Of these it is the concept of disease that has had the greatest influence on physicians (5), leading to what is often referred to as the medical model of illness. This model assumes that a set of etiological circumstances gives rise to pathological changes which, in turn, produce manifestations—the symptoms and signs which serve as the everyday evidence on which physicians act.

If adverse health experiences can be arrested or reversed—which has been the prime aim of clinical medicine—all to the good. If they persist, however, the medical model becomes inadequate because it fails to provide a problem-solving framework against which a physician can set his appraisal of the consequences. These may be referred to collectively under the title of disablement, but they may also be differentiated according to their varying impact on life experience. This leads to extension of the disease sequence in the following manner:

Disease or disorder, the intrinsic situation
↓
Impairment, wherein the experience is exteriorized as the individual becomes aware that he is in some way unhealthy or unusual; impairment is a biomedical concept relating to abnormalities of body structure and appearance and of organ or system function, whatever their origin, and it may be regarded as representing disturbances at an organ level
↓
Disability, wherein the experience is objectified as it takes form in regard to the execution of common activities; disability is a more functionally-oriented concept, reflecting the consequences of impairments in terms of activity performance, and it represents disturbances at the level of the person
↓
Handicap, wherein the experience is socialized as the individual comes to be placed at a disadvantage relative to others; handicap is a social concept, reflecting the adverse or disadvantageous valuation attached to an individual's performance or status when these are compromised by impairments or disabilities.

Identification of this sequence (2) contributes to problem-solving because the options for intervention vary between the different levels. Thus, whereas impairments are primarily the concern of conventional medical services, disabilities fall within the ambit of rehabilitation endeavors, and handicaps can be tackled by social policy and welfare provisions.

ASSOCIATED CHARACTERISTICS

If one approaches the challenge from the standpoint of handicap, one is able to perceive that the disabled are notable for the many disadvantages they tend to have in common. The shared nature of many of their problems assists the quest for social remedies with fairly wide application. However, if attention is focused on disability, one is in danger of getting lost in diversity. Certainly, the different social and cultural situations of people with disabilities are important, but placing too much emphasis on their dissimilarities is unhelpful to efforts at seeking more general solutions that could be incorporated in future policy (6).

The two most important intrinsic influences on disablement experience are age and the nature of the underlying disease or disorder. Unfortunately, it is not possible to present a completely integrated picture because information has to be derived from different sources. Between these sources there is considerable variation, both in regard to orientation to particular classes of impairment, such as mental, sensory, or physical, and in relation to organizational aims and methods of ascertaining those affected. These differences create barriers that can be insuperable; for example, it is not really possible to cross the age divide between children and adults so as to synthesize data into a comprehensive appraisal, and in what follows children have largely been neglected for this reason. Inevitably, these difficulties exert an adverse influence on policy development, so that provision has tended to be *ad hoc* and piecemeal and, therefore, too often inequitable.

The overall effect of age varies according to the demographic structure of the population considered. In developed countries such as the USA, in which the toll of childhood mortality is relatively small and an appreciable proportion of people survive to old age, approximately 1 in 10 of the impaired are young adults (less than 45 years of age), 1 in 3 are middle-aged, and more than half are 65 years old or more. Because of their greater longevity there tends to be an excess of women overall, but under retirement age impairment is usually encountered at slightly higher rates in males. The frequency of impairment is most striking in a group now commonly referred to as the "old old," those over the age of 75 years, in whom multiple pathology and an increased likelihood of living alone (through widowhood) contribute to severe levels of dependence. At the level of severe disability, the predominance of the elderly is therefore even more marked, as can be seen in Figure 1.1.

Failure to appreciate the influence of age leads to serious misconceptions, most notable among which is the notion we have designated as the fit disabled, epitomized by the stereotype of a young adult in a wheelchair. Certain underlying disorders, conspicuously those that are nonprogressive and which are often associated with fairly localized lesions, such as poliomyelitis or the effects of trauma (e.g., amputation or paraplegia), leave the rest of the body unaffected so that remarkable compensatory development may be possible. It is persons with this type of problem, who tend to be fairly young adults, who may be regarded as the fit disabled.

The larger part of disablement is accounted for by chronic diseases such as vascular disorders of the nervous system (including stroke), heart and chest disease, and arthritis. Because of both the nature of the underlying disease processes and the ages at which people become vulnerable to these conditions, the victims have much less potential for compensatory development, leading us to refer to them as the frail disabled.

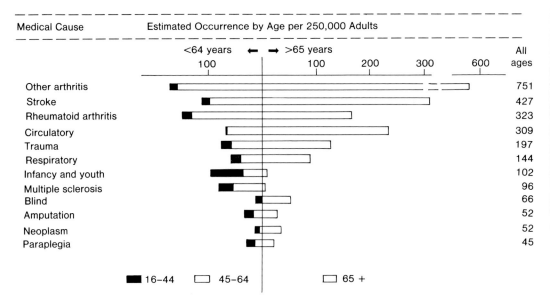

Figure 1.1.   Age distribution of the severely disabled.

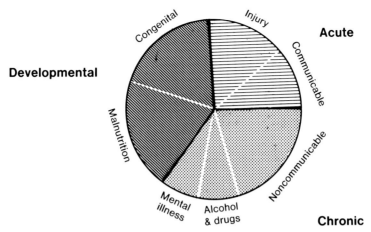

Figure 1.2.   Causes of disability worldwide (WHO estimate of population affected, 500 million; prevalence, 1 in 10).

A similar distortion is evident in appreciation of disablement occurring in those under retirement age. In fact the mean age of these so-called younger disabled is over 50 years, with just over one-half aged 55 to 64 and a further quarter of the impaired being in the immediately preceding decade. As a result, the inappropriately designated degenerative conditions, such as stroke, dominate the picture even before retirement. Even in those needing institutional care the average age is older than is commonly imagined, age ceilings for admission notwithstanding, although in this environment a concentration of chronic neurological disorders is encountered, reflecting the differential impact of different types of impairment, especially those affecting control as opposed to energy or mechanical difficulty, upon the ability to sustain self-care.

FREQUENCY AND SEVERITY

World horizons must be taken more into account. The World Health Organization estimates that approaching 500 million people are disabled, a prevalence of 1 in 10, and of these one-third are children and four-fifths live in developing countries. The principal classes of underlying causes for this state of affairs are shown in Figure 1.2. The tragedy is

Table 1.1.
Estimated Frequency of Major Classes of Impairment and Severe Disability in Adults

Class of Impairment	% Frequency of Occurrence in the General Population	
	Impairment (All Degrees)	Severe Disability
Mental (retardation and illness)	10.1	1.2
Sensory (vision and hearing)	15.9	0.5
Physical (congenital, traumatic, and other)	8.3	1.8
All classes	34.3	3.5

heightened when it is realized that so much of this burden could be avoided, with a large part of malnutrition, trauma, and infection being preventable—in theory, at least.

In developed countries the potential for primary control or prevention is not as great because the pattern of disabling illness is different. Table 1.1 is based on British experience (7), but the burden is not dissimilar throughout the industrialized world. The most striking thing in Table 1.1 is the overall frequency of impairment (34%), yet this percent is almost certainly an underestimate when full account is taken of visual impairment and similar problems. The balance between different classes of impairment changes appreciably when attention is concentrated on those who are severely disabled, physical problems moving from third to first place so as to account for half the overall burden. At least a third of the population are impaired in some way, one in three of the impaired are disabled to some extent, and one in three of the latter experience such severe restriction in activity as to be placed at a considerable disadvantage in relation to their peers.

Within the major classes shown in Table 1.1, approximately one-fifth of mental impairment is due to mental retardation, and a similar proportion applies among the severely disabled. Of those with sensory impairments, at least two-thirds have visual problems at both levels of severity. Even at the impairment level, trauma accounts for only one-ninth of all physical problems, and congenital lesions for only an eightieth, while for severe disability, other types of conditions, predominantly the chronic disorders of later life, account for 93% of the total.

The extent to which people are affected spans a spectrum from those at one end, who have some detectable impairment which nevertheless causes little or no disturbance of overall function, to those at the other extreme who are severely disabled and are at a profound disadvantage. The extremes are not too difficult to define, and their connotations are, respectively, people at risk but generally without current needs for support and people with high dependency needs. It is the middle of the spectrum that is problematic, which is why the inappropriate stereotypes have emerged and why society is uncertain about how to grapple with priorities and needs.

We have attempted to illuminate this problem by relating the frequency of selected physical disorders to the amount of impairment and disability they cause (3). The results are shown in Figure 1.3, based not on analyses of conventional groupings of conditions, such as the chapter headings of the *International Classification of Diseases*, but on a restructuring of the source data so as to preserve individual causes of known importance while aggregating the remaining conditions into reasonable-sized groups according to the similarity of the conditions in medical terms, the severity of the disabilities caused, the age and sex distribution of the persons

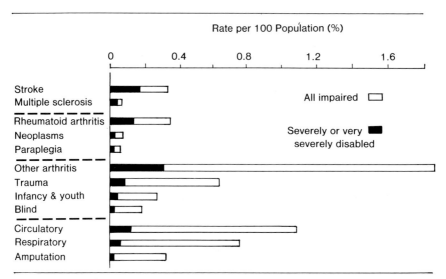

Figure 1.3. Interplay between severity and prevalence (for selected causes of disablement in adults) (Reproduced with permission from: PHN Wood and EM Badley (3).)

afflicted, and the extent to which conditions tended to coexist with each other (8) (many of the groupings are self-explanatory, but our original publication should be consulted in order to ascertain the basis for the other groupings).

The advantage of displaying the data in this way is the ease with which relative frequency and severity can be taken into account simultaneously. The four classes of severity were determined by the proportions of the impaired who were at least severely disabled—more than 50% for those suffering from stroke, parkinsonism, and multiple sclerosis; more than 25% in regard to rheumatoid arthritis (RA), neoplasm, and paraplegia, as well as in what we termed geriatric conditions; more than 15% with other arthritis (predominantly osteoarthrosis (OA)), trauma, infancy and youth, visual impairment, and genitourinary conditions; and less than 15% with the other groups. The contrast between RA and OA exemplifies the point—although individuals with RA tend to be more severely disabled, there are more people in the population severely disabled by OA because of its greater overall frequency.

TRENDS

One of the most taxing challenges is to assimilate changes occurring in one's everyday experience (9). This is particularly true in regard to the disease burden, which has undergone considerable alteration over a period of a few decades. The seeds of change were sown around the turn of the century, as most industralized countries began to succeed in conquering a large part of pestilence and other major acute life-threatening scourges. Inevitably, though, the solution of one set of major problems has served to reveal fresh ones which, by their very nature, tend to be more intractable.

Extension of average life span has allowed an alarming burden of chronic and disabling illness to emerge among those who would formerly have been likely to perish in childhood. The dominance of these maladies has been enhanced by demographic changes, an increase in the size of the population at risk due to there being more vulnerable older people. The problems have been further exaggerated by the way in which sophisticated technology and care have permitted the survival with reduced competence of those formerly doomed to earlier death. One important consequence has been repeated and continuing calls on services to ameliorate the difficulties. Of individual causes of disability, trauma has lost its commanding position as World War II has receded into the past, the continuing tide of road traffic accidents notwithstanding.

During the same period societal expectations have also changed. Disease has come to be seen in a different light, and the value attached to it has changed as a result. In particular, illness and disability are no longer so readily accepted as part of life's inescapable taxes. Improved health care and more enlightened welfare provisions have been developed in response to these attitudes. At a more individual level the plight of the sick and disadvantaged now tends to excite greater sympathy, leading to demands for a more sensitive appraisal of illness phenomena and a greater encouragement of personal autonomy than has been associated with traditional medical outlooks. Relationships that have not assimilated these developments lead to failures in so-called compliance, when looked at from the physician's point of view, and to considerable dissatisfaction on the part of people with disabilities—who, as a result, have often sought more sensitive assistance elsewhere, notably through the establishment of self-help groups.

CONSEQUENCES

Handicap or social disadvantage may be the common end result of diverse adverse health experiences. Handicap arises not just from biomedical factors, such as those previously mentioned, but also from the interaction of these factors with the individual's personal attributes, the environment in which he is located, and the resources he is able to command in terms of material wealth, support from family and friends, and welfare facilities. Many of these will be considered in greater depth elsewhere in this book, but a few general comments are necessary in this context.

Individual characteristics exert a very potent influence, not only in regard to coping strategies but also in relation to adaptability for redeployment of activity. The latter is very evident in blue collar workers, in whom limited education and expertise in physical skills can make vocational rehabilitation of the physically disabled very difficult—problems now exacerbated by the trend towards higher levels of unemployment. The role of the environment has received much emphasis, especially as concerns ease of access to public facilities, including buildings, and opportunities for participation in group activities, epitomized by the Wheelchair Olympics. While such measures are much to be welcomed, though, it must be recognized from what has been said about the frail disabled that only a proportion of people with disabilities are likely to benefit from such developments.

Three aspects of resources call for special comment. First, disablement experience is often associated with downward social mobility and poverty, due to exhaustion of resources in the process of coping with chronic illness and recurring medical expenses. Secondly, increased geographical mobility has led to family dispersion and this, with factors such as urban renewal, has tended to reduce the individual's social network for support, circumstances that are especially likely if the affected person is elderly. Thirdly, public policy has too often equated disadvantage with dependency, particularly such as arises from disabilities affecting the ability to work or for self-care. As we have tried to show elsewhere, the freedom of the individual to be self-sufficient is illusory unless full account is taken of his interdependence with his family, his environment, and social institutions or agencies.

CONCLUSIONS

The considerations raised in this chapter provide an indication of part of the knowledge base necessary for an approach to rehabilitation of people with disabilities. There are three areas in which our understanding remains sadly deficient. The first concerns the natural history of conditions giving rise to disability; surprising though it may seem, there is a dearth of good descriptive material on the unfolding of disablement and on the ways in which this is influenced by the underlying disease, other biomedical factors, and behavioral and societal responses to the experience. The second, which is not unconnected, is that the means for assessing outcome are very primitive, yet there is a need to appreciate "as much about outcomes of disease as about diagnosis of disease, and at as detailed, scientific, and sophisticated a level" (10). The third concerns the fact that our long-term hopes should center on averting the antecedent causes of disablement by developing effective means for the prevention of chronic diseases.

The basic skills of rehabilitation relate to comprehensive assessment of all dimensions of the individual's disablement experience and to the ability to work constructively with others in seeking the solution of problems encountered. Ways in which these skills may be acquired will be considered elsewhere in this book, but they have also been the subject of a recent review (11).

Both knowledge and skills are essential, but they are likely to be applied imaginatively and effectively only if they are reinforced by appropriate attitudes. These attitudes influence the aims identified for rehabilitation (12) and are determined not only by appreciation of the nature of the problems and how they arise but also by more personal and idiosyncratic attributes such as religious, political, and philosophical biases. Such biases have tended to contaminate much thinking about rehabilitation, and readers need to be constantly alert to their diverse manifestations. An obvious example has been the strong and often unhelpful influence of the puritan work ethic, difficult though it is to distance oneself from prevalent societal prejudices. A perhaps more topical instance is the strength of feeling about sexuality and disablement, some of the unjustified assumptions about which we have recently tried to display (13). The pernicious aspect of so many attitudes is that they themselves determine so many of the disadvantages people experience— as Antonio says in *Twelfth Night*, "in nature there's no blemish but the mind; None can be call'd deform'd but the unkind."

References

1. Wood PHN, Holt PJL: The development of strategic guidelines for regional planning of rehabilitation services. *Int Rehabil. Med* 2:143–152, 1980.
2. World Health Organization: *International Classification of Impairments, Disabilities, and Handicaps—A Manual of Classification Relating to the Consequences of Disease.* Geneva, WHO, 1980.
3. Wood PHN, Badley EM: *People with Disabilities—Toward Acquiring Information Which Reflects More Sensitively Their Problems and Needs,* monograph 12. New York, World Rehabilitation Fund, 1981.
4. Wood PHN: The language of disablement: a glossary relating to disease and its consequences. *Int Rehabil Med* 2:86–92, 1980.
5. Wood PHN: Advances in the classification of disease. In Smith A: *Recent Advances in Community Medicine* vol 2, Chap 13. New York, Churchill Livingstone, 1982, pp 169–183.
6. Wood PHN, Badley EM: An epidemiological appraisal of disablement. In Bennett AE: *Recent Advances in Community Medicine,* vol 1, chap 9. New York, Churchill Livingstone, 1978, pp 149–173.
7. Wood PHN, Badley EM: Setting disablement in perspective. *Int Rehabil Med* 1:32–37, 1978.
8. Badley EM, Thompson RP, Wood PHN: The prevalence and severity of major disabling conditions—a reappraisal of the Government Social Survey of the handicapped and impaired in Great Britain. *Int J Epidemiol* 7:145–151, 1978.
9. Wood PHN, Bury MR, Badley EM: Other waters flow—an examination of the contemporary approach to care for rheumatic patients. In Hill AGS: *Topical Reviews in Rheumatic Disorders,* vol 1, chap 1. Littleton, Mass., John Wright, P.S.G., 1980, pp 1–23.
10. Blaxter M: The future of rehabilitation services in Great Britain. *Int Rehabil Med* 2:199–209, 1980.
11. Wood PHN, Chamberlain MA: Undergraduate medical education in rehabilitation. *Int Rehabil Med* 5, in press, 1983.
12. de Blécourt JJ, Wood PHN, Badley EM: Aims of rehabilitation for rheumatic patients. *Clin Rheumat Disord* 7:291–303, 1981.
13. Williams GH, Wood PHN: Sex and disablement: what is the problem and whose problem is it? *Int Rehabil Med* 4:89–96, 1982.

CHAPTER TWO

The Nature of Disability and Handicap

R. L. KIRBY

Although only 2 decades ago the evaluation of disability was described by the American Medical Association as "an administrative, not a medical responsibility" and although the family physician still knows less about disability than most lawyers and social workers, there is growing recognition of the clinical usefulness of disability evaluation.

Improvements in acute and infant care have allowed patients with more severe illnesses to survive. Unfortunately, many of these individuals are left with residual disabilities. The family physician is confronted daily with patients requiring him to estimate the nature, extent, and temporal expectations of a disability and to take steps to minimize it.

While the *International Classification of Diseases* (now in its 9th Edition) provides a relevant classification based on causes and manifestations, there is a tremendous amount of useful information which is ignored by this conventional classification. Recognizing this, in 1980 the World Health Organization (WHO) published the first *International Classification of Impairments, Disabilities, and Handicaps*.

IMPAIRMENT

The WHO definition of impairment is "any loss or abnormality of psychological, physiological or anatomical structure or function," regardless of etiology. Examples include joint pain, limitation of motion, ataxia, dyspnea on exertion, anxiety, premorbid personality, or susceptibility to fractures, falls, fits, and diabetic reactions. Many of the subsequent chapters in this text deal with such impairments of the neuromusculoskeletal system, sometimes called the features or manifestations of disease.

DISABILITY

The WHO definition of disability is "any restriction or lack (resulting from an impairment) of ability to perform an activity in the manner or within the range considered normal for a human being."

Activities of Daily Living

"Activities of Daily Living" (ADLs) is the most commonly used term to describe such whole person performances. The terms are defined by the task (e.g., writing) rather than the region (e.g., hand function), as it is possible to have no arms and yet write with one's feet. Ordinarily, there is little concern about how a task is completed as long as it is done reliably, safely, and at an acceptable cost in time, energy, and subsequent pain. The functions described are behavioral, that is, observable and measurable. The categories that most ADL lists have in common are illustrated in Figure 2.1.

Sufficient categories exist to adequately describe subtleties, but not so many as to preclude remembering them all, or requiring a checklist for the routine clinical evaluation in the physician's office. There are unavoidable areas of overlap, so that a given ability, such as donning trousers after a bowel movement, might be assigned to more than one category, such as dressing and personal hygiene.

This language of whole body function is unambiguous, widely accepted, and translatable into several languages or disciplines without loss of meaning. There is no need to translate the expressions of performance limitations to patients, families, social workers, paramedical disciplines, or other physicians.

Hierarchy

Within any ADL category some tasks are ordinarily more difficult than others, and one can construct a hierarchy of dif-

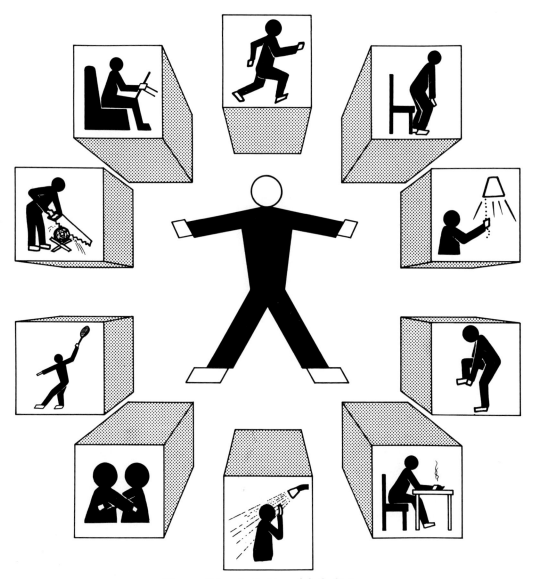

Figure 2.1.   Activities of daily living.

ficulties. Having determined a patient's position on this ascendancy of capabilities, one may ordinarily assume that the patient can perform less difficult items with ease but cannot perform more difficult ones. A patient with severe osteoarthritis of the hips may just be able to rise from a toilet seat. One may assume that he can rise easily from a tall stool but is unlikely to be able to get out of an unmodified bathtub.

One usually confirms this assumption by enquiring about one or two more and less difficult items as the hierarchy may vary subtly from one disorder to the next. While an individual with severe osteoarthritic hips may walk but not hop, a patient with an amputation may hop but not walk. However, such minor variations in hierarchical order seldom present practical difficulty.

Assistance

Assistance to functional performance may take the form of persons, medications, or aids and appliances. Most normal individuals are dependent upon an amazing assortment of gadgets (from coffee mugs to washing machines) for their standard of living. Much of the progress in the rehabilitation of the severely disabled is due to advances in technical aids.

Although the aid, appliance, or medication may be readily available, reliable, and affordable, the individual is nevertheless slightly less mobile and independent than a person who requires no such assistance. This is reflected in ADL rating scales, such as those discussed in Chapter 4 (see Table 4.1).

Total independence may be an inappropriate goal for many individuals. For a patient with severe rheumatoid arthritis, the demands of independence on inflamed joints may be harmful. In such circumstances, dependence on a visiting nurse for twice weekly bathing or a homemaker for heavy housework may be preferable to a poorly thought out and unreasoning drive for complete personal independence.

Limiting Factors

Limiting factors are those that preclude a higher level of function. Although they may be difficult to identify, they are of particular importance since the therapeutic strategy is aimed at correcting or bypassing these factors. For instance, an individual with difficulty in transferring to the upright position from a standard height toilet, due to inability to flex the knees beyond 70°, may be treated by attempting to gain more flexion range. If this is impractical or impossible, then the addition of an elevated toilet seat may allow toileting and transfer independence.

Limiting factors may be intrinsic or extrinsic. Intrinsic limiting factors are usually the clinical manifestations, features, or impairments resulting from a disease. Extrinsic limiting factors are those in the environment (e.g., architectural barriers) which preclude functioning at the limits of one's intrinsic capabilities. The latter will be discussed later under "Handicap."

The Degree of Disability

Disability may be defined as the discrepancy between an individual's current functional capacity and normal functional capacity, as expressed by the equation:

$$D = \frac{NFC - CFC}{NFC} \times 100\%$$

where D is disability, NFC is normal functional capacity, and CFC is the individual's current functional capacity.

Normal functional capacity should ideally be that particular individual's normal level, but when this is unavailable or inappropriate, then the functional capacity of one's peers is used. This approach permits us to consider disabled an individual who was significantly more able than his peers, such as a champion swimmer slowed—although not necessarily to the point of losing—by a shoulder ailment. Such an individual should only realistically be compared to his own previous performances, which would be well documented. For an individual disabled since birth, such as a patient with cerebral palsy, comparison with normal values is more appropriate.

Unfortunately, the range of normal functional abilities is wide, and normal values are not generally available. It is therefore conventional to describe the individual's current functional capacity, rather than attempting to estimate the disability. This is not only practical but also humanistically preferable, as it emphasizes the positive residual abilities—what is left, not what has been lost.

If the concept of disability is to have any clinical (as distinct from epidemiological and administrative) relevance, then a further distinction needs to be made, that of "significant" disability. Normally, one's functional capacity exceeds his requirements, and an individual is said to have functional reserve. Significant disability is the discrepancy between functional requirements and actual capabilities. If one needs or wants to perform a task and is incapable of doing so, then one is said to have a significant disability, a relationship which may be expressed by the equation:

$$ SD = \frac{RFC - CFC}{RFC} \times 100\% $$

where SD is significant disability, RFC is required functional capacity, and CFC is current functional capacity.

Significant disability, therefore, is intimately related to an individual's goals and aspirations. It is the proportion of one's existence invalidated by the disability. As such, it demands the full attention of the physician and rehabilitation team.

A very small loss of functional capacity, such as a slowing by 1 second in the running of the 100-meter sprint, may be a very significant disability to a competitive sprinter when success or failure is measured in hundredths of a second. Conversely, a severe disability, such as inability to walk, may be only mildly significant to a symbol-oriented individual such as a philosopher.

Indeed, loss of functional capacity may occasionally be an asset, rather than a significant disability, if there are secondary gain factors such as freedom from responsibility and financial worries, or if the loss provides a stimulus to a changed outlook on life.

HANDICAP

The WHO defines handicap as "a disadvantage for a given individual resulting from an impairment or a disability that limits or prevents the fulfillment of a role that is normal (depending on the age, sex, and social and cultural factors) for that individual."

Handicap thus reflects interaction with and adaptation to the individual's surroundings and community and concerns such dimensions as social integration and economic self-sufficiency. An individual with a below-knee amputation may be physically capable of driving a truck, but may be precluded from doing so by licensing authorities. Handicaps are inherently less quantifiable than disability and less modifiable by the medical and rehabilitation community, except through their efforts in the sociological and political arenas.

DIAGNOSIS

Diagnoses are not biologic entities but are mere categories in which we place patients for practical reasons. The diagnostic process is not complete until sufficient information has been accumulated for management.

The performance implications of a diagnosis should be consciously considered and formalized rather than camouflaged as "a feel for the patient." In so doing the physician adds considerable depth to his understanding of a patient. To the physician, a patient with recurrent dislocation of the shoulder may represent a simple problem of joint stability. To the patient however, the functional consequences of the instability are of paramount importance—what he is prevented from doing safely, such as skiing, scuba diving, and sailing.

Information on functional performance abilities and requirements is too critical to management to leave it half-buried in the data base—a mere qualifier of symptoms of no more significance than the date of onset. A separate category (whether one wishes to call it a problem, disease, or syndrome) is warranted if independent explanation, investigation, treatment, or prognosis is required. Full diagnostic status for the functional performance domain seems justified, a conclusion that the WHO seems to endorse. The functional assessment should lead to a functional diagnosis.

Despite the obvious causal relationship between the etiologic, anatomic, and functional diagnosis, no one component is either necessary or sufficient to the diagnosis of the others. Even with the most consummate etiologic or anatomic diagnosis, one can make only an educated guess about the functional limitations. Many factors influence final performance—physical impairments, motivation, emotional state, fatigue, and pain—frustrating attempts to predict functional capacity. The simultaneous occurrence of

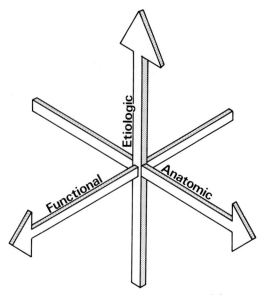

Figure 2.2.   The three dimensions of diagnosis.

two or more impairments may not produce additional functional difficulties, as one impairment may preempt the other. An individual with hemiplegia who requires an amputation on the same side, may have his overall ambulation function improved by the second impairment, with a passive prosthesis preferable to spastic equinovarus.

The functional diagnosis is not only the third type, but the third dimension of diagnosis (Fig. 2.2), fleshing out an otherwise impersonal picture and implying totality and a sense of completeness in the preception of the patient and his problem.

CHAPTER THREE

Clinical Evaluation

Neurological Evaluation

G. H. KRAFT

In general, medical rehabilitation is most concerned with two broad areas of disabilities—neurological and musculoskeletal.

The neurological examination from the rehabilitation viewpoint is concerned not only with the etiology and location of a lesion but also with the functional effect of the deficit produced. In addition, this examination carefully assesses changes in the interaction between the neurological and musculoskeletal systems due to disease.

It must be emphasized that this type of neurological examination requires a knowledge of the natural history of many disorders. Since the physician now performing the examination may see the disorder late in the disease process, typical neurology textbook descriptions may not be valid. In addition, complications should be anticipated so that they can be prevented during the rehabilitation program. For example, a stroke may be described in a classical text as a condition producing one-sided weakness. To the physician practicing rehabilitative medicine, however, other problems which may

occur later might be more urgent, such as shoulder subluxation, shoulder-hand syndrome, decubitus ulcers, joint contractures, and problems produced by increased tone and spasticity.

UNIQUE QUALITIES OF THE REHABILITATIVE NEUROLOGICAL EXAMINATION

Integration of Neurological and Musculoskeletal Examinations

Although the musculoskeletal examination is discussed separately later in this chapter, one must never perform a neurological examination without taking into account the interaction between the neurological and the musculoskeletal systems. This interaction is important in the diagnosis and management of conditions caused by pathology in one system, giving rise to secondary pathology in the other system.

For example, a physician may carefully evaluate a patient with a headache. If the examination is normal, the patient may be diagnosed as having a "tension headache," and muscle relaxants may be prescribed. In other patients, examination may reveal a tender greater occipital nerve which might be surgically sectioned, resulting in temporary relief. Yet, for a complete understanding of the pathophysiology, the musculoskeletal system must be included as part of the examination and the interaction of the neurological and musculoskeletal systems understood. Much of what manifests itself as tension headache in some patients or greater occipital neuropathy in others is primarily a disease of the skeletal system, producing a secondary disorder of the muscular system and tertiary disorder of the nervous system. This condition, the *cervical spondylosis triad*, is primarily due to underlying degenerative changes in the cervical spine, leading to attempts by the body to reduce neck motion by increased muscular splinting. This splinting, initially a protective mechanism, may cause myogenic pain and, if severe enough, can produce sufficient compressive force on the greater occipital nerves to produce the typical pains of greater occipital neuralgia.

This example demonstrates the importance of the integration of findings from neurological musculoskeletal examinations with an understanding of the natural history of disorders.

Functional Evaluation

Whereas other medical examinations evaluate a patient with regard to a disease process, the rehabilitative examination also evaluates the patient in terms of functional deficit. For example, two medically similar patients may have had strokes; one has left hemiplegia and the other, right hemiplegia; the former shows a marked perceptual deficit, the latter aphasia. To a physician concerned only with medical management, treatment of the two would be rather similar. However, from the rehabilitative perspective, the patients are very different. Verbal communication with the patient with left hemiplegia will be possible, but the per-

ceptual deficit may make retraining difficult. On the other hand, rehabilitation of the patient with right hemiplegia may require communication with gestures and pantomime. Entirely different mechanisms of retraining will be needed with the two patients.

The concept of functional evaluation involves several aspects:

(a) *Activities of Daily Living (ADL)* assessment. Evaluation of a patient's ability to carry out day-to-day self-care skills is an important measure of function.

(b) Ambulation evaluation.

(c) Behavioristic components of a patient's disorder. The physician should determine the degree to which learning of pathological behavior contributes to a patient's problems.

Special Expertise in Examination of the Motor Unit

The physician who has an in depth understanding of kinesiology and an understanding of clinical electromyography is able to understand peripheral movement disorders in an unique way. He is especially competent to assess disorders of the motor unit.

TECHNIQUES OF THE PHYSIATRIC NEUROLOGICAL EXAMINATION

Several of the manifestations of neurologic disease mentioned here are discussed in more detail in Chapter 10.

Intellectual, Perceptual, and Communication Evaluation

This is an extremely important component of the physiatric neurological examination, and functional deficits in this sphere can occur in the absence of motor or sensory abnormalities detected on routine testing. Intellectual functions can be tested by assessing orientation, memory, numerical ability, general information, and judgment. An assessment of the capacity for new learning will give the examiner an idea of the ease with which the patient may be retrained.

In brain-damaged patients, the ability to appreciate space, distance, movement, and form need to be assessed. When such *perceptual* functions are diminished, the patient's capacity to perform basic physical functions may be impaired. Perceptual deficits can be assessed by having the patient copy a square, triangle, or Maltese cross to determine how well he reproduces the figure and recognizes his errors. Perceptual deficits of this type are usually associated with damage to the right cerebral hemisphere and consequent left hemiplegia. On the other hand, symbolic functions such as abstract reasoning, language, and numerical ability are generally associated with left hemispheric lesions and are seen in right hemiplegia.

It is useful for the student to conceptualize evaluation of the higher central nervous system functions in terms of language and actions. Each of these, in turn, can be divided into output or input impairments.

LANGUAGE IMPAIRMENT

Dysfunction in this sphere is known as *asphasia* (see Chapter 10). The most obvious form is the output disorder known as *expressive aphasia*. This can further be subdivided into *verbal aphasia*, where there are problems with spoken language, *agraphia*, the inability to express thoughts in writing, and *anomia*, the loss of the ability to name objects.

A patient may also demonstrate input aphasia, known as *receptive aphasia*, which is the inability to understand spoken words. Commonly, the patient may show *global aphasia*, the condition in which both expressive and receptive aphasia are present.

IMPAIRMENT OF ACTIONS

Output dysfunction of actions is known as *apraxia*, or "motor planning problems." A patient who is able to carry out simple motor tasks but not integrated motor activities is said to have *ideational apraxia*. The patient who has problems performing all motor tasks, even simple ones, is considered to have *motor apraxia*.

Agnosia is a disorder of the input side. *Astereognosis* is the condition in which a patient is unable to identify an object placed in his hand. This may be present in the absence of motor or sensory deficit on specific modality testing. Since normal function requires hand use without looking at the object handled, astereognosis produces a major impairment. *Neglect* is another type of impairment in which a patient may actually be unaware of an extremity and, consequently, may have little functional use from it. *Extinction* is neglect in which the patient has good sensation on unilateral testing, but with bilateral simultaneous stimulation does not detect the stimulus (e.g., visual, tactile) on one side.

It is obvious that these subtle deficits, which may not be detected on routine modality-specific examination, might produce severe impairments of a patient's function. Only by specific testing can they be detected and treatment strategies be devised to correct for them.

Cranial Nerve Examination

Cranial nerves II, III, and VII are of greatest importance in the physiatric neurological examination. For examination of other cranial nerves, see Table 3.1.

CRANIAL NERVE II (OPTIC NERVE)

The type of visual loss points to the site of a lesion (Fig. 3.1). Loss of half of the vision in one eye is *hemianopsia*; loss in corresponding halves of both eyes is *homonymous hemianopsia*. Congruous homonymous hemianopsia is produced by a lesion in the occipital lobe; temporal lesions are less congruous. *Central sparing* is seen in occipital lesions because there is double arterial supply to the area of central vision (which explains sparing if the lesion is vascular), and because the macular fibers sweep laterally and are diffuse at the occiput (explaining sparing with space-occupying lesions).

Table 3.1.
Cranial Nerve Examination

Nerve	Examination
I	Sense of smell
II	Visual acuity, visual fields, optic nerve, pupillary response to light (afferent)
III	Eye movements, pupillary response (efferent) to light and accommodation, ptosis
IV	Eye movements (superior oblique)
V	Facial sensation, muscles of mastication, corneal reflex (afferent), jaw jerk
VI	Eye movements (lateral rectus)
VII	Facial muscles of expression, lacrimation, taste
VIII	Hearing, balance
IX	Gag reflex (afferent)
X	Gag reflex (efferent), vocal cord
XI	Trapezius, sternocleidomastoid function
XII	Tongue muscles

CRANIAL NERVE III (OCULOMOTOR NERVE)

There are two components: motor and parasympathetic. Motor fibers innervate the extrinsic eye muscles: eyelid levator, superior, inferior, and medial rectus, and inferior oblique. The parasympathetic fibers supply the pupillary constrictor and ciliary muscles (which, when contracted, cause the lens to become more convex and thus to adapt for accommodation). Complete paralysis results in *ptosis*, *pupillary dilatation*, *iridoplegia* (rigidity of pupil), *cycloplegia* (paralysis to accommodation), and rotation of the eye outward and downward.

Disturbance in *conjugate* eye movements is caused by supranuclear pathology in either the frontal or occipital lobes, or in the pons. *Nystagmus* is an abnormal back-and-forth movement of the eyes. It can be caused by either neuromuscular weakness, which is elicited by extreme positions in gaze (causing the rapid component to be in the direction of gaze) or

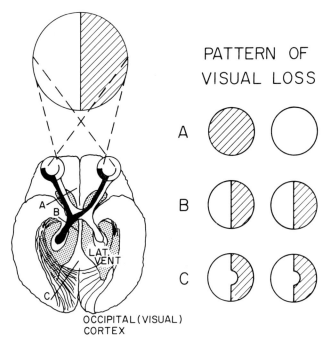

PATTERN OF VISUAL LOSS

Figure 3.1. A lesion of one optic nerve will produce total loss of sight in one eye, leaving the other eye unaffected. Any lesion central to the optic chiasm produces hemianopsia. This figure demonstrates the types of visual loss produced by lesions as A, B and C (see text).

central pathology in the region of the fourth ventricle or the cerebellum, leading to horizontal, vertical, or rotary nystagmus.

Horner's Syndrome

This disorder consists of constriction of the pupil, ipsilateral absence of sweating, ptosis, enopthalmos, and flushing. This is due to interruption of the sympathetic supply coming from the C8 through T7 nerve roots and is an important observation in the physiatric neurological exam-

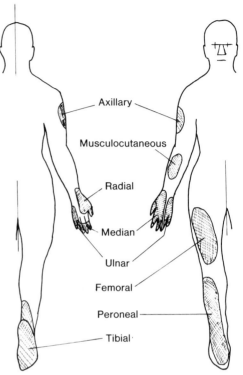

Figure 3.3. Areas of exclusive cutaneous innervation of important peripheral nerves. Other areas are supplied by overlap of more than one nerve, or by the other peripheral nerves.

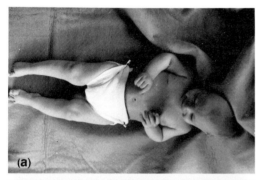

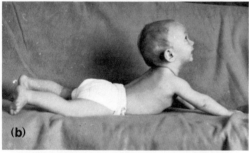

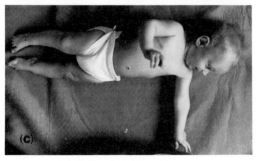

Figure 3.2. Tonic neck reflexes in a child aged 7 months. (Reproduced with permission from: B Gowitzke and M Milner: *Understanding the Scientific Basis of Human Movement*, ed 2. Baltimore, Williams & Wilkins.)

ination since it occurs with avulsion of these roots in brachial plexus injuries or in spinal cord injury at this level.

Argyll Robertson Pupil

Pupils react to accommodation (constriction for near objects) but not to light; classically, a sign of syphilis but also seen in other CNS diseases.

Adie's Pupil

Pupils react very slowly to either light or accommodation; associated with decreased deep tendon reflexes (DTRs).

Dilated and Fixed Pupil

This condition is seen following intracranial pathology due to swelling and pressure on cranial nerve III.

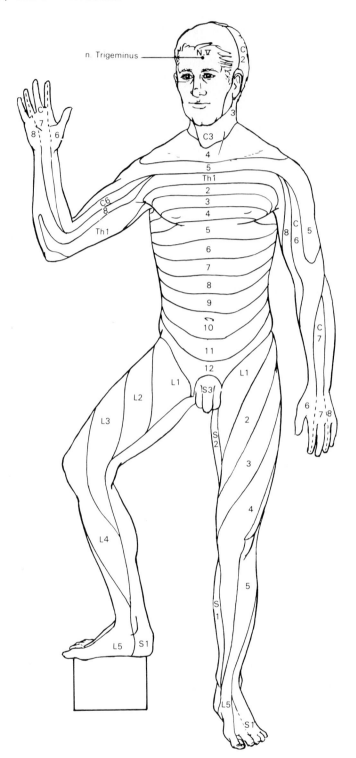

Figure 3.4.   Sensory dermatomes. (Reproduced with permission from: V. C. Nwuga. *Manipulation of the Spine.* Baltimore, Williams & Wilkins.)

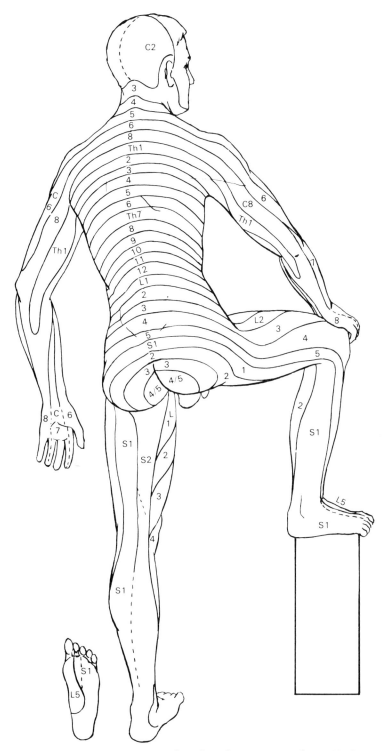

Figure 3.5. Sensory dermatomes. (Reproduced with permission from: V. C. Nwuga. *Manipulation of the Spine,* Williams & Wilkins.)

CRANIAL NERVE VII (FACIAL NERVE)

There are three components to this nerve: motor, sensory, and parasympathetic. The level of the lesion can be determined as follows:

Upper Motor Neuron

Facial paralysis will be unilateral with sparing of the forehead muscles, as cortical innervation of the forehead is bilateral.

Lower Motor Neuron Lesion Distal to Junction of Chorda Tympani

Taste will not be impaired but total unilateral facial paralysis will be present.

Lesions from Cerebellopontine Angle to Ganglion

Lesions in this region will cause decreased lacrimation and tearing in addition to facial paralysis. Lesions from the ganglion to the chorda tympani junction will cause decreased lacrimation and paralysis but with unimpaired tearing.

Cerebellar Examination

Cerebellar dysfunction can be tested with the *finger-to-nose* and *heel-to-shin* tests. The patient is asked to alternately touch his nose and the examiner's finger. In cerebellar disease, as the patient's finger approaches the target, an intention tremor will be observed, and past-pointing will occur. Cerebellar disease effect on the lower extremity can be demonstrated by having the patient run his heel up and down the opposite shin. Cerebellar function must be intact for this to occur without overshooting.

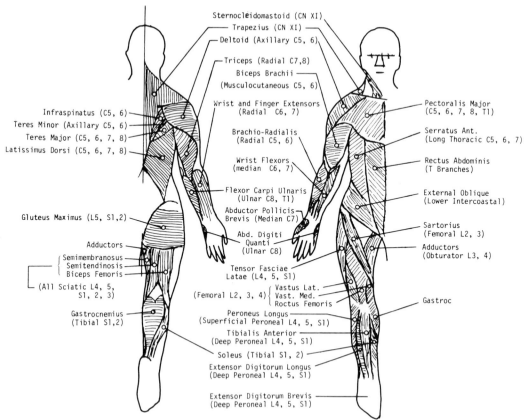

Figure 3.6. Frequently tested muscles. The name and location of each muscle are shown. The peripheral nerve innervating each muscle and nerve roots supplying it are in parentheses.

Reflexes

DEEP TENDON REFLEXES (DTRs)

The most commonly tested are the *biceps, triceps, brachioradialis, quadriceps,* and *ankle (Achilles)* or *triceps surae* DTRs. These are generally increased in upper motor neuron diseases and reduced in diseases of nerve roots, peripheral nerves, or muscle. DTRs are elicited by sharply tapping the tendon of insertion. Increased DTRs produce *clonus,* such as the alternating flexion and extension of the foot on forced ankle dorsiflexion, and the *Hoffman reflex,* brisk flexion of the fingers upon flicking the fingernail. More cephalad upper motor neuron pathology is associated with the *jaw jerk,* a sudden closing movement of the jaw upon tapping the slightly open lower jaw.

SUPERFICIAL REFLEXES

These are normal. The most important of these are the *abdominal skin reflex,* in which scratching the periumbilical skin produces periumbilical muscular contraction, and the *plantar skin reflex,* where stroking the sole of the foot produces toe flexion. Both of these are lost in pyramidal tract disease because the reflex arc, which probably includes the cortex, is interrupted at the higher level. The *bulbocavernosus reflex,* where pinching the glans penis evokes a contraction of the external anal sphincter, and the *anal reflex,* where stimulation of the perianal skin produces an external sphincter contraction, require intact S3 and S4 reflex arcs. Their absence confirms pathology at these levels.

PATHOLOGICAL REFLEXES

The most important of these is the *Babinski reflex,* in which firm stroking of the plantar surface of the foot causes dorsiflexion of the large toe. The Babinski reflex is present only with upper motor neuron lesions. The *snout reflex,* a puckering of the mouth on stroking the lips, is seen in disorders such as diffuse cerebrovascular disease, encephalopathies, senility, and alcoholism.

POSTURAL REFLEXES

There are a number of these abnormal reflexes, in which change in one part of the body produces change in another. They are used primarily in evaluating children with cerebral palsy. Examples are the *tonic neck reflex* (Fig. 3.2) and the *crossed extensor reflex.*

Sensory Examination

Sensory abnormalities to pinprick, light touch, heat, vibration and proprioception should be sought. They may be identified in terms of:

PERIPHERAL NERVE INNERVATION

Figure 3.3 demonstrates the exclusive cutaneous regions supplied by frequently tested peripheral nerves.

Table 3.2.
Grading System for Muscle Strength

Numerical Grade	Descriptive	Criteria
0		No muscle contraction can be seen or felt
1	Trace (T)	A palpable or visible flicker of muscle contraction can be identified but no movement at the joint is produced
2	Poor (P)	With gravity eliminated the muscle can move the joint through the entire available range of motion
3	Fair (F)	The muscle can move the joint through the available range of motion against gravity
4	Good (G)	Full available range against gravity and some resistance is possible.
5	Normal (N)	Full available range against gravity and full resistance by the examiner.

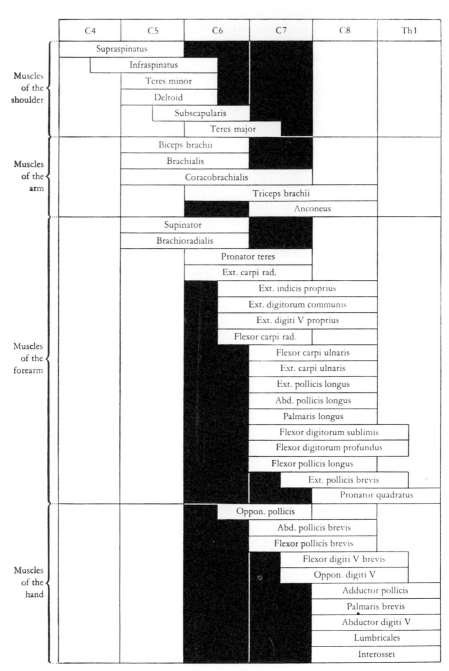

Figure 3.7.   Segmental innervation (myotomes) of the upper limb muscles. (Reproduced with permission from: V. C. Nwuga. *Manipulation of the Spine*, Williams and Wilkins.)

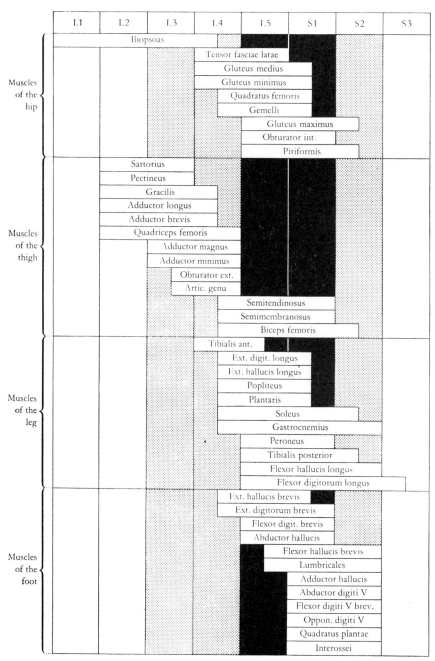

Figure 3.8. Segmental innervation (myotomes) of the lower limb muscles. (Reproduced with permission from: V. C. Nwuga. *Manipulation of the Spine*, Williams & Wilkins.)

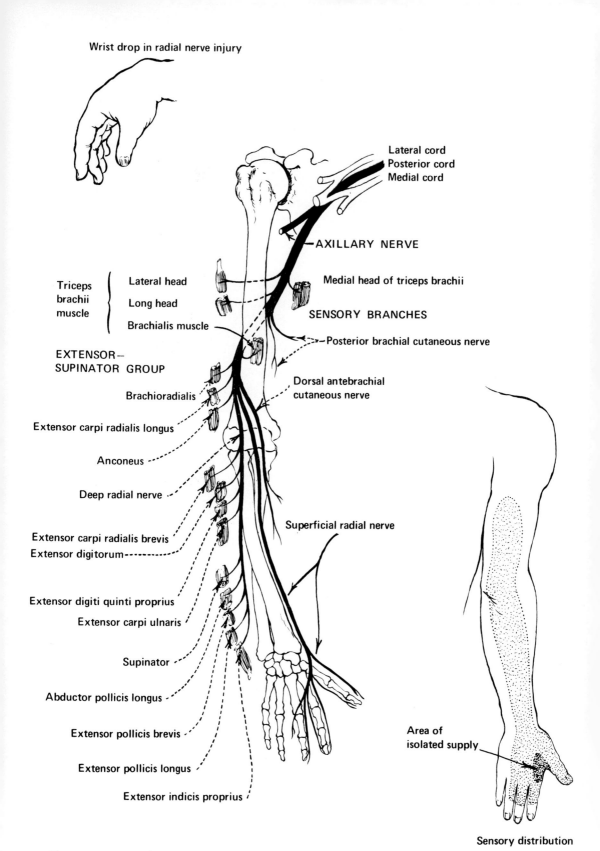

Wrist drop in radial nerve injury

Lateral cord
Posterior cord
Medial cord

AXILLARY NERVE

Medial head of triceps brachii

Triceps brachii muscle { Lateral head / Long head }

Brachialis muscle

SENSORY BRANCHES

Posterior brachial cutaneous nerve

EXTENSOR− SUPINATOR GROUP

Dorsal antebrachial cutaneous nerve

Brachioradialis

Extensor carpi radialis longus

Anconeus

Deep radial nerve

Superficial radial nerve

Extensor carpi radialis brevis
Extensor digitorum

Extensor digiti quinti proprius
Extensor carpi ulnaris

Supinator

Abductor pollicis longus

Extensor pollicis brevis

Extensor pollicis longus

Extensor indicis proprius

Area of isolated supply

Sensory distribution

Figure 3.9. Distribution of radial nerve. (Reproduced with permission from: C. A. Trombly and A. D. Scott. *Occupational Therapy for Physical Therapists.* Baltimore, Williams & Wilkins.)

30

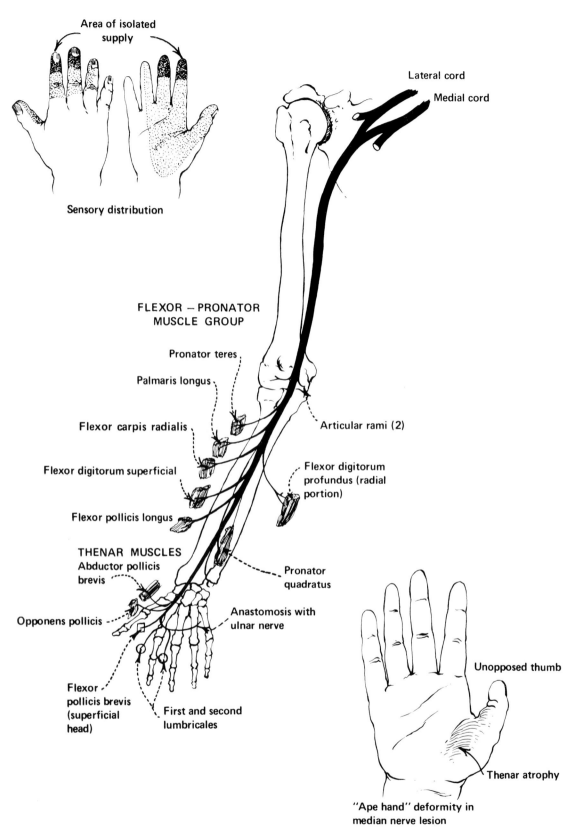

Figure 3.10. Distribution of median nerve. (Reproduced with permission from: C. A. Trombly and A. D. Scott. *Occupational Therapy for Physical Therapists.* Baltimore, Williams & Wilkins.)

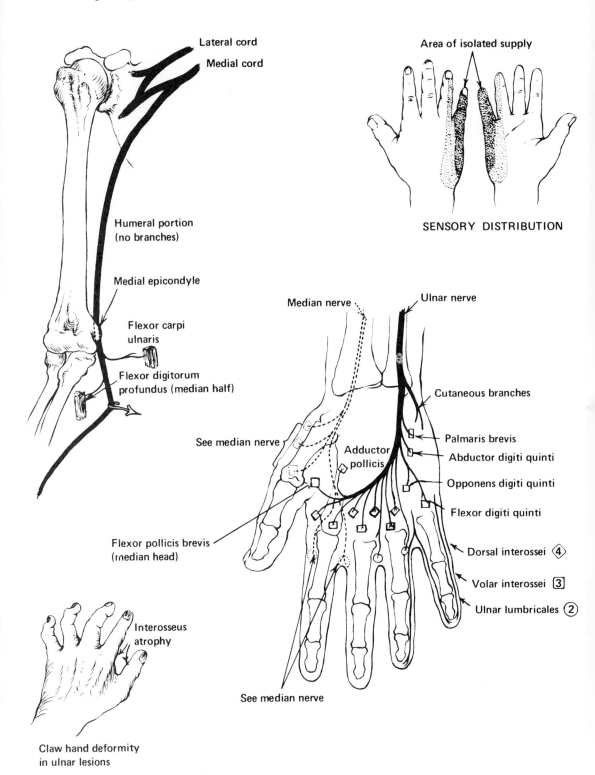

Figure 3.11. Distribution of ulnar nerve. (Reproduced with permission from: C. A. Trombly and A. D. Scott. *Occupational Therapy for Physical Therapists.* Baltimore, Williams & Wilkins.)

NERVE ROOT INNERVATION

Dermatomal areas supplied by cervical through sacral nerve roots are shown in Figure 3.4 and 3.5.

Motor Examination

Neurological weakness can be caused by upper motor neuron or motor unit diseases. The examiner can identify upper motor neuron weakness by noting overflow contraction of other muscles upon attempted contraction of a weak muscle. Weakness caused by nerve or muscle disease does not produce this.

The examiner should be familiar with: the peripheral nerve innervating each muscle (Fig. 3.6); the nerve roots supplying each muscle; Figures 3.7 and 3.8 summarize the innervation of muscles which may require testing. Figures 3.9–3.11 illustrate the type of motor and sensory information necessary to evaluate peripheral nerve lesions. Muscle strength should be quantified. A nominal scale for standardized muscle testing is illustrated in Table 3.2.

The examiner may gain additional information by palpation of clinically affected muscles. For example, in acute radiculopathies, muscles supplied by the affected nerve root may be tender. In myopathies, muscles may have a doughy or fatty consistency, and in neuropathies they may have identifiable string-like bands.

Clinical Evaluation of the Musculoskeletal System

R. L. KIRBY

Patients with disorders of the musculoskeletal system require much the same approach to clinical evaluation as patients with problems of other organ systems. This chapter will deal with elements of the clinical evaluation which are specific to, or are of particular interest in, patients with musculoskeletal disorders.

This chapter covers both the screening evaluation and the problem-solving approach to musculoskeletal disorders. Table 3.3 lists clinical evaluation items which do not fall into either of these two categories, but nevertheless are of importance by virtue of a relationship between them and musculoskeletal disorders.

THE SCREENING CLINICAL EVALUATION OF THE MUSCULOSKELETAL SYSTEM

If a patient's presenting complaint is a localized problem (e.g., left knee pain), the musculoskeletal screen is used to briefly ensure that no other musculoskeletal problems exist, whether associated or unrelated to the presenting complaint. When the patient's presenting complaint is unrelated to the musculoskeletal system, the screening evaluation attempts to identify occult problems (e.g., limb length discrepancy, scoliosis) which are common, serious, and in which early identification alters outcome.

Table 3.3
Clinical Evaluation Items of Particular Interest in Patients with Musculoskeletal Disorders

History of Present Illness
  see Problem-solving section
History of Past Health
  infancy
    developmental delay
    congenital hip dislocation
    clubfoot
  adolescence—scoliosis
  hospitalizations—residual contractures
  injuries
    residual joint instability
    residual limb length discrepancy
  rheumatic fever—Jaccoud's arthritis
  tuberculosis—tuberculous spondylitis
  diabetes—neuropathic joint disease
  bleeding diathesis—hemophiliac arthropa-
    thy
Family History
  ankylosing spondylitis
  muscular dystrophy
  scoliosis
Personal-Social-Vocational
  education
  job history
  architectural barriers
  financial and personal resources
Habit Data
  medications
  prescribed exercise
  therapeutic aids and appliances
Functional Enquiry and Physical Examination
General
  fatigue—inflammatory polyarthritis
  weight—degenerative joint disease
  fever—infective arthritis
Head and Neck
  headaches—from cervical spine
Eyes
  bifocals—cervical sprain
  visual loss—complicating steroids, chloro-
    quin
  halos—complicating chloroquin
  pain—episcleritis of rheumatoid
  redness
    iritis of ankylosing spondylitis
    conjunctivitis of Reiter's syndrome
  dryness
    sicca of rheumatoid
Ear, Nose, and Throat
  hearing loss—of Paget's
  tinnitis—of salicylate toxicity
  earache—from jaw joints
  dental problems
    from sicca
    jaw joint problems
  dryness—sicca of rheumatoid
  taste change—complicating penicillamine
  ulcers
    of granulocytopenia
    of Behcet's syndrome

Respiratory
  dyspnea
    rheumatoid lung
    progressive systemic sclerosis
  pain—pleurisy of rheumatoid
  tumor—hypertrophic osteoarthropathy
Cardiovascular
  pain—pericarditis of rheumatoid
  dyspnea—aortic insufficiency of ankylosing
    spondylitis
  claudication—neurogenic
  Raynaud's—of collagen vascular disease
Gastrointestinal
  dysphagia—progressive systemic sclerosis
  pain ⎫ of drug-induced
  hematemesis ⎬ peptic ulcer
  melena ⎭ disease or gastritis
  diarrhea—enteropathic arthritides
Genitourinary
  urethritis
    septic arthritis
    Reiter's syndrome
  flank pain—stones of uric acid
  outflow obstruction—skeletal metastases
Breast
  masses—skeletal metastases
Skin
  rash
    psoriatic arthritis
    of vasculitis
    of gold, penicillamine therapy
  calcification—progressive systemic sclerosis
  lumps
    rheumatoid nodules
    gouty tophi
Hematologic
  anemia
    of chronic disease
    drug-induced blood loss
  lymphadenopathy—regional inflammation
  splenomegaly—of Felty's syndrome
Endocrine
  growth and development
  menopause—osteoporosis
  temperature intolerance—thyroid myopa-
    thy
Neurologic
  sensory—nerve entrapment
  balance—falls and fractures
  spasticity—contractures
Musculoskeletal
  see screening and problem-solving sections

THE INTERVIEW

FUNCTIONAL PERFORMANCE

This is a screening inventory searching for difficulties with activities of daily living.

> *Initial Open-Ended Question*—"Do you have any difficulties performing activities in your daily life?"
>
> *Follow-up Question*—If the answer is no, then to be sure, enquire: "So you don't have any difficulties getting around? ... you can climb 2 flights of stairs, run and so forth? ... no trouble getting in or out of the bathtub? ... clipping your toenails? ... washing your back? ... putting on your socks or tying your shoes? ... trouble performing your duties at work? ... trouble with any of your hobbies or sports? ... one question for each of the ADL categories (see Chapter 2).

REGION SCREEN

This is a screening inventory to identify any current or previous musculoskeletal problems in the various body segments.

> *Initial Open-ended Question*—"Any trouble with the muscles, bones, or joints anywhere?"
>
> *Follow-up Question*—If the answer is no, then ask: "No swelling, morning stiffness, aches or pains, clicking, grinding, or weakness anywhere?"
>
> *Follow-up Question*—If the answer is still no, draw the patient's attention to each region in turn: "Nothing in your neck ... jaw ... shoulders ... elbows ... wrists ... hands ... upper back ... lower back ... hips ... knees ... ankles ... or feet?"

THE PHYSICAL EXAMINATION

Since the screening musculoskeletal examination places heavy loads on the cardiovascular system, it should not be performed in patients with recent myocardial infarction, exercise-induced cardiac dysrhythmia, or unstable hypertension.

FUNCTIONAL PERFORMANCE

The observation of the patient's function begins from the moment the physician meets the patient. He observes how the patient moves, stands, sits, removes his coat, or other garments during the interview and examination.

If in the course of this "surreptitious" evaluation the patient has not sufficiently demonstrated to the physician's satisfaction that he moves well, smoothly, and without pain or limitations, the physician should ask the patient to perform a series of tasks which place simultaneous demands on the muscles, bones, and joints in several regions and simulate some of the complex actions which constitute the Activities of Daily Living. For instance, one might observe the patient walking back and forth in the examination room with an ordinary gait, on heels and toes, crouching to pick an item from the floor, reaching behind the head and then behind the back, and rapidly opposing the thumb to each finger in turn.

REGION SCREEN

The physician briefly examines each body region for features of musculoskeletal disease. In evaluating the bones, one looks for obvious deformities, discomfort, and limb length discrepancies. In screening the joints, a passive range-of-motion examination usually suffices. For muscle, the muscle strength is assessed. One rapid technique is to have the subject place the arm or leg in the air with each joint held in midrange. The patient is asked to resist any forces by the examiner who systematically and forcefully attempts to flex-extend, abduct-adduct, and internally-externally rotate each joint in turn. Although this technique only assesses isometric strength, a normal subject can be rapidly screened.

The physician must be alert to features not on this abbreviated "agenda." For instance, when checking the elbow range, one may detect a rheumatoid nodule near the olecranon. The screening examination should not take longer than 5 minutes in a normal subject, and it is unusual for a significant musculoskeletal problem to be missed.

Should the screening musculoskeletal evaluation reveal nothing of note, the examination is complete. If an abnormality is identified or even slightly suspected, the problem-solving approach is used.

PROBLEM-SOLVING APPROACH TO THE MUSCULOSKELETAL SYSTEM

Once a problem has been identified, either by the patient volunteering it or through the screening evaluation, the physician will explore by further questions and examinations until he is satisfied that the problem is either insignificant or until he has reached a three-dimensional diagnosis—understanding the cause, structures involved, and functional implications of the problem (Fig. 3.12).

The problem-solving approach consists of formulating a hypothesis, deriving the logical consequences of the hypothesis, and then proceeding to test them. The experienced physician will have only a few hypotheses which can be quickly evaluated. The less experienced will require a step-by-step assessment of the structures involved in that musculoskeletal region to provide the necessary information.

For instance, in evaluating a patient with medial knee pain (Fig. 3.13) the physician may suspect that a recent partial tear of the medial collateral ligament is at fault. If this hypothesis is correct, then one would expect swelling, bruising, and tenderness to palpation, and a valgus stress on the semiflexed knee should produce medial joint pain. If none of these features are present, the physician forms a new hypothesis, such as a medial meniscus tear, and then proceeds with specific maneuvers to assess the logical consequences of this hypothesis.

Generally, the etiologic diagnosis is made from the history, particularly from the circumstances and rate of onset. The implications for functional performance will have been partially assessed by the screening evaluation, although the precise extent of the limitation remains to be determined (e.g., the walking distance) and the apparent limiting factors to that functional category (e.g., knee pain), remembering that subjective estimations of performance abilities are at best rough

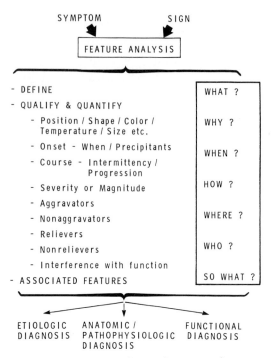

Figure 3.12.   Analysis of positive features to achieve a 3-dimensional diagnosis.

indicators, and sometimes are frankly misleading.

As with most other body systems, the musculoskeletal system has a limited repertoire of responses to the myriad combinations and permutations of etiologic insults to which it is subjected. The remainder of this chapter will consist of identifying what these features are, and some of the clinical maneuvers the physician can use to identify whether or not the feature is present. Minor modifications of approach are necessary for each anatomical region. While all important principles are discussed, a thorough coverage of specific maneuvers is beyond the scope of this chapter. The reader is referred to Hoppenfeld (1) and d'Ambrosia (2).

CLINICAL FEATURES OF BONE DISEASE

Bones should be examined from end to end, both at rest and under stress.

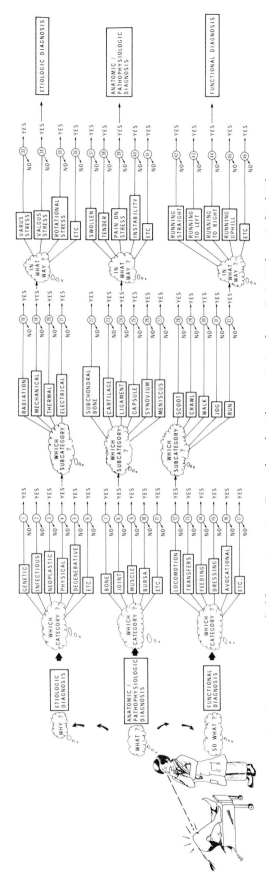

Figure 3.13. Algorithm for assessing medial knee joint pain. (Reproduced with permission from: R. L. Kirby, Medical Education 15:106–109, 1981).

ABNORMAL NUMBER

Bones, or portions of bones, may be absent (e.g., congenital amputation), or duplicated (e.g., supernumerary digits or an additional rib).

ABNORMAL SIZE

The bone may be enlarged, such as the limb hypertrophy related to the increased blood flow of arteriovenous malformation. The bone may be reduced in size, as with the neurologic reduction of muscle pull on bones in poliomyelitis.

Clinically, the length is more practical to measure than the diameter or circumference, and one usually screens several bony segments at the same time, such as the full leg length. If shortening of the full limb is present, then measurement of the individual segments which make it up is performed.

Particularly difficult to detect is symmetric abnormality of bone size, such as in patients with a generalized growth disturbance or in whom the limb–trunk ratio is abnormal. The most dramatic examples are achondroplastic dwarfism or Marfan's syndrome.

ECTOPIC BONE

In addition to true extra bones as described above, bone may occur in abnormal locations, such as myositis ossificans, where bone occurs in muscle, as a complication of trauma. Calcification (e.g., the calcinosis cutis of progressive systemic sclerosis) does not constitute abnormal bone.

DISCOMFORT

Particularly pain-sensitive portions of bone are periosteum and endosteum. Problems producing pain through pressure, traction on, distension of, and infiltration or inflammation of these structures include subperiosteal hematoma, hypertrophic osteoarthropathy, tumor, fracture, and osteomyelitis.

Bone pain is usually described as deep and aching, occasionally throbbing, and often worse at night. It has been suggested that venous pooling and interosseous hypertension is responsible for night pain.

Bone pain may sometimes be reproduced or exaggerated by direct pressure (tenderness), by traction by a muscle attached to the involved bone, by activating muscles which indirectly produce movement at the site of pathology (e.g., contraction of the hip abductors produces pain in the presence of a subtrochanteric fracture of the femur), by manually moving one portion relative to the other (e.g., in an incompletely united fracture), and by longitudinally transmitted force or the "anvil" sign.

DEFORMITY

Deformity is an abnormality of bone configuration, by virtue of a localized alteration in size, shape, or continuity. The ease with which one can detect bony deformity depends upon severity, and the amount of soft tissue cover. Deformities may be lumps (e.g., exostosis), depressions (e.g., following osteomyelitis), malalignment or angulation (e.g., from malunion of a fracture), or a smooth bend (e.g.; rickets).

ABNORMAL MOBILITY

Any clinically detectable motion between segments of the same bone is abnormal. The excessive motion is most commonly due to recent trauma producing fracture or epiphyseal separation. Occasionally, abnormal mobility occurs in the form of a pseudoarthrosis, either congenital or due to fracture nonunion.

CREPITUS

Crepitus is a nonmusical sound, often palpable. Crepitus may be of varied origin (joint, bone, or musculotendinous) and is not always abnormal. The characteristics of the crepitus (its site, pitch, and method of reproduction) often allow one to distinguish between normal and abnormal, and to determine the anatomic origin. Crepitus of bony origin (excluding subchondral bony crepitus due to joint damage, or crepitus produced by tendon moving over bony prominence) is usually "grinding" and related to abnormal mobility.

CLINICAL FEATURES OF JOINT DISEASE

The components of a joint which can be clinically distinguished in medium-sized or superficially placed joints are synovium, ligamentous and capsular restraints, and intervening structures. Joints should be examined at rest, and during loaded and unloaded motion.

Synovium

REDNESS

Erythema over joints implies increased blood flow and synovitis is a common cause. The absence of erythema does not exclude joint inflammation, particularly if the joint is deeply buried or the inflammation is mild.

HEAT

Similarly, heat over a joint is usually due to synovitis, although synovioma or vascular malformation may also raise local temperature. Extracapsular inflammation (e.g., cellulitis) may also produce heat, as may an elastic wrap or splint by preventing normal cooling.

STIFFNESS

Stiffness or "gelling" is increased resistance to joint movement *within* the available range of motion. Stiffness may be due to nonarticular disease such as parkinsonism or myofascial pain states. The stiffness of joint pathology is usually due to inflammation of synovium and capsule. This is a local phenomenon—the knees may be stiff while the ankles remain supple.

Characteristically, stiffness is present after inactivity (e.g., bedrest), and improvement is seen after a warm-up period.

The degree of inflammation is proportional to both the length of the "limbering up" period and the length of time immobile before stiffness is perceived.

DISCOMFORT

Synovium is insensitive to pain. Although pathology does produce discomfort, it is usually by involvement of the adjacent well-innervated capsule and ligaments.

Tenderness due to synovitis is usually diffuse and poorly localized. Also, there is pain at the extremes of motion in any plane. If significant synovial fluid accompanies the synovitis, intraarticular pressure elevations contribute to the passive tension in capsule at the extremes of motion.

SWELLING

Swelling due to synovial disease may be fluid or soft tissue. The well-demarcated boundaries of the swelling permit exclusion of extracapsular swelling (e.g., fat, hematoma, or edema).

Small amounts of intracapsular fluid (synovial fluid, blood, or pus) can be displaced from one portion of the joint to another. If sufficient fluid is present, it can be made fluctuant either by expressing fluid from other portions of the joint space or by examining the joint at the extremes of motion where intraarticular pressure is greatest. Pressure on one portion of such contained fluid produces pressure throughout that fluid, detectable by a distant palpating finger or producing ballottment (e.g., of the patella). Soft tissue (e.g., synovitis or synovioma) usually feels "doughy" and cannot be made fluctuant or be as rapidly displaced as fluid.

Ligamentous and Capsular Restraints

BRUISING

Bruising implies extracapsular blood. A hemarthrosis produces no discernible bruising unless there is an associated capsular rent. Purplish bruising may occur over a joint or at a distance by tracking along tissue planes. Later, with breakdown of the blood, the discoloration yellows.

DISCOMFORT

Capsule and ligaments are well innervated. Ligamentous tenderness is localized. The pain of a mild or moderate ligamentous sprain will be aggravated by joint motions which produce tension in that ligament. With complete disruption of the ligament little or no discomfort is produced, as no tension is generated in the affected structure. Unpleasant apprehension is seen at impending joint subluxation or dislocation.

ALTERED RANGE OF MOTION

The normal freedom of motion at a joint is determined by local anatomy—the shape of bone and articular surfaces and the placement of soft tissue restraints such as capsule, ligament, and musculotendinous complexes. Both rotational (around axes) and translational (along planes) motions may be either lost or increased, due to shortening or lengthening of ligamentous-capsular restraints, respectively.

INTERRUPTED MOTION

Triggering or catching of ligament over bony prominences or spurs may interrupt smooth joint motion.

Intervening Structures

It is difficult on clinical grounds alone to distinguish between meniscus, hyaline cartilage, and subchondral bone. They share clinical features and will be considered together.

DEFORMITY

Significant loss, particularly asymmetrical loss, of intervening structures permits joint deformity (e.g., genu valgus). Deformity may also be due to prominent osteophytes at the joint margin, or a tensely filled meniscal cyst.

DISCOMFORT

Meniscus and hyaline cartilage are relatively insensitive to pain. Although pathology in these structures does produce discomfort, it is usually due to interrupted motion or pressure on sensitive soft tissue or subchondral bone. When tenderness is present, it is usually well localized (e.g., over a posterior meniscal horn tear).

Pain on loading may be present. For instance, with loss of meniscus and hyaline cartilage in the lateral compartment of the knee, a valgus force applied to the knee will produce lateral compartment discomfort. If the pathology is well localized (e.g., due to osteochondral flap fractures, loose body, or deranged meniscus), then the pain on loading may only be present through a small portion of the total joint arc. When bone ends are denuded of hyaline cartilage and the motion is accompanied by axial load, then pain on motion occurs.

Discomfort due to damage in intervening structures may sometimes be distinguished from that originating in capsule and ligament by comparison between motion with distraction and motion with compression. Unloaded motion tends to produce pain with soft tissue involvement, whereas loaded motion results in pain with either soft tissue or intervening structure pathology. The Apley "grinding" and distraction maneuvers are examples of this phenomenon at the knee.

ALTERED RANGE OF MOTION

Loss of joint motion may be due to derangements of intervening structures (e.g., meniscal tear, loose body). Increased motion or instability may be due to their loss or collapse. For instance, valgus instability of the knee may be due to loss of lateral compartment hyaline cartilage and collapse of subchondral bone in a patient with rheumatoid arthritis.

INTERRUPTED MOTION

Interrupted motion may be due to roughness or irregularity of intervening structures, and is usually aggravated by loaded motion and minimized by unloaded motion.

CREPITUS

General comments on crepitus were made earlier. Crepitus due to damage of intervening structures may be snapping, clicking, clunking, sandy, or grinding in nature, and is usually more prominent during loaded motion.

CLINICAL FEATURES OF MUSCULOTENDINOUS DISEASE

The components of the musculotendinous unit which can be clinically distinguished in medium-sized or superficially placed muscles are the muscle belly, tendon-related structures, and muscle attachments to bone. Muscle should be examined at rest and during passive stretch and active contraction.

Muscle Belly

ALTERED BULK

Muscle bulk may be reduced (e.g., the atrophy of disuse) or increased (e.g., the pseudohypertrophy of Duchenne muscular dystrophy). Moderate abnormalities of muscle size can be detected on inspection, although measurement of circumference is more sensitive.

ALTERED SHAPE

The shape of the muscle belly may be altered by bony displacement, intramuscular hematoma, herniation of the muscle belly through its fascia, or rupture of the musculotendinous unit with "bunching."

ALTERED CONSISTENCY

Detected by palpation, consistency may be reduced (e.g., in disuse atrophy after a prolonged immobilization in a cast) or increased (e.g., by fibrous replacement of Volkmann's ischemic contracture).

DISCOMFORT

The muscle belly is relatively insensitive to pain except by distortion or damage to its fascial envelopes and in some characteristically sensitive areas (see Chapter 11, subchapter on *Myofascial Pain States*).

Discomfort may be reproduced by palpation, passive stretch, or active contraction. Sometimes, repetitive activity will be necessary (e.g., the exercise-induced anterior compartment syndrome of the leg).

ALTERED LENGTH

Increased passive length of the musculotendinous unit may be seen with chronic or repetitive stretch (e.g., in muscle imbalance). Shortening of the muscle may be due to sustained positioning, muscle imbalance, fibrous replacement, or adhesions between the muscle belly and underlying bone.

To assess the length of a muscle which crosses more than one joint, it is necessary to stretch the muscle across all joints crossed. For instance, to assess the length of the gastrosoleus, extend the knee fully and measure the ankle dorsiflexion range. If shortening is detected it may be distinguished from lost motion due to joint disease by slackening one of the joints crossed—this allows increased motion in the other. Using the gastrosoleus example, if ankle dorsiflexion increases substantially when the knee is flexed, then muscle shortening is present.

When the shortened muscle crosses only one joint, one must rely on discomfort and passive tension in the involved muscle at the limit of motion.

WEAKNESS

The force generated by muscle cannot be measured directly but can only be inferred from a measure of torque (tendency for rotation to occur) at a joint. This varies with the joint angle, the position of other joints crossed by the muscle, and the rate of shortening. By strength, we mean the maximum torque that can be generated by contracting muscle. The term is not synonymous with power which is defined as the work performed per unit of time.

The most commonly used grading system for the clinical assessment of muscle strength is that developed by the Medical Research Council in 1943 (Table 3.2).

The physician should use mechanical advantage to overcome very strong muscles. For instance, when assessing the strength of shoulder abductors, apply force to the wrists rather than to the elbows. Another trick is to alter the position of the joints crossed by the muscle. For instance, the elbow flexors may be overcome in a strong patient by assessing them with the elbow nearly extended. In this position the muscle is disadvantaged on the length-tension curve, and the angle of insertion of biceps is such as to provide more of a joint stabilizing than a rotational force.

Alternatively, muscle contractility may be quantitatively assessed by asking the patient to perform movements against resistance repetitively (e.g., pushups), or by sustained contractions (e.g., holding the arms out straight). In some situations (e.g., myotonia congenita or myasthenia gravis) improvements or deteriorations in strength may be seen with repetitive contractions.

Reduced output may be due to reflex inhibition from pain, impaired consciousness or cooperation, rather than reduced strength. In such situations, muscle contracts in a rachety fashion. In true weakness, significant effort is often accompanied by postures and contractions of other muscles which assist the weakened muscle.

When assessing patients with upper motor neuron disease, muscle strength may be misleading, as muscle may be firing strongly but may be under little voluntary control.

ABNORMAL CONTRACTIONS

Abnormal contractions of muscle include such clinical signs as myoedema (localized bulging of muscle after percussion), myokymia (involuntary sinuous contractions of a few muscle fascicles at a time), fasciculation (isolated irregular involuntary contractions of motor units), myotonia (difficulty stopping a contraction), protective muscle spasm (distinguished from a cramp by its appropriateness), and cramp (a spontaneous and uncontrolled contraction of an entire muscle).

A discussion of central nervous system abnormalities of contractility such as spasticity, rigidity, tremor, myoclonic jerks, altered speed, or control of contractions is beyond the scope of this chapter.

Tendon-Related Structures

The tendon-related structures include the tendon, tendon sheath, sesamoid bone, and retinacular or other soft tissue pulleys.

ALTERED SHAPE

The shape of tendon or tendon sheath can be altered by nodules, synovial proliferation, or effusion in the tendon sheath.

DISCOMFORT

Discomfort can be brought out by direct palpation (tenderness), by the application of tension with passive stretch or active contraction, or by active or passive movement of tendon.

The discomfort may be at a particular portion of the excursion of the musculotendinous unit due to mechanical impingement of the pain-sensitive section on tendon tunnels or bone producing a "painful arc". Conversely, the primary pathology may be in the underlying bone, such as the irritation of extensor tendons over an ulnar styloid eroded by rheumatoid arthritis.

If the discomfort is contributed to by active muscular contraction, reflex inhibition may occur (e.g., the "drop sign" of supraspinatus tendonitis).

DISLOCATION AND SUBLUXATION

If recent, and acute (e.g., with lateral dislocation of the patella), there may be considerable discomfort and apprehension at any attempt to reproduce the dislocation. In the dislocated position the musculotendinous unit may provide forces which perpetuate the deformity (e.g., extensor finger tendons chronically dislocated between the metacarpal heads aggravating ulnar deviation in rheumatoid arthritis).

RUPTURE

Rupture usually occurs near junctions such as the origin, insertion, or musculotendinous junction. It may occur where wear is greatest or blood supply is minimal. After rupture, the muscle belly shortens excessively, producing a deformity.

Complete rupture can be identified by determining that the muscle belly is functioning but that no tension is produced in the musculotendinous complex. When discomfort interferes with contraction, manual compression of the muscle belly produces some shortening (e.g., Thompson's sign for ruptured tendo achillis) or passive joint motion may be used to produce tension in normal musculotendinous complexes.

INTERRUPTED MOTION

Interrupted motion may be due to reflex inhibition, tendon tracking abnor-malities, triggering of tendon over bony prominences, or triggering in a tendon tunnel due to a localized discrepancy between tendon size and tunnel capacity.

CREPITUS

Crepitus due to triggering is usually of a snapping quality while that due to inflammation in tendon or tendon sheath is more "sandy" or "crunchy."

Attachments

The attachments, or entheses, of the musculotendinous unit to bone are the origin and insertion.

ALTERED SHAPE

The attachments may be prominent through swelling of the tendon or underlying bone (e.g., tibial tubercle).

CONSISTENCY

On palpation, an inflamed tendinous attachment may feel soft and boggy.

DISCOMFORT

Although discomfort may be present at rest, it can usually be reproduced or aggravated by direct pressure at the attachment (tenderness), by passive stretch, or by active contraction by the muscle belly.

Suggested Reading

1. Hoppenfeld S: *Physical Examination of the Spine and Extremities.* New York, Appleton-Century-Crofts, 1976.
2. D'Ambrosia R: *Musculoskeletal Disorders: A Regional Examination and Differential Diagnosis.* Philadelphia, Lippincott, 1977.

CHAPTER FOUR

Special Diagnostic Procedures

Body Fluids

P. S. TEPPERMAN

The practice of Rehabilitation Medicine, as in any medical discipline, requires selective use of laboratory investigations. Based on clinical symptoms and signs obtained through a careful history and physical examination, additional objective evidence of disease processes may be obtained from laboratory investigations. Such examinations may be useful for diagnostic purposes, following the course of an illness, assessing the effect of therapeutic intervention, and monitoring potential adverse effects of treatment. The following section is devoted to a brief overview of blood, urine, and spinal and synovial fluid investigations commonly of specific value to the physiatrist, with a brief mention of amniotic fluid from amniocentesis.

BLOOD

Hematology

Evaluation of *hemoglobin, hematocrit,* and *red blood cell indices,* as well as *cell morphology* on routine blood films, is needed to identify the presence and type of anemia, such as the anemia of chronic disease, drug-induced blood loss, or aplastic anemia. Recognition of anemia is important in the prescription of an exercise program and may in addition disclose the need for further studies such as serum B_{12} to confirm the etiology of a neuropathy (i.e., pernicious anemia). *White blood cell indices,* including count and differential, are important in diagnosis of infectious processes such as septic arthritis or osteomyelitis or in detection of drug-induced granulocytopenia. *Erythrocyte sedimentation rate (ESR)* is a valuable nonspecific indicator of inflammation which is useful in screening for both infective (e.g., septic arthritis) and inflammatory (e.g., rheumatoid arthritis) disorders.

Biochemistry

Many chemical investigations are of particular value in medical rehabilitation. For example, evaluation of *bone biochemistry* (serum calcium, alkaline phosphatase, and inorganic phosphate) may assist the diagnosis of metabolic bone disease or the early detection of primary or secondary bone tumors. *Blood sugars* (fasting, 2 hours pc, and glucose tolerance test) will provide not only a diagnosis of diabetes mellitus but might also suggest the etiology of an otherwise "idiopathic" peripheral neuropathy. *Renal function* (BUN, creatinine) should be followed carefully in the patient with a neurogenic bladder. *Creatine phosphokinase* (CPK) elevation assists in the diagnosis of myopathy. *Liver enzymes* (Gamma GT, SGOT, SGPT, LDH) must be assessed periodically in those patients on treatment with phenatoin (Dilantin®) for seizures or dantrolene sodium (Dantrium®) for spasticity. *Acid phosphatase* elevation may provide the first clue to the etiology of a secondary bone tumor in a male (*i.e.*, prostatic malignancy). *Uric acid* levels are important in the diagnosis of gouty arthritis. *Serum protein and immunoelectrophoresis* may provide a diagnosis of multiple myeloma in a patient with an elevated ESR presenting with back pain, and also may be of use in patients with autoimmune disorders affecting neuromuscular, musculoskeletal, or other structures. Special studies, such as *serum copper* and *ceruloplasmin* studies, might lead to the diagnosis of a reversible dementia such as Wilson's disease.

Serology

Serological assessments are particularly important in the diagnosis of collagen diseases. These include *rheumatoid factor (latex fixation), antinuclear factors,* and *LE cell preparations.* A false positive *VDRL* may be encountered in many collagen disorders but one must keep in mind the true positive VDRL in the patient presenting with posterior column signs or mental status impairment (*i.e.*, neurosyphilis). An important clue to the diagnosis of seronegative spondyloarthropathies (*e.g.*, ankylosing spondylitis, psoriatic spondyloarthritis, Reiter's disease) may be provided by *HLA typing,* where B27 is usually positive.

URINALYSIS

Urinalysis is a simple noninvasive procedure which is readily available and frequently valuable in medical rehabilitation. This includes routine urinalysis (*i.e.*, dipstick) and microscopic assessment of a single voided specimen as well as urine cultures and chemical analysis of 24-hour urine collections.

Perhaps the greatest use is apparent in management of the neurogenic bladder for diagnosis of urinary tract infection as well as following the long-term effects on renal function.

Urine studies will also facilitate diagnosis of other disease processes. For example, abnormalities in *urine calcium* and *hydroxyproline* excretion provide valuable clues in the diagnosis of metabolic bone disease. The presence of *Bence Jones protein* in the urine of a patient presenting with intractable back pain often leads to the diagnosis of multiple myeloma. *Red blood cell casts* may be the first indication of systemic lupus erythematosus with renal involvement.

SPINAL FLUID ANALYSIS

Examination of cerebrospinal fluid (CSF) provides the clinician with useful diagnostic information in many neurological disorders. CSF is most often obtained by lumbar puncture. Although invasive, this is a relatively simple procedure contraindicated only by clinical evidence of increased intracranial pressure, local infection at the puncture site, or poor patient cooperation.

Cerebrospinal fluid may be evaluated for appearance, pressure, content of protein, chloride and sugar, cells (RBC, WBC, and other), micro-organisms, serology, and immunoglobulins.

CSF is normally clear with an opening pressure of about 120 mm of water. Protein content varies between 15 and 40 mg%. The CSF glucose level ranges from 50 to 85 mg%.

Detection of intracerebral hemorrhage which extends into the ventricular system is often facilitated by the finding of blood in the CSF. Infection may be detected and classified (*e.g.*, pyogenic *vs.* aseptic meningitis) by white blood cell count and morphology as well as specific cultures. A significant decrease in CSF glucose and chloride is observed in pyogenic or tuberculous meningitis. A positive VDRL will be obtained in neurosyphilis. Immunoglobulin studies assist in the diagnosis of multiple sclerosis (elevated IgG and oligoclonal bands). Tumor cells may be detected on cytological studies. Elevation of CSF protein is frequently apparent with inflammatory disorders such as meningitis, encephalitis, multiple sclerosis, and syphilis as well as intracranial tumor.

SYNOVIAL FLUID ANALYSIS

Evaluation of synovial fluid is a valuable aid in the diagnosis of arthritic conditions. In the presence of joint effusion, fluid may be easily obtained by arthrocentesis. A strict sterile technique must be observed to avoid infection, the only serious complication of joint aspiration.

Synovial fluid can be analyzed for (a) gross appearance (color, clarity), (b) viscosity, (c) mucin clot formation, (d) biochemistry (glucose and protein content), and (e) microscopic appearance (cytology, crystals, inclusions). It may also be cultured to detect micro-organisms.

On the basis of the above evaluations, synovial fluid may be divided into three diagnostic categories.

Group I (normal, traumatic, osteoarthritis) exhibits generally clear yellow fluid with high viscosity, good mucin clot formation, and a small number of white blood cells. Traumatic fluid may contain many red blood cells. Osteoarthritic fluid often exhibits numerous cartilage fragments.

Group II is inflammatory fluid. This is characteristically cloudy with decreased viscosity and fair to poor mucin clot formation. A considerable increase in white blood cells (polymorphs) is apparent. Such fluid is found in rheumatoid arthritis and other inflammatory arthropathies, including crystalline-induced arthritis, wherein fluid will often contain monosodium urate (gout) or calcium pyrophosphate (pseudogout) crystals.

Group III fluid is septic. It is very cloudy, turbid, or frankly purulent, with low viscosity and poor mucin clot formation. There is usually a marked increase in white blood cell count over that seen in inflammatory fluid. Glucose content is low, and micro-organisms can usually be cultured.

AMNIOTIC FLUID

Meningomyelocele is a relatively common condition encountered in pediatric rehabilitation. Analysis of amniotic fluid for α-fetoprotein is a valuable diagnostic technique for the prenatal detection of this disorder.

References

1. Bannister R: *Brain's Clinical Neurology*. London, Oxford University Press, 1969.
2. McCarty DJ Jr: *Arthritis and Allied Conditions*. Philadelphia, Lea & Febiger, 1979.
3. Wintrobe MM, Thorn GW et al: *Harrison's Principles Of Internal Medicine*. New York, McGraw-Hill, 1980.

Diagnostic Imaging Techniques

J. LESZCZYNSKI

The concept of radiography as the sole diagnostic imaging technique is now obsolescent. New imaging techniques include computerized axial tomography scanning, nuclear medicine, diagnostic ultrasound, and thermography. Soon, nuclear magnetic resonance and positron emission imaging will be added. Techniques such as invasive angiography are now less frequently used, and pneumoencephalography is rarely performed. The decision to use a particular imaging technique, the appropriate sequence, the extent of the examination, the benefits and risks to the patient, and the cost implications require sound judgement based on clinical experience.

RADIOGRAPHY

A systematic visual scan of the components of a radiograph—soft tissues, bone, and visceral elements—is essential in evaluation.

Definitions

In *plain radiography*, part of the body to be investigated (e.g., the knee joint) is interposed between the source of radiation described as x-rays (roentgen rays) in the x-ray tube and a sensitized film in a cassette. The shadow picture or radiograph is the result.

In *tomography*, the x-ray tube and film cassette movements allow focal planes to be created as sharp and focused images (e.g., the nidus of an osteoid osteoma) of variable thickness while nonfocal plane objects become blurred and nondistracting.

The primary criterion in *computer tomography scanning (CTS)* is the creation of an accurate cross-sectional image using the shortest feasible scanning time. The thickness of such an image varies from 5–10 mm. In a CT scanner, the x-ray tube and detector cells rotate synchronously, or the cells may be stationary around the periphery of the scanner. The image is a pictorial display of a thin slice of anatomy (e.g., of the lumbar spinal canal). Each CT picture consists of thousands of computer picture elements arranged in rows and columns (matrix). The conversion of the matrix of numbers into a picture produces a display of internal anatomy based on the individual organ's capacity to absorb radiation (Fig. 4.1). CTs may be enhanced by concurrent use of a radiopaque contrast medium.

Angiography consists of images of contrast medium flowing rapidly through a pulsating vascular system. It must be obtained with high spatial and contrast resolutions. Computer-enhanced images of intravenously injected contrast media are now feasible but are not widely available, and the artery to be studied (e.g., the common carotid) must be entered by needle or catheter with the risk of dislodging an atheromatous plaque. The risk is justified, however, when a surgically remedial localized stenosis is suspected.

In *myelography*, a radiopaque contrast medium is injected into the subarachnoid space of the spine and reflects the flow of cerebrospinal fluid and outlines the spinal cord (Fig. 4.2). It is most commonly used before discectomy but can confirm spinal cord malformations or neoplasms as well.

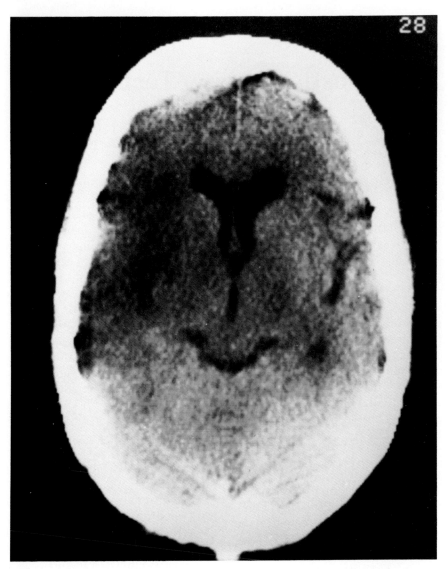

Figure 4.1. CT scan. A low density lesion is seen here, involving the right frontoparietal region associated with some compression of the lateral ventricle. The posterior fossa is clear. The described findings are due to a large infarct in the right middle cerebral artery distribution.

Many patients feel unwell for a few days after a myelogram, and a few develop a chemical arachnoiditis. The water-soluble contrast, although providing better definition and less arachnoiditis, causes seizures if it is allowed to flow intracranially. For this reason, oil-based contrast is used for high cervical myelography.

Cineradiography applies the principles of a movie film to record dynamic events of an organ system frequently using a contrast medium. For joint movements, fluoroscopy is preferred because of the lower dose of radiation. It may be recorded on videotape.

Xeroradiography, by use of a specially charged film, produces excellent contrast in soft tissue, such as an amputation stump.

Arthrography is performed by the introduction into the joint of contrast material(s), usually carbon dioxide and a wa-

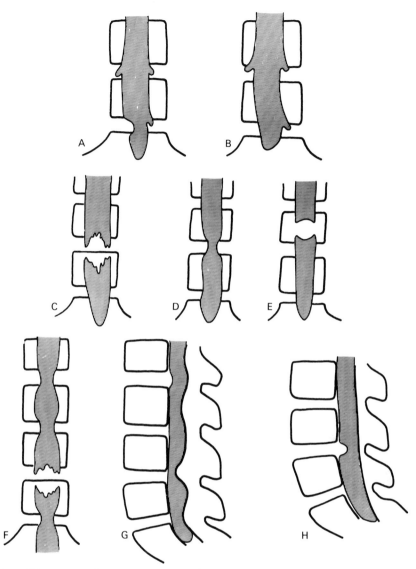

Figure 4.2. Diagrammatic representation of commonly seen myelographic defects. (A) Lumbosacral disc rupture with indentation of the oil column. (B) Cutoff of the first sacral root sleeve due to a lateral disc rupture. (C) Sequestration of a large fragment of disc material at the L4-L5 level. (D) Annular constriction of the oil column at the L4-L5 level. This radiographic appearance is produced by a diffuse annular bulge of the L4-L5 disc and is *not* due to a bilateral disc protrusion. (E) An intrathecal tumor will produce a characteristic defect delineated by a meniscus. Frequently, this defect is in relation to a vertebral body on x-ray, rather than to the disc space. (F) Compression of the cauda equina from a posterior lesion such as a spinal stenosis may produce a complete block in the oil column on the anteroposterior view, but the true site of the lesion will be revealed by studying the lateral view (G) where it can be seen that there is a marked posterior indentation. (H) Anterior indentations of the oil column are frequently seen on the lateral view, but these are rarely of clinical significance. (Reproduced with permission from I. McNab: *Backache*. Baltimore, Williams & Wilkins)

ter-soluble radiopaque agent. The agents outline radiolucent structures, such as a torn meniscus.

NUCLEAR MEDICINE

The use of imaging devices with a rectilinear scanner and scintillation camera. A shielded sodium iodide crystal moves mechanically across the field of interest, increments a specific but constant distance down the patient, and then moves back across and scans the distribution of radioactivity. The readout system moves in synchrony with the detector and presents the processed information for visual interpretation. *Technetium-99* (^{99}Tc) pertechnate imaging is the commonest used for brain flow and scan studies or other

vascular work. It is injected intravenously, and the radiation dose is low.

^{99}Tc methylene diphosphonate is the most commonly used bone scanning agent, although gallium can also be used if infection or neoplasm are suspected. Joint scans also can be used as a measure of localized inflammation, using agents that are detected either in the vascular synovium or in the adjacent bone (Fig. 4.3). The inflammatory phase of *spondyloarthropathies* is well shown by technetium-99 scanning. The advantage of a technetium-99 bone scan is that it demonstrates the current level of inflammatory activity in the joints as the intensity of uptake is related to osteoblastic cell activity whereas x-rays document the end result of the total disease process.

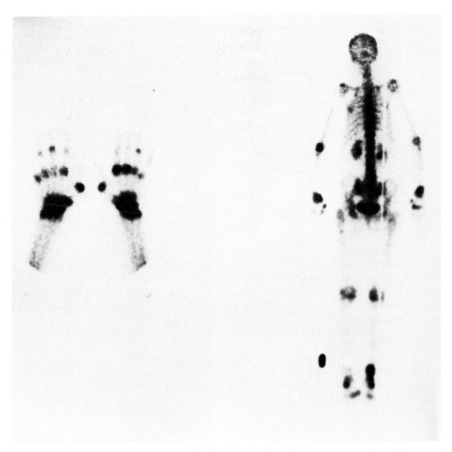

Figure 4.3. Bone scan. In this patient with rheumatoid arthritis, increased activity can be seen around many joints, reflecting increased turnover in juxtoarticular bone.

In *septic arthritis* a technetium bone scan is invaluable in making an early diagnosis and a *gallium-67* scan even more specific because of its selective uptake by leukocytes. Late x-ray changes show extensive joint destruction and perhaps bony fusion.

DIAGNOSTIC ULTRASOUND

Sound waves greater than 20,000 Hz are mechanical wave phenomena which require a medium for their propagation. The velocity of the waves depends on the density and compressibility of the medium. The formation of images of internal body structures is based upon the "sonar" (sound navigation and ranging) principle. It is used to determine the location of an object within a medium by measuring the time interval between the production of an ultrasonic pulse and the detection of its echo resulting from the reflection off the structure's surface. A popliteal cyst, a complication of synovitis of the knee, can be demonstrated by ultrasound (Fig. 4.4). There is neither risk nor discomfort.

THERMOGRAPHY

Infrared rays are emitted from the skin and are directly equivalent to the skin temperature. Using electronic screening devices, pictorial heat maps (thermograms) of whole areas of the body can be made. Thermography is noninvasive and without hazard. It has been used in diagnosis and prognostic assessment of disease. Thermographic maps of the body in musculoskeletal disorders may show areas of local increased vasodilation ("hot spots") or vasoconstriction ("cold spots").

APPLICATIONS
Musculoskeletal System

Osteoarthritis. Radiography provides a shadow image of bones, joints, and soft

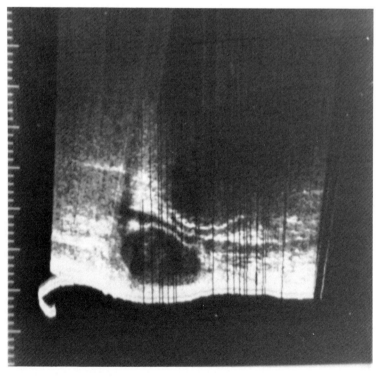

Figure 4.4. Diagnostic ultrasound. A fluid-filled 4-cm mass, a popliteal cyst, is present on the posterior aspect of the lower femur.

tissues. The commonest abnormality is *osteoarthritis* (OA) or *degenerative joint disease* (DJD). The radiological features are: joint space narrowing due to cartilage loss, subchondral bone sclerosis and cyst formation, and presence of osteophytes. In the hands, these features are typically seen in the distal interphalangeal (DIP) joints (Heberden's nodes) and in the proximal interphalangeal (PIP) joints (Bouchard's nodes), but *not* in the metacarpophalangeal (MCP) joints. In the foot, the metatarsophalangeal (MTP) joint of the big toe, the bunion joint, is the commonest site of OA. In the knees, there is usually radiographic evidence of OA in the patellofemoral and medial tibiofemoral joints. The latter leads to genu varum or bow leg deformity. To demonstrate genu varum or genu valgum, knee radiographs are obtained with the patient standing. Although calcification of knee cartilages may be seen in OA it is one of the diagnostic signs of *chondrocalcinosis* (pseudogout). In the hip joints, there is early osteophyte formation on the superolateral aspect of the femoral head and inferior aspect of the acetabulum with an upward displacement of the head. OA also frequently involves the cervical and lumbar spine at C5-6-7 and L4-5-S1 levels. Radiologically, there is disc space narrowing, marginal osteophytes, and narrowing and sclerosis of posterior facet (apophyseal) joints (Figs. 4.5 and 4.6).

Osteopenia (Bone Thinning). This condition is frequently noted especially in the elderly and bedridden but also in the postmenopausal female and in patients on corticosteroid medication. Radiologically, there is thinning of cortical bone and loss of bony trabeculae. Compression fractures occur especially in vertebral bodies. It is radiologically difficult to distinguish between the osteopenia of osteoporosis and osteomalacia. Bone densitometry may be used as an objective measure.

Rheumatoid Arthritis. This condition is the classic example of an inflammatory arthritis. Its radiological hallmark is erosion of cartilage and bone with early peri-

articular osteopenia due to inflammatory hyperemia. Erosions are characteristically seen in a symmetrical distribution in the small joints of the fingers with involvement of the metacarpophalangeal (MCP) and proximal interphalangeal (PIP) joints but usually *not* the DIP joints (Figs. 4.7 and 4.8). However, any other joint may show evidence of involvement. Erosions are seen at the attachment of the synovial membrane and appear as punched out areas varying in size. The end result may be a complete destruction of the joint or a bony ankylosis. Examples of other inflammatory erosive arthritides are ankylosing spondylitis, psoriatic arthritis (Fig. 4.8), and gout. A "Baker's cyst" may be identified by arthrography (Fig. 4.9).

Spondyloarthropathies. These are inflammatory joint conditions which involve the axial skeleton and include ankylosing spondylitis. The diagnostic radiological features are erosions of sacroiliac (SI) joints, later fusion (Fig. 4.10). The inflammatory phase is well shown by technetium-99 scanning with increased uptake in the SI joints. Late radiographic changes in the spine are an ossification of the ligaments, including the anterior and posterior longitudinal ligaments and the "bamboo spine."

Gout. This condition characteristically involves the MTP joint of the big toe with evidence of soft tissue swelling and "punched out" erosions and occasionally a calcified tophus (a subcutaneous collection of sodium urate crystals).

Osteomyelitis. Technetium-99 bone scanning is of major diagnostic value, and radiographs show changes of periosteal elevation and separation some days after clinical onset. Late appearances show thickened cortical bone or an infarcted fragment of bone, a sequestrum.

A *sinogram* is useful in delineating the tract in a discharging point on the skin and the underlying bone which may be the site of chronic osteomyelitis. A radiopaque contrast medium is injected into the tract and serial radiographs taken.

Heterotopic bone formation. This is

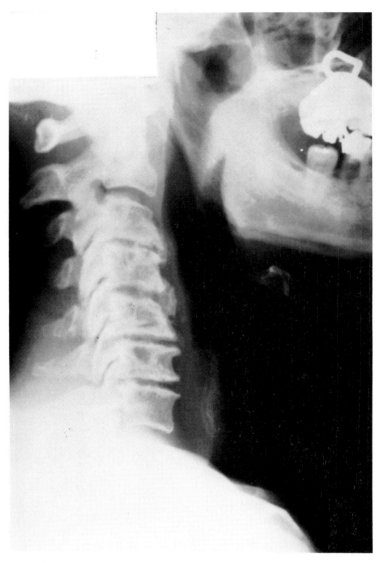

Figure 4.5.   Cervical spine. Degenerative disc narrowing is particularly evident at the C3-4 level, and although the disc space at C4-5 is only slightly reduced in width, there is a fairly large block of bone present anteriorly at this disc space. Degenerative changes are again evident at C5-6 and C6-7 levels, with marginal osteophytosis which, in the case of the lower levels, encroaches upon the intervertebral foramina. There is also marked lipping present at the neurocentral joints of the midcervical spine.

seen in traumatic paraplegia and quadriplegia. Early diagnosis is made by a technetium bone scan which clearly shows areas of bone formation. The clinical appearances can be confused with deep vein thrombosis and can be positively excluded by a *venogram* which displays the deep and superficial venous systems of the lower limb by a contrast medium injected into a vein of the foot. Areas of thrombosis or vein compression are seen. Heterotopic bone formation is seen typically in the hip region, and radiographs are quite striking (Fig. 4.11).

Fractures. Radiographs play a major role in the assessment and progress of healing of bone fractures with auxiliary use of tomography or technetium scans to

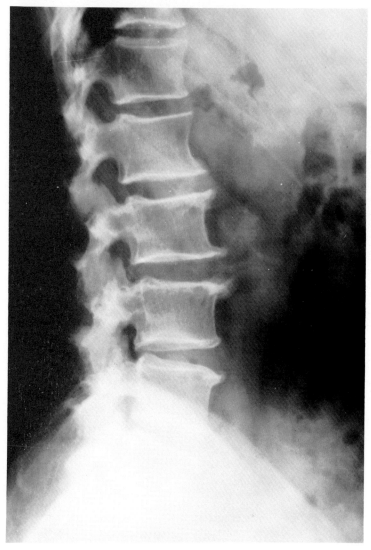

Figure 4.6. Extensive hypertrophic fringing is present, but the disc spaces are nevertheless well maintained.

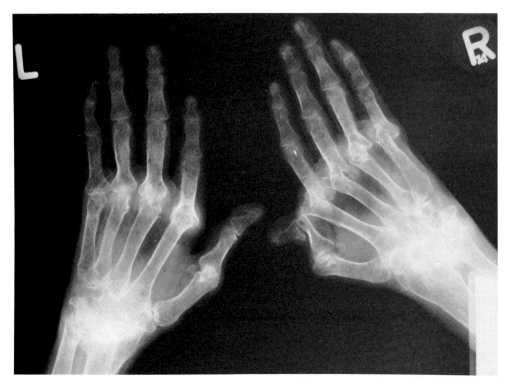

Figure 4.7. There is marked osteopenia with subarticular erosion and subluxation involving principally the metacarpophalangeal joints, especially on the right side. The terminal phalanx of the right thumb is subluxated. There is also marked narrowing of both wrist joints with some subarticular sclerosis and probable fusion between several of the bones.

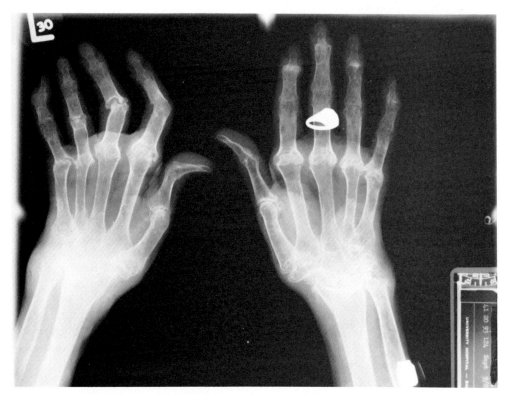

Figure 4.8. Hands and wrists. Marked osteopenia of the regional bones. There are erosive changes of the radial and ulnar styloids, as well as the inferior radioulnar processes. There is narrowing of the radiocarpal joints as well as the transcarpal joints; erosive changes are noted of the MCP and IP joints, as well as hyperextension of the distal digit of the left first finger and subluxations at the MCP joints. The erosive changes of the distal IP joints is suggestive of psoriasis. There is a lateral deviation of the left phalanges.

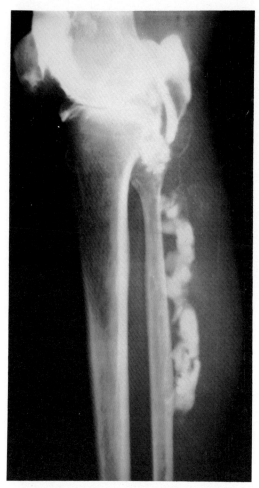

Figure 4.9. Arthrogram—right knee. In the initial tap of the knee joint, 30 ml of bloody synovial fluid were withdrawn. Thirty ml of contrast media were introduced, and films were taken. There is irregularity of the supra-patellar bursa and of the synovial cavity itself; this is probably on the basis of synovial thickening and hypertrophy. On the initial film prior to extension, there is an almost normal appearance to the posterior aspect of the joint. However, with flexion a definite extension is outlined which appears to have a discrete neck. This should represent a Baker's cyst. From this area there is extravasation of contrast medium to the region of the midportion of the calf. This should represent a ruptured Baker's cyst.

demonstrate fractures difficult to visualize and microfractures. The radiographs of bones in infants, children, and adolescents show cartilage at the growing ends of the long bones (epiphyses) with second-ary ossification centers. Ossification usually ceases by the early 20s.

Scoliosis and Kyphosis. These are curvatures of the spine and should be assessed by serial radiographs to monitor progression or response to treatment.

Neurological System

The commonly used imaging techniques include radiographs of the skull, brain scan, computerized axial scanning (CTS) (Fig. 4.1), echoencephalograms, and angiography.

CTS (which may be combined with an intrathecal injection of a contrast medium) is of great value in assessing changes in the size of the brain (cerebral atrophy), dilatation of the ventricles (cerebral atrophy and hydrocephalus), tumors, and cerebral infarcts (Fig. 4.1). CTS of the spinal column demonstrates spinal cord and radicular compression by intervertebral disc protrusion, bone, or tumors.

Angiography is used in the investigation of the internal and external carotid (carotid angiography) and the basivertebral (aortic arch angiogram) arterial systems. It demonstrates aneurysms, arteriovenous malformations, and vascular tumors, as well as atheromatous plaques, ulcers, and narrowing or occlusion of an artery. The procedure is not without risk to the patient.

Genitourinary System

These procedures are used in the investigation of the paralyzed bladder and its complications, due to spinal cord injuries, stroke, or multiple sclerosis.

The *intravenous pyelogram* allows a sequential viewing of the excretion by the kidneys of a contrast medium administered intravenously. Sequential x-rays visualize the kidneys, minor and major collecting renal systems, renal pelves, ureters, and bladder. It is a method of estimating kidney function, the presence of renal, ureteric or bladder stones, prostatic enlargement, congenital anomalies and trauma.

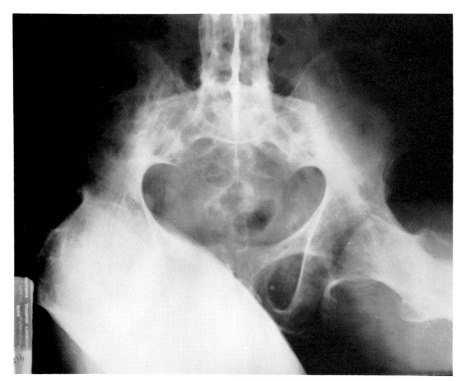

Figure 4.10. Advanced ankylosing spondylitis. There is a bony ankylosis at the hips and some generalized demineralization. The lower portion of the lumbar spine exhibits the classical bamboo appearance; also there is obliteration of both sacroiliac joints and "bearding" at the ischial and iliac crest regions.

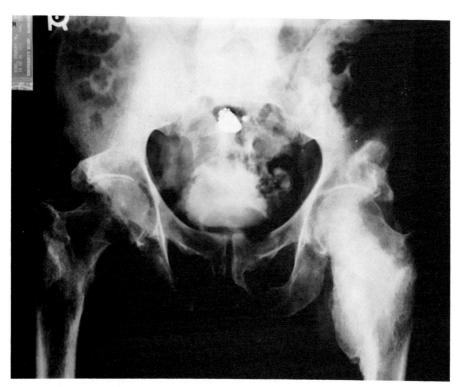

Figure 4.11. Extensive soft tissue ossification in the region of the left hip and upper femur. There is also a small area of ossification extending laterally from the superior right acetabulum, representing heterotopic bone formation.

A *voiding cystourethrogram* provides a sequential radiographic study of bladder filling, using a contrast medium and voiding through the urethra. It may show vesicoureteral reflux. Recently, *urodynamic studies* combine measurements of bladder volume and pressure and electromyographic activity of the external sphincter.

References

1. Coulam CM, Erickson JJ, Rollo FD, James EJ: *The Physical Basis of Medical Imaging*. New York, Appleton-Century-Crofts, 1981.
2. Shanks SC, Kerley P: *A Textbook of X-ray Diagnosis*, vol XI. Philadelphia, W.B. Saunders, 1971.
3. Husband JE, Golding SJ: *Computed Tomography of the Body: When Should It Be Used?* Brit Med J 284:4–8, 1982.

Electrodiagnosis

D. O. WIECHERS

Electrodiagnosis is the application of different neurophysiological techniques to aid in the diagnosis of various disorders affecting the neuromuscular system. In some countries there is a specialty of medicine known as Clinical Neurophysiology. Generally, electrodiagnosis is an integral part of the specialty of Physical Medicine and Rehabilitation, and expertise is necessary to become board certified.

The most common neurophysiological techniques employed clinically are: (a) calculation of peripheral nerve conduction velocity, (b) the search in a muscle for free fibrillating fibers 18–21 days after a suspected peripheral nerve compromise, and (c) the recording and analysis of motor unit action potentials—searching for disintegration or reorganization of the motor unit either in neuromuscular diseases or following peripheral nerve injury. Therefore, an in depth understanding of the motor unit and its pathophysiology is essential in electrodiagnosis.

Several neurophysiological techniques that are of use in specific instances in clinical practice will not be discussed here. The student is directed to textbooks of electromyography for information regarding single fiber EMG, macro EMG, and visual, auditory, and somatosensory evoked potentials (1, 2).

The electrodiagnostic examination begins with a history and a physical examination. The specific electrodiagnostic studies to be performed are then selected by the differential diagnosis and used to confirm or reject the clinical impression. The electrodiagnostic examination is almost never routine. Which peripheral nerve or which muscle to study is totally dependent on the findings as the examination proceeds. It is very common for the examination to change direction several times during the course of study in order to make the correct diagnosis. It is not uncommon to begin an examination looking for a peripheral nerve compromise and end the examination 1 or 2 hours later with a diagnosis of motor neuron disease. For this reason diagnostic electromyography can only be performed by a physician knowledgeable of neuromuscular disorders.

THE MOTOR UNIT

The motor unit is comprised of an α motor neuron located in the anterior horn, its axon, and all the individual muscle fibers that are attached to the axon. Motor units come in many sizes (3). Some have only a few muscle fibers, such as the extraocular muscles; others have hundreds, like the hip extensor muscles. The diameters of some axons are very large and heavily myelinated and are capable of conducting impulses at about 60 m/second (4). Smaller diameter axons have less myelin and conduct impulses at a rate of 45 m/second.

At the neuromuscular junction, the impulse is transmitted by the chemical mediator acetylcholine. Difficulties in transmission can result in several muscle fibers of a motor unit not receiving the message to contract, resulting in fatigue or weakness, as is seen in myasthenia gravis or botulism.

With successful neuromuscular transmission, individual muscle fibers depolarize, and the impulse is propagated down the muscle fiber at 4–7 meters/second (5).

If we record the depolarization of an individual muscle fiber with a special single-fiber electrode, we obtain a biphasic wave of about 1 millisecond in duration (Fig. 4.12). If we now record the depolarizations of all the muscle fibers of a motor unit within about a 1-mm recording area of the standard monopolar or concentric electrode (Fig. 4.12), we obtain usually a triphasic wave with a duration of about 3–8 msec. The standard monopolar or concentric electrodes have a recording surface of about 0.1 mm^2 and, therefore, they are recording the algebraic summation of the individual biphasic depolarization of 2–12 muscle fibers of that motor unit (2, 6). The way in which the normal physiology of the motor unit is altered by certain pathological processes determines what is recorded in disease states.

THE INSTRUMENT

The basic electromyograph is composed of a preamplifier that has a uniform re-

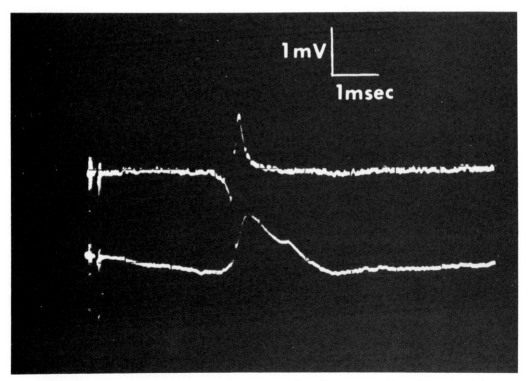

Figure 4.12.   A single fiber potential compared with a motor unit action potential.

sponse to frequencies from at least 2 Hz to 10,000 Hz with an input impedance of about 100 megohms (8). It is a differential amplifier or a difference amplifier that records only the electrical activity that is not common to the two recording electrodes, called the active and the reference electrode (Fig. 4.13). The electrical signal is then displayed visually on an oscilloscope and through a loud speaker. The signal may also be fed into a computer for analysis or stored on magnetic tape.

Electrodes for routine electromyography (EMG) are monopolar or concentric (Fig. 4.14). Monopolar electrodes (active) are stainless steel wires coated with Teflon with an exposed recording tip of approximately 0.1 mm². A second monopolar electrode, or a surface electrode of approximately 1 cm in diameter, is the reference electrode. Concentric needle electrodes are hollow needles through which a platinum wire is passed and in-

sulated from the needle canula. The tip of the platinum wire is the recording surface and is usually of approximately 0.03 mm² (6). The cannula of the needle is the reference electrode.

A physiological stimulator is necessary for determining nerve conduction velocities. The stimulator should have adjustments for intensity and duration to ensure supramaximal stimulation. The stimulator should be isolated from the ground, and the sweep of the oscilloscope should be triggered by the stimulator.

NERVE CONDUCTION TECHNIQUES

Nerve conduction studies are usually performed first in the electrodiagnostic exam after the history and physical.

A peripheral nerve in the extremity can be thought of as a conduit. Within this conduit or peripheral nerve run thousands of axons. Some run distally to mus-

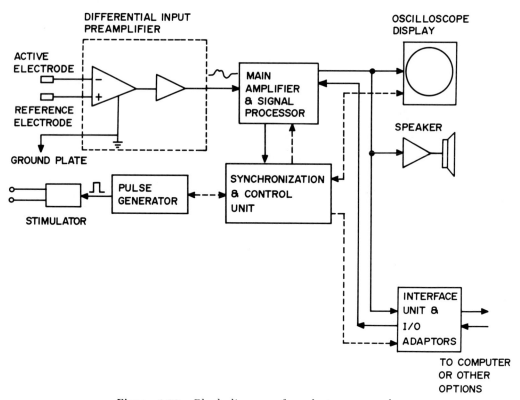

Figure 4.13. Block diagram of an electromyograph.

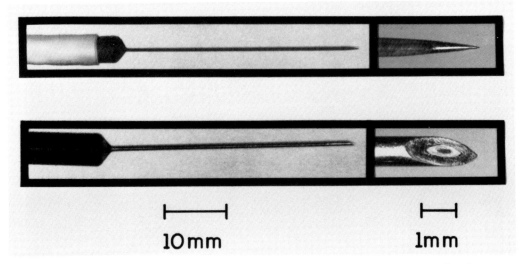

10mm   1mm

Figure 4.14.   EMG needle electrodes—upper, monopolar; lower, concentric bipolar.

cle fibers from α motor neurons. Some run proximally from sensory endings carrying light touch, vibration, temperature, etc. Others run proximally carrying I_a afferent fibers from muscle spindles.

Supramaximal stimulation of a peripheral nerve will then result in the depolarization of all of its motor and sensory nerve fibers. Stimulation of the digital nerves (pure sensory) allows the recording of the depolarization of the axons proximally at several points along the peripheral nerve (orthodromic stimulation) (Fig. 4.15) (9). By measuring the time in milliseconds from stimulation to the peak of the sensory response (latency) in at least two locations and subtracting the proximal latency from the distal latency, we get the time of conduction between two recording sites. The measured distance between the recording sites, divided by their conduction time, will give the sensory conduction velocity.

Supramaximal stimulation of a peripheral nerve proximally in an extremity will result in the depolarization of all of the muscle fibers of a distal muscle which is innervated by that peripheral nerve. With a surface electrode placed over the motor point of the muscle and a reference electrode over the distal tendon of the muscle,

we can record the total muscle depolarization, or "M" wave (Fig. 4.16). Dividing the distance between two points of stimulation along the peripheral nerve by the difference between the times (proximal—distal latencies) to the beginning of the depolarization (M-wave) will give the motor conduction velocity of the fastest-conducting motor units in that peripheral nerve (10).

The *motor nerve conduction studies* routinely performed are on the facial, radial, median, ulnar, femoral, tibial, peroneal, and medial and lateral plantar nerves (10).

The *sensory nerve conduction studies* routinely performed are on the radial, median, ulnar, lateral antebrachial cutaneous, lateral femoral cutaneous, saphenous, medial cutaneous branch of the superficial peroneal, and sural nerves (9).

The *Achilles reflex* is frequently recorded and analyzed electrically. Recording the reflex in this manner is called the "H" reflex (10). The I_a afferent nerve fibers from the muscle spindles in the gastrocnemius or soleus muscles are stimulated in the tibial nerve in the popliteal space. Following stimulation, the impulse travels up to the spinal cord and monosynaptically stimulates an α motor neuron at

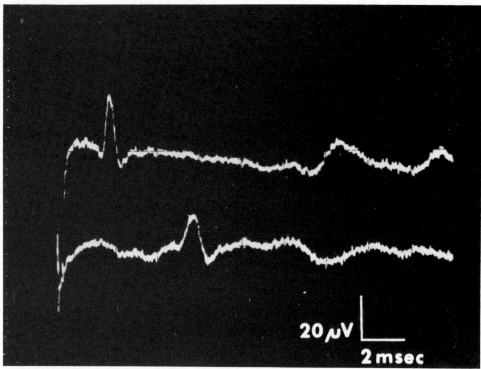

Figure 4.15. Sensory nerve action potential recorded from median nerve at the wrist and elbow with the stimulus applied through a surface electrode to the digital nerves.

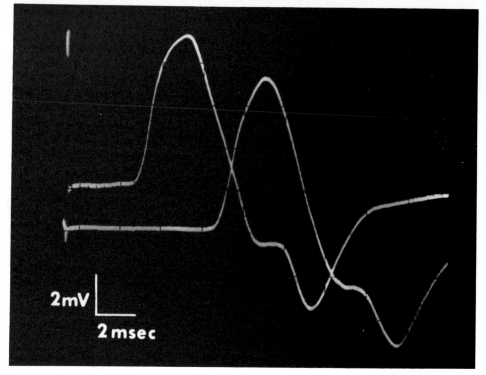

Figure 4.16. Motor nerve stimulation producing a muscle evoked potential (M-wave), stimulating ulnar nerve at the wrist and at the elbow and recording from the abductor digiti quinti.

the S1 level. The depolarization (H-wave) of the gastrocnemius or soleus is then recorded some 20–30 milliseconds after I_a afferent stimulation. Since the tibial nerve in the popliteal space is a conduit with not only I_a afferent fibers but also axons from α motor neurons, some motor units are stimulated directly, and a small M-wave is obtained preceding the H-wave at low intensity of stimulation (Fig. 4.17).

Ideally with proper stimulation techniques we would see no M-wave and a large H-wave. If our intensity of stimulation increases, we get more M-wave and less H-wave. The size of the M and H waves varies with stimulation, like opposite sides on a teeter-totter, since ideally they are both the same size.

Increasing the intensity of stimulation of the tibial nerve in the popliteal space to supramaximal results in an M-wave of maximal size and no H-wave. With continued supramaximal stimulation, a small new wave is seen prior to when the H-

wave was previously observed. This "F" wave is produced when a few of the motor units are capable of backfiring (10). The impulse is carried antidromically (backwards) up the motor unit to the α motor neuron with supramaximal stimulation of its axon. With supramaximal stimulation, a single α motor neuron is capable of refiring or backfiring 0.1 to 20% of the time and returning a new impulse down its axon (1). Since only a few motor units in a whole muscle are capable of backfiring with each distal stimulation, the size of a recorded F wave from the motor point of the muscle is small relative to the M wave and H wave, and it varies in size and shape with repetitive stimulation.

ELECTROMYOGRAPHY

Electromyography (EMG) is the intramuscular recording and analysis of motor units. Almost any muscle in the body can be studied, and there are five basic steps for each muscle examined (12):

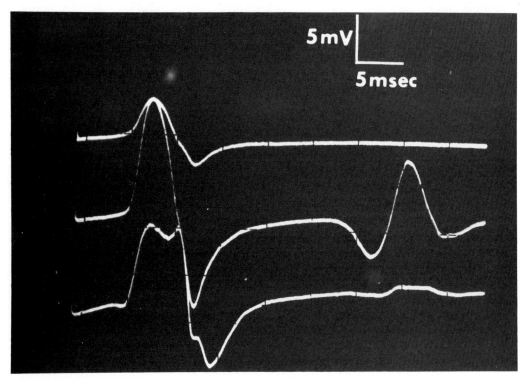

Figure 4.17. Late waves "H" and "F" produced by increasing the intensity of stimulation.

Step 1—Muscle at rest
Step 2—Insertional activity
Step 3—First recruited motor units and recruitment of low and medium threshold motor units
Step 4—High threshold motor units with maximal contraction
Step 5—Determination of which other muscles require examination to rule out certain diagnoses, summary of the findings, assessment and evaluation, and rendering of the final diagnosis.

Muscle at rest is normally electrically silent (Step 1). When the electrode is inserted into a muscle (Step 2), there is a depolarization record from those muscle fibers that are injured or impaled by the electrode (insertional activity). Electrical silence returns in the normal state (13).

Step 3 is the recording of individual motor units with analysis of their amplitude, duration, rise time, number of phases, and stability on repetitive voluntary firing (14). The motor unit potential recorded (Fig. 4.18) can take any size or shape, depending on where in the motor unit territory we record the algebraic summation of the depolarization of the individual muscle fibers (15). It is, therefore, most important to move the electrode into the electrical center of the motor unit by maximizing the amplitude and minimizing the rise time of the positive-to-negative spike component of the potential.

Quantitative analysis of 20 first recruited motor unit action potentials in a muscle is a necessity when the normalcy of the first recruited motor unit action potentials seen with voluntary contraction is unclear. The amplitude, duration, and percentage of units with greater than five phases or polyphasic potentials varies from muscle to muscle, with the patient's age, and with the strength of contraction in normal people (14). The parameters of the motor unit are affected by the electrode type, and the lead-off or recording surface of the electrode, the frequency or band pass of filters, and the input impedance of the preamplifier (6).

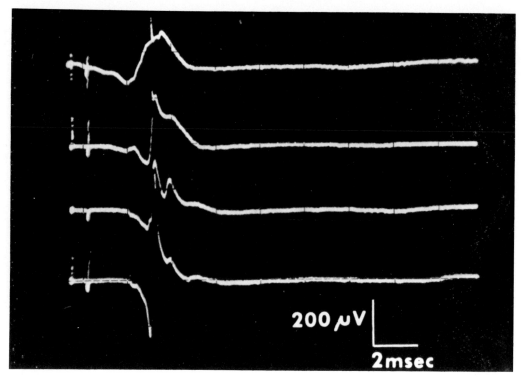

200 μV

2msec

Figure 4.18. Changes in a motor unit potential's parameters with shifting of the electrode position.

As the patient increases the strength of contraction in a muscle, the 2nd, 3rd, and 4th recruited motor units can be recorded and analyzed. At this point the oscilloscope screen tends to become full, and individual motor unit analysis becomes difficult. As the patient increases the strength of contraction, we rapidly reach maximum (Step 4) and now can analyze the full interference patterns visually and acoustically.

Step 5 is the analysis of the findings of this muscle. More importantly, it will determine the direction of the remainder of the examination, that is, which muscle should be studied next to prove or disprove a root level lesion, a peripheral nerve branch, or a peripheral neuropathy. This step is also critical in determining which further studies are needed to determine a distal or proximal myopathy, a motor neuron disorder, or a combination of a peripheral nerve compromise with an underlying peripheral neuropathy. The electrical findings are then combined with the history, physical, and laboratory data to arrive at a final diagnosis.

PATHOLOGY

Peripheral Nerve or Root Level Compromise

If a peripheral nerve is cut or severely traumatized, the axons of many motor units are compromised. This results in Wallerian degeneration, and the nerve fiber degenerates down to the muscle fiber with loss of the nerve terminal. The distal portions of the nerve, however, remain excitable for approximately 72 hours (16). Nerve conduction studies after 72 hours would demonstrate a loss of motor units in the muscle with supramaximal stimulation or a reduced amplitude of the evoked response (M-wave). If the injured motor units had the fastest conducting axons, then there would be slowing of the overall nerve conduction velocity across the injured area.

Some axons, when injured to a mild degree, are not altered anatomically but have a physiological block of conduction across the injured area which is called neuropraxia (17). The distal portion of the axon conducts normally, but when stimulated proximally, the depolarization wave will not pass through the neuropraxic segment. Conduction velocity determination across a peripheral nerve segment containing a lot of neuropraxic axons will be slow if the faster-conducting axons are affected. The conduction velocity through the portions of the peripheral nerve not containing the neuropraxic segments will be normal. If injury to an axon continues, anatomical changes occur, and the axon undergoes Wallerian degeneration (17).

The muscle fibers that lose contact with their α motor neurons undergo changes. The whole muscle fiber membrane develops receptor sites for acetylcholine and becomes hypersensitive. The resting membrane of the muscle fiber now begins to undulate, beginning at negative 70 to 80 μV and increasing in amplitude until negative 55 μV or threshold is reached (18). The single-muscle fiber then depolarizes spontaneously, which is called a fibrillation potential. It takes 18–21 days for the muscle fibers of an injured motor unit to fibrillate if the axon is injured at the root level and less time if the axon is transsected closer to the nerve terminal and muscle fiber.

The recording of a fibrillating muscle fiber is the spontaneous occurrence of a biphasic wave with an initial positive deflection of about 1–2 msec in duration and 25–200 μV in amplitude. These are recorded when the muscle is at rest. With insertion of the electrode into a muscle that has fibrillating fibers, we can provoke a positive-shaped potential called a positive sharp wave, which will have the same clinical significance as fibrillation potentials but require mechanical stimulation for production (Fig. 4.19). Positive sharp waves can be provoked in muscles just before individual muscle fibers spon-

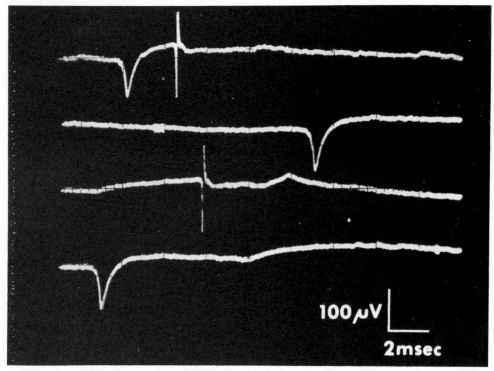

Figure 4.19.   Fibrillation potentials (very short duration) and positive sharp waves. (Note: in electrophysiology tracings, positive is downward.)

taneously start fibrillating (19). They are therefore frequently the earliest abnormality recorded in a mild radiculopathy or nerve injury. The positive sharp waves, however, are the most frequently misread abnormality on EMG since motor units can have any size or shape, depending on where in the electrical territory of the motor unit we are recording. Voluntary motor units can have the exact size and shape as positive sharp waves and can be easily misinterpreted by novice electromyographers. The difference between voluntary motor units and the true provoked positive sharp wave is the regular frequency of firing of the voluntary motor unit.

Denervated muscle fibers will continue to fibrillate for a long period of time before they atrophy and become nonfunctional. Fibrillating fibers can, however, be reinnervated by two mechanisms. The first is the regrowth of the injured axon at about 1 mm/day (20). When the regrowing axon comes into direct contact with the fibrillating muscle fiber, a new neuromuscular junction is formed. The second method of reinnervation is by terminal axon sprouting (21, 22). A functioning noninjured motor unit that is in close proximity can send out a terminal axon branch or sprout, and if this branch contacts the fibrillating muscle fiber, a new neuromuscular junction will form. This can result in a whole area of a muscle fascicle being innervated by one motor unit and corresponds to fiber type grouping seen on biopsy.

When this new parent motor neuron fires, it now depolarizes more muscle fibers than it did previously, and the recorded motor unit action potential is of increased amplitude and duration with extra phases. Terminal axon sprouts that have grown to reinnervate the orphaned muscle fibers are initially unmyelinated, and impulse transmission to this axon sprout is tenuous and frequently fails. Transmission down this unmyelinated terminal axon sprout is frequently slowed, and getting the impulse across the newly formed neuromuscular junction can be difficult. The result of these transmission difficulties early in reinnervation can be seen as "instability" in the motor unit size and shape when analyzed carefully on repetitive voluntary discharges. As the reinnervated motor unit matures over the next 3–4 months, the motor unit becomes stable (23).

In summary, with a peripheral nerve or root level compromise we see an EMG that demonstrates fibrillating muscle fibers and positive sharp waves, and a dropout or loss of motor units with recruitment. As time passes, we will see reinnervation motor units or motor units of increased amplitude and duration and an increased percentage of polyphasic potentials in the affected muscles.

Peripheral Neuropathy

From a neurophysiological point of view, we can look at peripheral neuropathies as two basic types: axonal and demyelinating.

These types relate to the initial pathology. As the disorder progresses, the process usually becomes combined, and features of both pathological disorders may be seen.

Axonal peripheral neuropathy is simply a loss of axons in the peripheral nerve or conduit. The death of an axon is no different from a traumatic injury to an axon from a neurophysiological point of view. If the axon is from a motor unit, then the muscle fibers of that axon will fibrillate and hopefully become reinnervated by terminal axon sprouting from neighboring motor units. As the disorder progresses, more and more axons are lost. If the fastest conducting motor units are lost, slowing in motor conduction velocity will be seen. If the fastest conducting motor units are not lost, then the only abnormality seen on nerve conduction studies will be a reduction in the amplitude of the recorded total muscle depolarization or M wave. The EMG of distal muscles in an axonal peripheral neuropathy may be the most helpful to confirm the diagnosis. With axon loss, free fibrillating muscle fibers will be recorded. With reinnervation, motor units of increased amplitude and duration will be seen. Recruitment becomes abnormal and demonstrates a loss of motor units per strength of contraction which will become more pronounced as the disease process progresses.

Demyelinating peripheral neuropathy is a disorder of the insulation, myelin, on the axon of the peripheral nerve. The myelin sheath facilitates fast axon conduction. In this disorder, segments of an axon lose their insulation, referred to as segmental demyelination, with the slowing of conduction by approximately 30–40%. This is easily detected by nerve conduction techniques because the fastest fibers are myelinated and, therefore, the conduction velocity slows early in the disorder. With enough loss of myelin, the axon will die and its muscle fibers will fibrillate, although later it may be reinnervated. As the disease progresses, it can become increasingly difficult to differentiate axonal from demyelinating peripheral neuropathy.

Motor Neuron Disorders

There are many disorders that have a specific affinity for the α motor neuron—e.g., poliomyelitis, amyotrophic lateral sclerosis, and the hereditary forms of progressive spinomuscular atrophy. When the α motor neuron is affected, the whole motor unit becomes unstable and frequently will spontaneously fire, with the generator potential being in the distal portions of the anterior horn cell (24).

These spontaneous discharges of a whole or portion of a motor unit are called fasciculation potentials. Fasciculation potentials by themselves are normal and occur with exercise and overwork, and abuse of caffeine, nicotine, and other stimulants. They occur so frequently in disorders of the motor neuron that a diagnosis of motor neuron disorder is rarely made in their absence. Death of the α motor neuron results in its muscle fibers fibrillating and perhaps later being reinnervated.

As the disorder progresses, more and more motor units are lost. Recruitment of motor units becomes distorted. As the fastest-conducting motor units are lost, the motor conduction velocity will begin to demonstrate mild slowing while the sensory conduction velocities remain unaffected (25).

Myopathies

Myopathies are disorders which affect the muscle fibers of a motor unit. The result is an overall loss of muscle fibers per motor unit. When recording a motor unit in a myopathy, there may only be one or two muscle fibers in the recording area of the electrode. The recording of this motor unit is a potential of small amplitude, short duration, and a highly polyphasic shape (26).

Early in the course of the disease, there is weakness in specific muscles due to fiber loss. Recruitment becomes abnormal as more motor units are needed to fire to give a specific resistance. This results in early recruitment of higher threshold motor units. An increased number of motor units recruited per strength of contraction is a hallmark of muscle disease. As the disease progresses and more muscle fibers are lost, a large area of muscle develops that is electrically silent. In end-stage muscle disease, there are a few motor units left in localized areas of muscle.

References

1. Wiechers D: Single fiber EMG. In Johnson E: *Practical Electromyography*. Baltimore, Williams & Wilkins, 1980.
2. Stalberg E, Young R: *Clinical Neurophysiology*. London, Butterworths, 1981.
3. Burke RE: Motor units: anatomy, physiology, and functional organization. In Brooks VB: *Handbook of Physiology*, sect. 1, The Nervous System and Sect II, Motor Systems. Washington, American Physiological Society, 1981.
4. Erlanger J: The interpretation of action potentials in cutaneous and muscle nerves. *Am J Physiol* 82:644–655, 1927.
5. Stalberg E: Propagation velocity in human nerve fibers *in situ*. *Acta Physiol Scand* 70 (Suppl 287):1, 1966.
6. Wiechers, DO, Blood, JR, Stow, RW: EMG needle electrodes: electrical impedance. *Arch Phys Med Rehabil* 60:364–369, 1979.
7. Thiele, B, Boehle, R: Number of single muscle fiber action potentials contributing to the motor unit potential. Rochester, Minn., Fifth International Congress of Electromyography, 1975. (abstr).
8. Reiner, S, Rogoff, J: Instrumentation. In Johnson E: *Practical Electromyography*. Baltimore, Williams & Wilkins, 1980.
9. Schuchmann, J, Braddom, R: Sensory conduction. In Johnson E: *Practical Electromyography*. Baltimore, Williams & Wilkins, 1980.
10. Braddom, R, Schuchmann, J: Motor conduction. In Johnson E: *Practical Electromyography*. Baltimore, Williams & Wilkins, 1980.
11. Trontelj, JV: A study of the F-response by single fiber electromyography. In Desmedt J: *New Developments in Electromyography and Clinical Neurophysiology*. Basel, Karger, 3:318–322, 1973.
12. Johnson, EW, Parker, WD: Electromyographic examination. In Johnson E: *Practical Electromyography*. Baltimore, Williams & Wilkins, 1980.
13. Wiechers, D, Stow, R, Johnson, E: Electromyography insertional activity mechanically provoked in biceps brachii. *Arch Phys Med Rehabil* 58:573–578, 1977.
14. Melvin, J, Wiechers, D: Measurement of motor unit action potentials. *Arch Phys Med Rehabil* 57:325, 1976.
15. Stalberg, E, Antoni, L.: Electrophysiological cross section of the motor unit. *J Neurol Neurosurg Psychiatry* 43:469–474, 1980.
16. Gilliatt, R: Recent advances in the pathophysiology of nerve conduction. In Desmedt J: *New Developments in Electromyography and Clinical Neurophysiology*, vol 3. Basel, Karger, 1973, pp 2–18.
17. Ochoa, J, Danta, G, Fowler, T, Gilliatt, R: Nature of the nerve lesion caused by pneumatic tourniquet. *Nature* 233:265, 1971.
18. Thesleff S, Ward MR: Studies on the mechanism of fibrillation potentials in denervated muscle. *J Physiol* 244:313, 1975.
19. Wiechers D: Mechanically provoked insertional activity before and after nerve section in rats. *Arch Phys Med Rehabil* 58:402–405, 1977.
20. Sunderland, S., Bradley, KC: Rate of advance of Hoffmann-Tinel sign in regenerating nerves. *Arch Neurol Psychiatry* 67:650, 1952.
21. Wohlfart, G: Collateral regeneration from residual motor nerve fibers in amyotrophic lateral sclerosis. *Neurology* 7:124, 1957.
22. Karpati, G, Engel, WK: "Type grouping" in skel-

etal muscle after experimental reinnervation. *Neurology* 18:447, 1968.
23. Hakelus, L, Stalberg, E: Electromyographical studies of free autogenous muscle transplants in man. *Scand J Plast Reconstr Surg* 8:211–219, 1974.
24. Conradi, S, Grimby, L, Lundemo, G: Pathophysiology of fasciculations in ALS as studied by

electromyography of single motor units. *Muscle Nerve* 5:202–208, 1982.
25. Wiechers, D, Warmolts, J: Anterior Horn Cell Disease. In Johnson E: *Practical Electromyography.* Baltimore, Williams & Wilkins, 1980.
26. Warmolts, J, Wiechers, D: Myopathies. In Johnson E: *Practical Electromyography.* Baltimore, Williams & Wilkins, 1980.

Biopsies of Musculoskeletal Tissues and Arthroscopy

R. L. KIRBY

Tissue biopsy is an important consideration in the investigation of musculoskeletal complaints. In most conditions the histologic findings are nonspecific and only "suggestive" or "supportive" of a diagnosis, adding little to the clinical evaluation and the less invasive investigative measures. However, in some disorders the histologic alterations are pathognomonic (Fig. 4.20).

The trend in musculoskeletal biopsy is away from open surgical biopsy and toward needle or perendoscopic biopsy under local anesthesia. Needle techniques performed at bedside are more convenient, generally requiring only sterile equipment, a drape, and gloves. Samples, although smaller, are usually adequate if appropriately oriented and fixed. If in doubt about the most appropriate histologic procedures or the fixation and transportation of the sample, consult the pathologist. Precautions and relative contraindications include allergy to local anesthetics, bleeding diathesis (including anticoagulant therapy), and vascular malformations or infection near the intended biopsy site.

MUSCLE BIOPSY

Muscle biopsy is usually performed

when a diffuse disorder of skeletal muscle is suspected, such as muscular dystrophy or polymyositis. In such an investigation one usually ensures that serum has been obtained for muscle enzymes (e.g., creatine phosphokinase) before invasive procedures, such as needle electromyography (EMG) and muscle biopsy, which elevate these enzymes.

EMG is usually performed before muscle biopsy as the electrodiagnostic findings may help in the selection of the biopsy site. However, since there is normally a mild focal inflammatory infiltrate in the muscle along the EMG needle track, in the investigation of a diffuse muscle disorder the EMG is performed on one side of the body and the muscle biopsy on the other.

In choosing a site for biopsy there are several other considerations. There should be a clinical or electrodiagnostic suspicion of involvement of the particular muscle in question, but the changes should not be too profound or only nonspecific end-stage changes may be found. Avoid small muscles, such as those of the thenar eminence, whose function may be impaired by biopsy. Neurovascular structures such as the axillary nerve in the posterior deltoid or the femoral artery be-

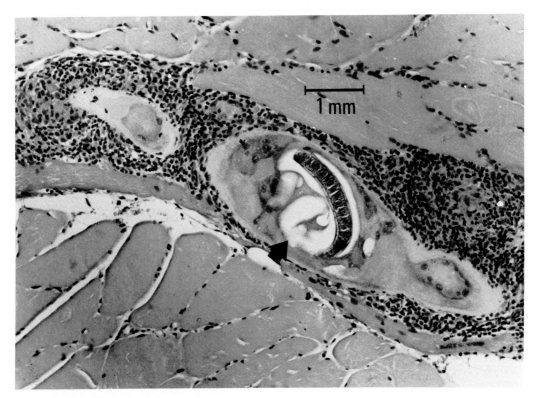

Figure 4.20.   Transverse section of the vastus lateralis obtained by needle biopsy. *Arrow* indicates a trichinella larva with surrounding muscle fiber necrosis and heavy mononuclear and histocytic infiltrate. (Reproduced with permission from R. L. Kirby *et al.*: *Archives of Physical Medicine and Rehabilitation* 63:264–268, 1982.)

neath the vastus medialis should also be avoided. Within a given muscle, generally biopsy at the junction of the middle and distal one-thirds of the muscle belly—if more proximal, one risks damage to the motor nerve to the muscle and, if more distal near tendon, the histology is difficult to interpret. All other factors being equal, choose a muscle with which the pathologist is most familiar, such as vastus lateralis or deltoid.

The most frequently used needle is the Bergström needle (Fig. 4.21). During insertion and removal, the lateral window is closed by a hollow inner sheath with a sharpened distal rim. The sheath is withdrawn; muscle is encourged to bulge into the window by finger pressure, needle manipulation, or suction; and the window is closed, snipping off 30–200 mg of tissue.

If insufficient muscle has been obtained, the procedure is repeated.

The obtained muscle should be handled cautiously to prevent mechanical artefacts—use a needle rather than coarse-toothed forceps. A common error is to use the wrong fixative; if the biopsy sample is placed in formalin, then no histochemistry or electron microscopy can be employed. Freezing in liquid nitrogen-cooled isopentane is used for the former (one has 15–30 minutes to get the sample to the laboratory for this) and a solution of 3% glutaraldehyde for the latter.

BONE BIOPSY

The usual indications for bone biopsy are to provide further information about either a localized bony abnormality (e.g.,

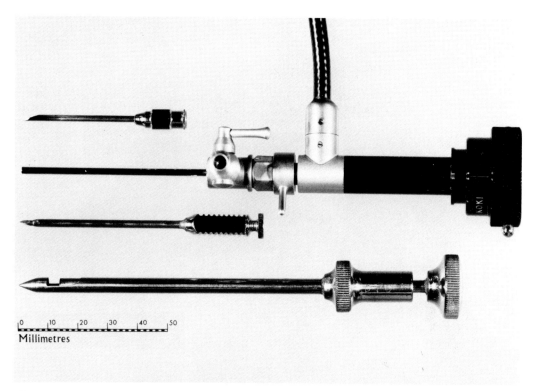

0   10   20   30   40   50
Millimetres

Figure 4.21.   The length and diameter of (from above down) a 14-gauge needle, a Watanabe no. 25 needle arthroscope, a Williams synovial biopsy needle, and a Bergström muscle biopsy needle are illustrated.

due to neoplasm) or a diffuse osteopenia (e.g., due to osteomalacia). Open biopsy is generally used for the former (excepting involvement of the vertebral body, where an attempt at needle biopsy under radiographic control may be made first) and needle biopsy for the latter, where the iliac crest is most often used.

Needle biopsies of the iliac crest may be performed with a Turkel's trephine needle. It is inserted perpendicular to the iliac crest, and its serrated teeth produce a cortical-cancellous-cortical bone sample. Since the cortical sections add relatively little to the pathologist's evaluation, a simpler technique is to use the small Jamshedi bone marrow biopsy needle. It is inserted near the posterior superior iliac spine parallel to the iliac crest and produces a long core of cancellous bone.

The sample should be transported to the laboratory in formalin buffered to a neutral pH; unbuffered formalin is acidic and will cause some demineralization of the sample. For the histology of bone tumors the samples are usually decalcified to facilitate thin sections (plastic embedding techniques and modern microtomes are now making thin sections of fully mineralized bone possible). In the evaluation of osteopenia, when the width of unmineralized osteoid is important (Fig. 4.22), undecalcified sections should be used. Alternately, the mineralization front may be marked before decalcification by exposure to silver nitrate.

The rate of bone turnover is sometimes estimated by the oral administration of one or more single doses of tetracycline days to weeks before the biopsy. The tetracycline labeling will fluoresce when exposed to ultra-violet light, and the amount

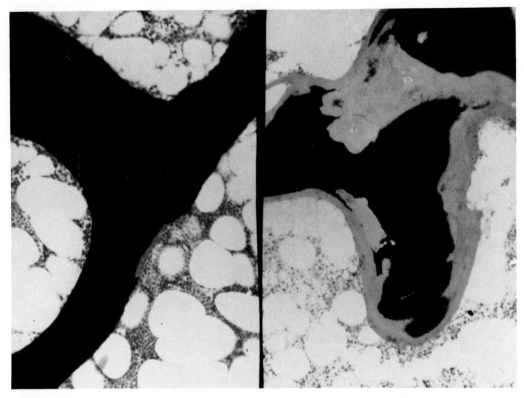

Figure 4.22. Bone biopsy. In this composite photograph a von Kossa stain has been used. On the left is normal bone and on the right a specimen from a patient with osteomalacia. The dark material is the mineralized bone. The lightly stained margin around the mineralized bone on the right is the unmineralized osteoid. (Courtesy of Dr. A. Covert, Dalhousie University.)

of bone laid down between the labeling and the biopsy can be measured.

SYNOVIAL BIOPSY

Synovial biopsy is of most use when investigating the patient with unexplained inflammatory monoarthritis. It is in this situation that one has the greatest likelihood of seeing a moderately specific histologic picture (e.g., synovioma, hypertrophic villonodular synovitis, tuberculous arthritis, crystal-induced synovitis). Occasionally, the synovial biopsy from a patient with seropositive rheumatoid arthritis will show the classical histologic appearance of nodules within the synovium. However, the diagnosis is usually clear without a biopsy.

Although needle biopsy is still used (Fig. 4.21), more often today the procedure is performed through the arthroscope. Open biopsy is preferred for small or deeply placed joints or biopsies of tenosynovium.

The biopsy material may be transported to the laboratory in formalin for standard histology. However, alcohol should be used when crystal-induced synovitis is suspected since formalin will dissolve uric acid crystals. If the synovium is to be cultured, as in suspected tuberculous arthritis, no fixative should be used.

ARTHROSCOPY

Takagi first introduced a cystoscope into the knee in 1918. The technique of arthroscopy was subsequently standardized by Watanabe. Yet, only in the last decade has it been widely used in North America. Techniques and equipment

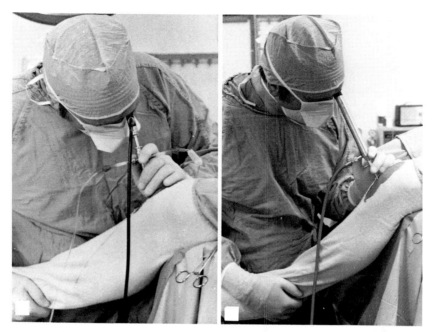

Figure 4.23.   Arthroscopist examining the interior of the knee with a Stortz 3.8-mm fiberoptic arthroscope. (Reproduced with permission from J. C. Kennedy: *The Injured Adolescent Knee.* Baltimore, Williams and Wilkins.)

have improved, particularly: optical systems, a wider range of arthroscope sizes (Fig. 4.21), the capacity to introduce operative tools through the arthroscope, the use of arthroscopy in joints other than the knee (e.g., ankle, shoulder, and elbow), and improvements for recording the results with photography or videorecording. There has been an increased use of local rather than general or epidural anesthesia with no consequent loss of accuracy or increase in the complication rate. There is also a trend towards performing this procedure in outpatient clean arthroscopy suites rather than in operating theaters (Fig. 4.23). Although the technique is most often performed by orthopedic surgeons with access to operating room facilities, the trends outlined have made the procedure more practical for rheumatologists and physiatrists.

There have been relatively few reported complications—equipment breakage, electrical injury, scoring of articular cartilage, discomfort in the joint after the procedure, hemarthrosis, effusion, precipitation of crystal-induced synovitis, and pulmonary embolism. Infective arthritis is rare, even though arthroscopy may be performed in settings of joint damage, immunosuppression, or debilitating illness, all of which are risk factors for infection.

The indications for the procedure, and the settings in which it has been found useful, include the assessment of acute knee injury, internal derangement of the knee joint, synovial biopsy under direct vision, follow-up after medical or surgical treatment, removal of loose or foreign bodies, and assessment of crystal-induced synovitis and, less often, inflammatory polyarthritis.

Locomotor Function Analysis

R. L. KIRBY

A 25-year-old housewife and mother of two has had a 2-year progressive course of stiffness and limitation of motion in the hand, wrist, knee, and metatarsophalangeal (MTP) joints. On examination there is moderate tenderness, swelling, and pain at the extremes of motion, which is moderately limited in all planes. Grip strength is reduced. She uses 2.4 gm of enteric-coated aspirin per day. Her hemoglobin is 11.0 gm%, ESR 45 mm/hour, latex fixation positive at 1:2540, and antinuclear factor is negative. X-rays reveal juxta-articular osteoporosis and small erosions at the joint margins. Her physician provides night-resting wrist and hand splints and institutes gold salt therapy. *What's wrong with this summary?*

A 45-year-old automechanic is struck by a drunken driver while driving home and sustains multiple injuries—fracture-dislocation of T12-L1 with partial paraparesis, pubic diastasis with an unstable left sacroiliac joint, an open comminuted fracture of the left femur, fracture of the right humerus severing the radial nerve, and a ruptured spleen. By the time he is transferred to the Physical Medicine and Rehabilitation Service he has had a splenectomy, internal fixation of his right humerus, and a midthigh amputation. He has lost 40 pounds and spent 9 weeks in bed. *Where does the rehabilitation team start?*

A team of researchers develop a new knee joint for artificial limbs. Others develop a pharmaceutical protocol to slow the progression of muscular dystrophy. Others a total ankle replacement for rheumatoid arthritis. *How do they measure effectiveness?*

By now you will have noticed that in all three situations the questions have something to do with measurement, documentation and, most importantly, functional performance. Let's consider the answers to the questions posed in these three situations.

In our *young mother with rheumatoid arthritis*, the information omitted was that she was no longer able to walk more than a block due to her MTP pain (making shopping almost impossible to do alone and precluding tennis, her favorite outlet). She was unable to get out of the bathtub by herself due to loss of knee flexion range, was having difficulty with small buttons due to discomfort and loss of motion in her fingers, and was unable to tie her shoelaces due to knee discomfort. She was also having difficulties in the kitchen with poor standing tolerance, difficulty carrying pots and opening jars, and difficulty writing due to pain and limitations in her fingers. Most of these items lend themselves to reliable measurement to assess the need for and success of therapeutic options such as shoe modifications, grab rails, bath seats, buttonhooks, elastic laces, high kitchen stool, wheeled dumbwaiter, and built-up pen.

Our *multiply-injured mechanic* requires intensive and long-term work on overcoming contractures of joint and muscle, strengthening weakened muscles, aerobic reconditioning, and working through all limited functional domains—locomotion, transfers, dressing, personal hygiene, and the use of hand tools. In each case, reliable measures of status permit the early recognition of plateaus in improvement, limiting factors, and their specific correction or bypass.

Our research teams all require reliable and valid measures of outcome—for instance, the knee flexion torque of the prosthetic knee, the shoulder abduction power of the patient with muscular dystrophy, and the walking distance at comfortable speed after ankle replacement.

These situations illustrate the settings in which locomotor function analysis can be a valuable adjunct to clinical evaluation and more familiar forms of investigation (e.g., blood, urine, x-ray).

What's available?

STRUCTURAL ANALYSIS

Flexibility. The range of motion of a joint can be determined by the use of a goniometer, or indirect measures such as toe touching can be used.

Posture. Posture is the relationship between one body segment and the next. Photographic techniques are the most popular, although linear measures (e.g., the occiput-wall distance in ankylosing spondylitis) are also useful.

Length. The determination of limb or segment lengths is usually performed with a tape measure, although calipers are more accurate.

Body Shape. Comparing the girths at a number of trunk, upper, and lower extremity positions to those of normal values can provide a measure of body shape. Moiré screen photography, which produces images which look like a contour map, can be used to identify and quantitate unusual prominences, such as a scoliosis hump.

Body Composition. The relative proportion of the body which is fat rather than lean mass can be determined using skin fold thickness and girth measurements with prediction equations. If no prediction equation exists for that patient population (e.g., the lower extremity amputee), then the subject should be weighed under water, permitting a more direct determination.

KINESIOLOGIC ANALYSIS

Kinesiology is the study of human movement, both the geometry of motion and the forces which produce it. All of the activities of daily living are accessible to kinesiologic analysis. Some of the more commonly used techniques are described.

Strength. Isometric strength can be measured by determining the amount of tension that can be produced in a cable (cable tensiometer), or the amount of force that can be delivered to a hydraulic device or other strain gauge apparatus. Isotonic strength can be determined using simple weights to establish the "single lift maximum." Some commercially available torquemeters provide a measure of isokinetic strength, where the joint crossed by the muscles is permitted to move at a predetermined angular velocity (e.g., 90°/ second).

Endurance. Either the length of time that muscular contraction can be sustained or the number of repetitions of a task can be measured.

Power. Power is work (force × distance) performed per unit time. Power measures require that measurable external work (not isometric) be performed and that time be recorded.

Muscular Contraction. The timing (and to a less reliable extent the magnitude) of muscular action during a motion can be recorded with surface or flexible indwelling fine wire electrodes. The signals can be transmitted to a recording device either by telemetry or through cables, depending on the necessity for freedom of motion during the task.

Body Point Tracking. Points on the body (e.g., the greater trochanter, lateral femoral epicondyle, and lateral malleolus) can be tracked through space, digitized, and combined with other measures to

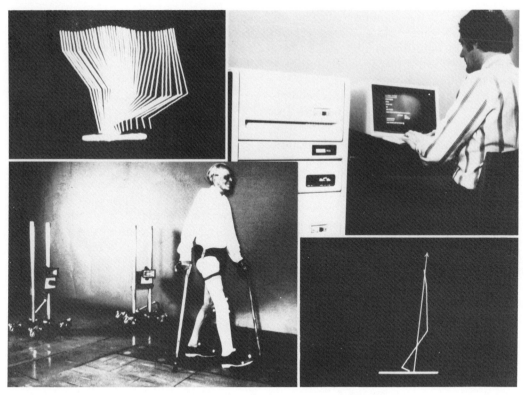

Figure 4.24. This composite illustrates an automatic data acquisition system utilizing infrared strobe videorecording. The equipment is shown in the *upper right* and *lower left insets*. On the *upper right* is a stick-figure output of the walking pattern from the waist down. At the *lower left* is a single stick-figure and a force vector representing the direction and magnitude of the ground reactive force. (Courtesy of the Vicon Division of Oxford Medical Instruments.)

permit computer analysis and display of linear and angular displacement, velocity, acceleration, and joint torques. Automated methods (e.g., with infrared photography or ultrasonic tracking) are becoming increasingly available and considerably reduce the time for data reduction and analysis (Fig. 4.24).

Force Measurements. The most common method for measuring force (e.g., during walking) is to use a force platform set into the walkway. Although force platforms are highly accurate, difficulties can be encountered (e.g., in getting the patient to step completely on the force platform without altering the walking pattern). Strain gauges have been used to instrument the pylons of artificial legs or shoes. Although as yet a less accurate approach, this frees the patient to walk the entire length of a walkway with force informa-

tion continuously recorded. Another method of measuring force is the use of an accelerometer which can be attached to an artificial limb.

Energy Cost. The energy cost of a task can be determined by measuring the oxygen consumption, if that task can be performed in a steady state way for approximately five minutes. The relative energy cost of doing the same task in different ways can be compared, for instance travelling a kilometer walking with crutches or using a wheelchair. Maximum oxygen consumption is a useful measure of physical fitness.

PROFILES OF FUNCTIONAL PERFORMANCE

The functional performance categories are described in Chapter 2. Within each category (e.g., locomotion), there is a hierarchy of activities ranging from the simple to the more difficult. Each task is performed in a standardized way. In quantitating these activities little attention is paid to how the individual accomplishes the task, as long as it is done in a reasonable time and safely. Any necessary aids, appliances, or physical assistance are noted, as are the apparent limiting factors to better performance. Nominal scales (Table 4.1) or measurements of time and distance may be used.

AMBULATORY MONITORING

Unfortunately, patients' estimates of their daily activity levels by interview or diary methods are frequently unreliable. A variety of devices are now available which can record events (e.g., the number of steps taken), or continuously record a physiologic or electronic signal (e.g., electrocardiographic, footswitch, or goniometric signals) by means of precision slow-motion tape recorders. Such devices are becoming increasing compact and socially acceptable.

LIMITATIONS

Quantitation is not without its problems, however. False positives and negatives exist as often in locomotor function analysis as they do in blood chemistry. Although there are many procedures available covering all aspects of locomotor function performance, there is neither widespread agreement on methodology nor normal values spanning the full spectrum of ages, races, and sexes.

Most performance tests take place in artificial surroundings which may be quite different from the individual's natural environment, and many quantitative methods encumber the patient with wires, markers, or other devices.

Furthermore, quantitation can spur some patients to unusual levels of performance (for which they may pay with increased pain the following day) while intimidating other patients. Locomotor function analysis can only detect what a

Table 4.1
Functional Performance Scale

Grade	Criterion
0	Completely unable to complete the task
1	Physical assistance necessary
2	Standby assistance or supervision necessary
3	Independent with aids or appliances
4	Independent without aids

patient *will* do in a test setting, which may be quite different from what he *can* do, and different still from what he *does* do without supervision and the external pressure to perform.

As with the use of blood, urine, and x-ray investigations, the physician must be careful not to overinvestigate the patient under his care. The cost to the health care system is one factor, but the time away from treatment for assessment is equally important.

Most of the investigations are mere quantitations of what an individual is able to do. However, some are stress tests to identify the amount of functional reserve or to precipitate limiting factors. Any stress test has the potential for catastrophe, such as a fatal cardiac dysrhythmia, the precipitation of an acute compartment syndrome, a fall and fractured neck of femur, or the aggravation of a subacute or chronic musculoskeletal condition. A physician capable of advanced cardiac life support should be readily available during testing.

Although individuals with a wide variety of backgrounds (e.g., engineers, kinesiologists, and physiotherapists) are required for the collection and initial analysis of data, it is important that the subject of any stress test be referred by a physician. The referring physician should have sufficient knowledge of the patient and the testing methods to be able to identify precautions or contraindications to stress testing.

SUMMARY

Quantitation permits the early detection of subtle abnormalities, and improvement or deterioration during the course of an illness or its treatment, and it permits the clinician to distinguish between alternate treatment options (e.g., between canes and crutches).

The techniques outlined are only methods by which clinical and research questions can be answered. The usefulness of these methods depends to the greatest extent on the ability of the physician to formulate a precise and testable hypothesis.

PART TWO

Therapeutic Tools

CHAPTER FIVE

Pharmacological Tools

Analgesics

S. C. COLACHIS, Jr.

Pain as a specific sensory experience involves receptors, conductors, and integrated cerebral mechanisms separate from those that mediate sensations of touch, pressure, cold, and heat (1). Pain perception depends on simple and primitive nerve connections. *Reaction* to pain, however, is modified by higher functions and depends on what the sensation means to the person in the light of past experience. Chronic pain can be seriously disabling and probably is related to emotional and behavioral phenomena (2, 3), rather than to acute pain.

Pure analgesics have a useful role in pain relief. The most potent analgesics, the narcotics, should be limited to severe, acute, or terminal problems. The use of narcotics in *chronic pain* problems is to be deplored, since there is little evidence to support its efficacy, and it is usually associated with addiction or habituation.

COMMON ANALGESICS FOR ORAL USE

Analgesic-Antipyretics

Acetylsalicylic acid (aspirin) is the most extensively used analgesic-antipyretic

and anti-inflammatory agent and is used as a standard for comparison of other drugs. It is very inexpensive. Because of the irritating effect of salicylic acid, buffered or enteric-coated derivatives are often used, and they are usually taken with meals. The salicylates alleviate pain both centrally (CNS) and peripherally. Salicylate is helpful in the nonspecific relief of pain due to headache, myalgia, neuralgia, and arthritis (4).

The salicylates block or inhibit prostaglandin synthetase activity (5). Prostaglandins inhibit gastric acid production. Aspirin affects the gastric mucosa. There is a back diffusion of hydrogen ions from the lumen of the stomach across the mucosal barrier that disrupts the capillary bed and produces microbleeding (5).

Para-aminophenol Derivatives

The coal tar analgesics, phenacetin and its active metabolite *acetaminophen* (Tylenol®), are effective substitutes for aspirin. They have no anti-inflammatory effect. Phenacetin is more toxic than acetaminophen and has been associated with renal papillary necrosis (5). Acute overdosage of acetaminophen can cause hepatic damage. Acetaminophen proves an able substitute for aspirin and its analgesic effects, particularly when aspirin is contraindicated (peptic ulcer) or allergy exists. It is common to use analgesics in combination forms; however, chronic use of any agents in combination with phenacetin and caffeine is to be condemned.

Narcotics-Opioid Analgesics

MORPHINE

Opioid is a term used to designate opium or morphine-like drugs. Their major effect is on the central nervous system and bowel. Recent studies have shown that the human body (and all vertebrates) produce similar substances called *enkephalens* and *endorphins* (4). There is probably no group of drugs to relieve pain or suffering of man that is as effective as the opium alkaloids. To date, no single drug has proven superior to morphine in the relief of pain. It is the standard against which all new analgesics are measured. Morphine produces analgesia, drowsiness, mood changes, and euphoria. The incidence of nausea and vomiting is common, as well as respiratory depression. With the relief of pain, the other sensory modalities, such as touch, vibration, hearing, and vision, are not affected. Relief of continuous dull pain is more effective than sharp intermittent pain. Its limitations are the addicting features and psychological dependence. Oral dosages of morphine are about 1/6 to 1/15 as effective as parenteral administration, which is given intramuscularly at 10 mg/70 kg of body weight.

CODEINE

Codeine or methylmorphine is available as codeine sulfate or phosphate. It is probably the most prescribed of the narcotic drugs. A dose of 120 mg of codeine (parenterally) is equivalent to 10 mg of morphine in producing analgesia, but it does have a high oral-parenteral potency ratio. It is 60% as potent as when given orally. An oral dose of 30 mg of codeine is equivalent in analgesia to 325–600 mg of aspirin; however, when the two drugs are combined, the effect is equal to 60 mg of codeine. About 10% of administered codeine is demethylated to form morphine, and its analgesic effect may be due to this conversion.

OXYCODONE

Oxycodone, a semisynthetic narcotic, is an ingredient in analgesic mixtures with aspirin, phenacetin, acetaminophen, or caffeine (e.g., Percodan® and Tylox®) and is a powerful reliever, but it is highly addictive, too. It is given orally and is as potent as morphine and is 10–12 times more potent than codeine.

Synalgos DC® is a semisynthetic narcotic analgesic related to codeine and is combined with a phenothiazine and nonnarcotic antipyretic-analgesic, aspirin and phenacetin. Its principal action is as analgesic and for sedation.

Mefenamic acid (Ponstel®), an analgesic agent, is indicated for relief of mild-to-moderate pain when therapy does not exceed 1 week.

Methadone is a synthetic opiate with the same qualities as *heroin*, an opiate derivative. The only major difference is that methadone, in regulated use, is legal. The physiological effects of both drugs is almost identical. It has effective analgesic activity, is efficacious orally, and is very useful in suppressing withdrawal symptoms in physically dependent persons on drugs such as heroin.

Meperidine (Demerol®) is a synthetic analgesic drug that is one-half as effective when given orally. Usually, 80–100 mg is equivalent to 10 mg or morphine parenterally. Although it produces sedation similar to that of morphine, slightly less euphoria, and equally depressed respirations, its duration of action is shorter than morphine.

Narcotic-like Agents

Propoxyphene (Darvon®) is a stereoisomer of methadone and a centrally acting narcotic analgesic agent. At equianalgesic doses, it is similar to codeine. Most studies have shown that 32 mg of propoxyphene is comparable to a placebo; higher doses are more reliable. Propoxyphene and aspirin (like codeine and aspirin) give a greater analgesic effect than either drug alone (6). Propoxyphene with acetaminophen is a popular analgesic (Darvocet-N-100®) that is not significantly toxic. Moertel (6) explored single-dose analgesics in a controlled double-blind study and found a 20% response equally to placebo and short-term analgesics.

Ethoheptazine (Zactane®) is chemically related to meperidine. It is relatively non-addicting but not impressive in producing analgesia.

Pentazocine (Talwin®) is a synthetic compound that, when given parenterally (30–50 mg), is equivalent to 10 mg or morphine. Orally (50 mg), it is similar in analgesic effect to 60 mg of codeine. Although originally intended to have no abuse potential, it is very addictive and produces severe contractures of tissue when given subcutaneously or intramuscularly.

Zomepirac sodium (Zomax®), an oral nonaddicting nonopiate analgesic, is one of the newer drugs for mild-to-severe acute pain. It has anti-inflammatory activity by virtue of its inhibition of prostaglandin synthetase activity. Its effectiveness as an oral analgesic (100 mg) was found to be greater than that of aspirin (650 mg) or codeine (60 mg).

Fenoprofen calcium (Nalfon®), 200 mg, has recently been used in acute pain. It has been on the market in higher doses (300–600 mg) as a nonsteroidal anti-inflammatory drug (NSAID), as most NSAIDs also have pure analgesic effects (see next section by Dr. Kantor). It is an effective analgesic for the relief of pain of moderate intensity, comparable to 60 mg codeine sulfate.

SUMMARY

Various powerful analgesics are available for use in medical rehabilitation; yet, they must be used with wisdom and in combination with sometimes better physical analgesic methods such as well-planned exercise, heat, and transcutaneous electrical stimulation (TNS). Whenever prescribed, analgesics should be governed by strict time and dosage quotas and a firm plan of action that takes into account the undesirable side effects that they all possess.

References

1. Finneson BE: *Diagnosis and Management of Pain Syndromes.* Philadelphia, W. B. Saunders, 1962, pp 3–5.
2. Cailliet R: *Soft Tissue Pain and Disability.* Philadelphia, F. A. Davis, 1977, pp 25–37.
3. Bonica JM: *The Management of Pain.* Philadelphia, Lea & Febiger, 1953.
4. Gilman AG, Goodman LS, Gilman A: *The Pharmacological Basis of Therapeutics,* New York, MacMillan, 1981, pp 494–526, 682–705.
5. Roth HS: *New Directions in Arthritis Therapy.* Littleton, Mass., PSG Publishing Co., 1980, pp 37–41.
6. Moertel CG: *Relief of Pain with Oral Medications.* Austr NZ J Med 6(1):1–8, 1976.

Anti-Inflammatory Drugs

T. G. KANTOR

Patients in rehabilitation services or outpatient clinics often have pain either as a result of their original problems or because of the modalities used to improve function. In many instances, narcotics are inappropriate because of their side effects and their tendency to produce tolerance and habituation. The "revolutionary" concept that inflammation is most often the basis for pain and that nonsteroidal anti-inflammatory drugs (NSAIDs) might therefore be general purpose analgesics has recently preoccupied the pharmaceutical industry. Many drugs formerly claimed to be exclusively anti-inflammatory and anti-arthritic are now claiming analgesia, and at least one bona fide NSAID only claims analgesia, although it could clearly be used for arthritis. The drugs in this class will be described in chemical groups and, as much as possible, in historic progression.

All of the NSAIDs reduce prostaglandin synthesis by interference with the enzyme cyclooxygenase. Prostaglandins are one group of chemical mediators of inflammation, and this feature has been considered to be paramount as an explanation for their efficacy. There are, however, many reasons to believe that the effect on prostaglandins is not an exclusive explanation for the activity of these drugs, and some drugs also modify the effects of other known mediators of inflammation such as kinins, complements, and O_2 radicals.

The adverse effects of these drugs are quite similar despite their diverse chemical groupings. The prostaglandin effect explains all the more important adverse effects of the entire group. All cause upper gastrointestinal intolerance with nausea, vomiting, and pyrosis, and all are responsible for a certain amount of salt and water retention—both of these effects are due to reduction of the locally produced prostaglandins in the stomach and kidney.

There is a very rare syndrome of true aspirin sensitivity in individuals who have a history of asthma and nasal polyps. Patients with these problems are almost invariably sensitive to other NSAIDs, which inhibit prostaglandin synthesis, and also to tetrazine dyes.

Anti-inflammatory drugs other than NSAIDs will also be discussed. The choice of which to use is often empiric since it is impossible to predict which one an individual patient will respond to or tolerate.

SALICYLATES

Aspirin, the prototype NSAID, has been available since 1893 as an analgesic (discussed in previous section) but its anti-inflammatory credentials were only established in 1943. Its analgetic dose is 650 to 1300 mgm every 4 to 6 hours. At doses over 4.0 gm daily, the anti-inflammatory effect on arthritis is readily apparent.

Unlike other NSAIDs, aspirin's elimination half-life becomes more prolonged with increasing doses and women achieve higher blood levels and more prolonged body residence time per unit dose. The analgetic blood level has never been established for aspirin, but it is generally agreed that over 15 mg% is a minimum to establish anti-inflammation. Salicylate blood levels are easily obtained.

At blood levels over 30 mg%, reversible tinnitus and reduction of hearing are almost always observed. Over 40 mg%, a respiratory alkalosis can occur, and higher blood levels not infrequently produce a metabolic acidosis with central nervous system effects.

In high doses, aspirin interferes with prothrombin production, and at doses starting with less than one tablet, interferes with platelet aggregation, which is also under prostaglandin control. Aspirin is therefore contraindicated in patients who have a bleeding diathesis, whether caused by disease or by pharmacological agents such as the coumarin derivatives. Interaction with oral hypoglycemic drugs can occur, increasing the hypoglycemic effect, and uric acid metabolism also is influenced by salicylates. Aspirin is strictly contraindicated in patients with active upper GI peptic ulceration and relatively contraindicated in those with a history of these conditions.

Salicylate preparations other than aspirin are marketed—various metallic salts of salicylate (sodium, aluminum, magnesium) and organic salts such as choline salicylate and salsalate are available. They are much kinder to the stomach but also less potent as analgesics and as anti-inflammatory agents.

PYRAZOLES

The phenacetin derivatives phenylbutazone and oxyphenbutazone constitute the available drugs in this group. They are potent anti-inflammatory agents and are presumably analgetic as well, although this property has not been formally tested. They inhibit prostaglandin synthesis.

Doses up to 600 mg daily in short-term courses of a week or less are excellent for acute musculoskeletal inflammatory conditions such as acute gouty attacks, tendonitis, and traumatic myopathies. Doses of 200 mg daily or less are useful and, some would suggest, are specific for the spondyloarthropathies such as ankylosing spondylitis, and certain forms of Reiter's syndrome and juvenile rheumatoid arthritis.

The potential side effects of these drugs limit their usefulness. In addition to the prostaglandin-related problems in the stomach and kidney common to all NSAIDs, these drugs can be responsible for profound and devastating bone marrow effects such as complete aplasia of any or all of the peripheral blood cells. They are the most potent salt-retaining compounds of all the NSAIDs. Their use is absolutely contraindicated for patients with upper GI peptic ulcer disease, hypertension, and congestive heart failure and for those with a reduction in peripheral blood cell elements other than the anemia of chronic disease.

PYROLES

These chemical entities include many NSAIDs. Indomethacin, tolmetin, sulindac, and zomepirac are all members of this group, and all are potent prostaglandin synthesis inhibitors. Indomethacin, tolmetin, and zomepirac all have a documented effect as all-purpose analgetic agents.

Indomethacin

This, the first introduced of the pyroles, has been shown in an oral dose of 50 mg to be equivalent to 650 mg aspirin in postoperative pain, possessing a very potent antiprostaglandin effect. At daily doses of 75 to 200 mg, it is a potent anti-inflammatory agent and has the same seeming specificity for the spondyloarthropathies as the pyrazoles.

The adverse effects are those expected in prostaglandin inhibition. In addition, a peculiar migrainous-like headache occurs not infrequently, especially after the first dose in the morning. Psychotomimetic effect may also occur and may be related to the serotonin-like chemical configuration of the drug. Night time doses of the oral drug (or suppository) may be very beneficial for patients with night time pain and morning stiffness of arthritis. A sustained release formulation claims an effective dose schedule of once or twice a day.

Tolmetin

This pyrole is probably analgetic, although weakly so, and has moderately potent anti-inflammatory properties. Its short half-life of 90 minutes requires a dosing schedule of 400 mg three or four times per day. Possibly because of the short half-life, adverse effects are less than with indomethacin's. It is one of the few NSAIDs cleared for use in children.

Sulindac

This pyrole has a peculiar pharmacology in that it is of itself nonactive but must be metabolized to the active sulfide form in the liver after absorption. The sulfide is a prostaglandin synthesis inhibitor and has a half-life of some 13 hours so that dosing of the parent drug for anti-inflammatory effect may be 150 or 200 mg every 12 hours. This allows better patient compliance.

A sulfone is also produced as a metabolite and may cause diarrhea in a higher proportion of patients than some other NSAIDs. Otherwise, its side effect pattern is that of other prostaglandin synthesis inhibitors.

Zomepirac

This drug, whose half-life is 3 to 4 hours, was unexpectedly found to have potent analgetic effect and was marketed as an analgetic. However, because of reports of toxic effects its manufacturer withdrew this product (Zomax®).

Other than the usual side effects of all NSAIDs, there seems to be slightly more central nervous system depressive reactions, but the drug will not substitute for narcotics in patients who are tolerant, and it causes no habituation of its own.

PROPIONIC ACID DERIVATIVES

Ibuprofen

This propionic acid derivative has a particularly wide range of dose schedule which attests to its relative safety and lack of adverse effects. In doses of 200 to 600 mg every 4 to 6 hours, the drug has been shown to have both analgetic and anti-inflammatory doses. Tolerated doses as high as 4200 mg daily have been reported.

Side effects are those expected of its inhibition of prostaglandin synthesis. Reduction of vision and kidney damage are also reported, but there is little evidence for the former, and the latter occurs less often than with any other NSAID.

Fenoprofen

This drug has a pharmacologic profile similar to ibuprofen but is clearly a different drug; 200 mg are equivalent to 650 mg of aspirin as an analgesic, and higher doses probably work better; 200 to 400 mg 4 times daily has anti-inflammatory effect, and higher doses could also be used. Fenoprofen has essentially the same side effects as ibuprofen, with a somewhat higher incidence of interstitial nephritis.

Ketoprofen

Ketoprofen possesses anti-inflammatory, analgesic, and antipyretic properties rather similar to aspirin, and has effective dosages and side effects similar to the above two propionic acid derivatives.

Naproxen

Naproxen is similar in all respects to the other propionic acids in its effect. At a dose of 250 mg every 12 hours, it usually confers an adequate anti-inflammatory effect because of its 13- to 14-hour half-life. A 375 mg tablet three times daily is considered to be possibly a more potent anti-inflammatory schedule. Its sodium salt (275 mg) introduced as an analgesic probably has no advantage over the parent compound. Both drugs reduce prostaglandin synthesis, and side effects are similar to other NSAIDs.

ANTHRANILIC ACIDS

Fenamates

Mefanamic acid and meclofenamic acid are examples of this prostaglandin synthesis inhibiting chemical group. As a short-term analgetic, mefanamic acid, in a dose of 250–500 mg every 6 hours, appears to be effective. However, there is a comparatively high incidence of diarrhea, rash, and elevation of BUN when the drug is used for more than a week and bone marrow toxicity has also been noted.

Meclofenamic acid in a dose of 100 mg three times daily has anti-inflammatory effect, but all-purpose analgesia has not been adequately tested.

DRUGS NOT AVAILABLE IN THE U.S.

At the time of writing, at least 20 other prostaglandin synthesis inhibitors, all of which have anti-inflammatory effects and presumably analgetic effects as well, are available in countries other than the United States. Of these, piroxicam and benoxaprofen will probably be the next introduced. Each has a potent anti-inflammatory effect, a half-life of up to 48 hours and will require only once per day dosing.

Piroxicam has a very narrow dose range. At 20 mg per day, satisfactory anti-inflammatory effect occurs. At 10 mg, there is little or no activity. At 40 mg, there is an unacceptable incidence of adverse GI intolerance, including peptic ulcer.

Benoxaprofen has its own problems and was withdrawn (as Oraflex®) from the market by its manufacturer. At a dose of 400 to 800 mg/day, satisfactory anti-inflammatory effect had been noted.

OTHER ANTI-INFLAMMATORY DRUGS

We have not mentioned corticosteroids as anti-inflammatory drugs as yet in this chapter because they should be considered last in the actual therapeutic situation. While their effects are considerably more potent than any of the NSAIDs, they have a high incidence of adverse effects, especially in the aged. Hypertension, change in cosmesis, lipid abnormalities, reduction of resistance to infection, diabetogenic potential, myopathy, osteoporosis leading to fracture and, possibly, peptic ulcer formation are all possible. If steroids seem indicated or other anti-inflammatory drugs are absolutely contraindicated, short-term high doses of 40 mgm (prednisone equivalent) or greater give a potent effect. If the dose is continued for more than 10 days, an attempt should be made to taper the drug. Doses of 10 mg prednisone or less may be maintained for a longer period with less risk of adverse effect. Alternate-day doses may reduce the suppression of the hypothalamic-pituitary-adrenal axis. Prednisone is preferred over the others because of its reduced myopathic effect. Parenteral doses of corticosteroids are available. "Pulse administration" of massive doses is still under investigation.

While gold, penicillamine, oxychloroquine, and various cytotoxic agents are used in rheumatology to reduce arthritic inflammation, they cannot be considered true anti-inflammatory agents. Several weeks may pass before an effect is seen. They require careful monitoring for adverse effects and should not be used except by specialists.

COMBINATIONS

Combinations of NSAIDs with opioids or opiates are rational for the reduction of pain since the former work in the periphery and the latter in the central nervous system. There is no reason to believe that any potential combination of the two groups would be deleterious, and they probably would be additive.

Reference

U.S. Pharmacopeia Dispensing Information, 1981. AMA Drug Evaluations, 1982.

Neuroactive Drugs for Neurological Impairment

L. S. HALSTEAD and J. CLAUS-WALKER

The term "neuroactive drugs" (NAD) was coined for those agents that affect one or more neurological structures of the body, such as autonomic or CNS. This group is important for several reasons in the pharmacological management of rehabilitation patients with severe neurological impairments: these patients may respond differently from neurologically intact individuals to a given medication; they often have complex, long-term neurological disorders which may require the simultaneous use of numerous NADs, increasing the risk of NAD interactions; and there is a large knowledge gap regarding the effect of many of these drugs in rehabilitation patients. Pharmacology textbooks describe responses observed largely in neurologically intact humans or animals and seldom deal specifically with the problems presented by patients with chronic neurological disorders. As these patients frequently receive NADs for extended periods of time, and while their short-term effects may be benign, the long-term effects may aggravate the underlying neurological impairment.

PRINCIPAL NEURORECEPTORS AND NEUROACTIVE DRUGS

Effective amounts of a neuroactive drug may either stimulate or inhibit a specific neuroreceptor. Knowledge of the principal pharmacological actions of a drug makes it possible to anticipate which receptors are likely to be stimulated or inhibited. There are many types of neuroreceptors scattered throughout the body, brain, and spinal cord. For most clinical purposes, however, it is necessary to be concerned with only five types: muscarinic and nicotinic cholinergic receptors, and alpha, $beta_1$-, and $beta_2$-adrenergic receptors. Table 5.1 summarizes the major anatomical sites of these neuroreceptors.

The clinical responses to a specific medication can be evaluated by its effect on the most distal receptors, in which the drug elicits its physiological action. This response is like a "final common pathway." Nearly all NADs have, in addition to a principal or primary effect for which they are prescribed, at least one neuroactive side effect. The "final common pathways" for medications with only one or two neuroactive effects are relatively straightforward. For example, propantheline (Probanthine®) is a single compound with two neuroactive effects. The principal effect is to inhibit cholinergic muscarinic receptors and thereby reduce neurally mediated bladder spasticity. However, as with all other anticholinergics, it has a secondary effect which causes sedation by inhibition of various brain receptors. Other drugs are more complex, especially those with several active components, and may have up to five neuroactive effects with as many "final common pathways." For example, the compound Dimetapp® contains two sympathomimetic amines and one antihistamine, which together produce four different neuroactive effects (Table 5.3). The primary effect of the amines is alpha adrenergic receptor stimulation while the side effect is CNS stimulation. The side effects of the antihistamine include inhibition of muscarinic structures and of various CNS receptors. Although the magnitude and clinical significance of both primary and secondary effects vary from patient to patient depending upon the drug,

Table 5.1
Anatomical Sites of Principal Neural Receptors[a]

Muscarinic Cholinergic
Blood vessels—mucosa, skeletal muscle, skin
Bronchial muscle
Eye—iris
Gastrointestinal tract—esophagus, stomach, small intestine, proximal colon, gall bladder, secretions, and sphincters
Genitourinary tract—detrusor, trigone, and internal sphincter
Glands—lacrimal, nasopharyngeal, salivary
Heart
Pancreas
Skin—eccrine sweat glands

Nicotinic Cholinergic
All autonomic ganglia and adrenal medulla
All skeletal muscles

α-Adrenergic
Blood vessels—abdominal viscera, mucosa, pulmonary, skeletal muscle, skin
Eye—iris
Gastrointestinal tract—sphincters
Genitourinary tract—ureters and urethra
Sweat glands—localized (apocrine)

β_1- and β_2-Adrenergic
Blood vessels—abdominal viscera, coronary, skeletal muscle
Bronchial muscle
Gastrointestinal tract—stomach, small intestine, proximal colon, secretions
Genitourinary—detrusor, ureter, and urethra
Glands—salivary
Heart

[a] There are multiple known and putative receptors throughout the brain and spinal cord. Interaction of these receptors results in a complex interplay of responses leading to excitation, inhibition, recruitment, and modification of other neural structures.

the dose, the route of administration, and other drugs taken by the patient, it is important to anticipate which organs the drug might affect. Table 5.2 summarizes the responses of the major effector organs to adrenergic and cholinergic stimulation.

INTERACTIONS OF NEUROACTIVE DRUGS ON NEURORECEPTORS

In addition to the "built in" unwanted side effects of single drugs, there are many kinds of drug interactions which can pro-duce adverse effects, especially in rehabilitation patients with neurological disorders. Among NAD, there are two types of interactions which are of special importance.

Additive interactions occur when two or more drugs produce similar modification on the same type of neuroreceptor. Often, this kind of interaction involves several chemicals which cause inhibition of CNS receptors, leading to daytime drowsiness and fatigue. This is especially likely to be seen in elderly persons or patients with brain injury who are taking an evening sedative like diphenhydramine (Benadryl®), along with one or more daytime medications with CNS depressive effects such as diazepam (Valium®) for muscle spasms or phenacetin with codeine for pain. Other examples involve medications which directly or indirectly reduce the stimulation of the same type of neuroreceptor. For instance, a male patient with spina bifida may be given phenoxybenzamine (Dibenzyline®) to relax the internal urinary sphincter while taking an antidepressant drug such as amitriptyline (Elavil®). Phenoxybenzamine *blocks* the α-adrenergic receptors, and amitriptyline depletes norepinephrine from sympathetic nerve endings which *decreases stimulation* of α-adrenergic receptors. Each drug alone can cause undesirable side effects, but together, they are more likely to produce signs of sympathetic insufficiency such as orthostatic hypotension.

Antagonistic interactions occur when the effect of one drug is reduced or canceled by a second drug. The most common neurological antagonistic interaction involves two drugs which bind to the same receptors to produce opposite effects. This type of interaction might occur when a patient taking guanethidine (Ismelin®) for hypertension is given a "cold remedy" such as Sinutab®. Guanethidine blocks the release of norepinephrine from sympathetic nerves, which *decreases* stimulation of α-adrenergic receptors, while the two sympathomimetic amines in Sinutab

Table 5.2
Responses of Effector Organs to Adrenergic and Cholinergic Stimulation[a]

Effector Organs	Adrenergic Stimulation		Cholinergic Stimulation	
	Receptor Type	Responses	Receptor Type	Responses
1. Adrenal medulla			Nicotinic	Secretion mostly of epinephrine and some norepinephrine
2. Arterioles of				
mucosa, skin,	α	Constriction	Muscarinic	Dilatation
skeletal muscle, and	α	Constriction	Muscarinic	Dilatation
abdominal viscera	β_2	Dilatation		
	α	Constriction		
3. Bronchial muscle	β_2	Relaxation	Muscarinic	Contraction
4. Gastrointestinal tract				
motility and tone	β_2	Decrease	Muscarinic	Increase
sphincters	α	Contraction	Muscarinic	Relaxation
secretion		Decrease	Muscarinic	Stimulation
5. Heart	β_1	Increased rate, contractility, conduction velocity, etc.	Muscarinic	Decrease rate, contractility, conduction velocity, etc.
6. Sex organs (male)		Ejaculation	Muscarinic	Erection
7. Sweat glands	α	Local secretion	Muscarinic	Generalized secretion
8. Urinary bladder				
detrusor	β_2	Relaxation	Muscarinic	Contraction
trigone and internal sphincter	α	Contraction	Muscarinic	Relaxation
9. Urethra[b]				
fibromuscular layer	β_2	Relaxation	Muscarinic	Contraction
	α	Contraction		
external sphincter			Nicotinic	Contraction
10. Uterus	α	Pregnant, contraction	Muscarinic	Variable
	β_2	Nonpregnant, relaxation	Muscarinic	Variable

[a] (Reprinted with permission from: L. S. Goodman and A. Gilman (eds). *The Pharmacological Basis of Therapeutics.* New York, MacMillian, 1975.
[b] Data from S. A. Awad, J. W. Downie, and H. G. Kiruluta. Pharmacologic treatment of disorders of bladder and urethra: a review. *Canadian Journal of Surgery* 22(6):515–518, 1979.

increase stimulation of α-adrenergic receptors. Clearly, one drug may cancel or modify the clinical effectiveness of the other.

CONSIDERATIONS IN THE SELECTION OF NEUROACTIVE DRUGS

An important guiding principal in prescribing medications is to identify the drug of choice for each particular clinical problem for each individual patient. In addition to the usual criteria used in selecting the best available drug, special considerations should be kept in mind when prescribing NADs to rehabilitation patients. These considerations all involve different strategies for minimizing undesirable and often avoidable side effects; four of these considerations are listed below with illustrations of how they might influence the current drug of choice in treating certain clinical problems.

The **first consideration** is to *avoid medication.* As in other areas of medicine, there are many times in rehabilitation when the best treatment is no medication at all. A good example is the mild-to-moderate depression seen at one time or another in virtually all rehabilitation patients who experience severe disabling illnesses. The use of antidepressant drugs in these patients presents a special problem, and the management of depression illustrates an important philosophical concept in rehabilitation medicine. The two main types of antidepressant drugs— tricyclic antidepressants and monoamine oxidase inhibitors—alter catecholamine metabolism, which can produce a number of adverse side effects. In addition, there is the danger that the drug will simply mask the symptoms of depression while the underlying causes remain untreated. In most of these patients, the depression is not endogenous but reactive and represents a normal and inevitable consequence of their illness. To treat them with an antidepressant drug fosters the belief that depression is undesirable and is caused by intrinsic or metabolic factors and places the therapeutic emphasis on a pill, not a program. Therefore, in the absence of a prior history of depression, formal and informal counseling, together with an active aggressive therapy schedule which emphasizes practical stepwise achievable goals, is probably the most effective approach to overcome depression for the majority of patients.

The **second consideration** is to assess the extent of side effects of comparable drugs on altered neural structures. The treatment of anxiety in patients with neurogenic bladder provides a good illustration. One of the major problems in treating this group of patients is that virtually all antianxiety agents have some anticholinergic effect which may interfere with satisfactory emptying of the neurogenic bladder. All of the phenothiazines (Thorazine®, Sparine®, Mellaril®, etc.), for example, produce this effect, which makes them undesirable in the management of anxiety. In addition, the phenothiazines possess a number of other neuroactive side effects which are undesirable in most rehabilitation patients with neurological disorders—especially when administered over an extended period of time. These include the slow depletion of neuronal

catecholamines, resulting in increased vasodilatation and orthostatic hypotension; altered central thermoregulation, resulting in decreased body temperature; and modification of other drugs, most notably to increase, prolong, and intensify the sedative effect of CNS depressants.

The benzodiazepines (Valium®, Serax®, etc.), which are now the most commonly prescribed antianxiety agents in the United States, also may have a fairly pronounced anticholinergic effect, with one exception—chlordiazepoxide (Librium®), which has relatively little or no anticholinergic effect and, thus, is unlikely to disrupt neurogenic bladder function. In terms of clinical effectiveness, none of the benzodiazepines has been shown to be superior to the others. For this reason, the absence of any significant neuroactive side effect gives the clinician a rational basis for selecting chlordiazepoxide as the drug of choice in treating anxiety in patients with neurogenic bladder.

The **third consideration** is the assessment of the optimal route of administration to effect treatment with minimal side effects. Most neuroactive medications are given orally or parenterally. However, alternate routes may offer important advantages, particularly because of fewer adverse systemic effects. This is especially relevant in treating neurologically impaired patients with cold symptoms. There are more than 100 medications available for treating uncomplicated symptoms due to mixed viral infections of the upper respiratory tract. Among these medications, however, there is no single product which is clearly superior by any objective measure, nor is there any evidence to support claims that any of these drugs is effective in altering the course of an infection. The only indication for prescribing such medications is to provide symptomatic relief. Although these drugs may not alter the course of the common cold, they are not harmless. In certain rehabilitation patients, such as spinal cord-injured patients, the adverse effects from these medications can be particularly serious. Most of the more commonly used oral medications, such as Actifed®, Sudafed®, Dimetapp®, and Ornade Spansule®, contain one or two potent sympathomimetic amines and, frequently, an antihistamine as well.

The *most common side effects* seen with the majority of these drugs are antimuscarinic symptoms and drowsiness caused by the antihistamines and CNS stimulation caused by the sympathomimetic agents. The antimuscarinic effects of particular concern in patients with neurological impairments are dry mouth, tachycardia, and decreased emptying of the neurogenic bladder. In addition to these side effects, there are a number of others which are less common but more serious, especially in the presence of altered neural control. Most of the commonly used cold medications enhance either directly or indirectly the effect and duration of endogenous catecholamines. In some patients, these drugs may contribute to the development of hypertension, and in spinal cord-injured patients with lesions at or above T_6, they may help precipitate hypertensive crises known as autonomic dysreflexia.

In view of the fact that the cold medications are ineffectual, except for relieving symptoms, and have a number of potentially adverse side effects, there are compelling reasons to use alternate safer methods such as the topical sympathomimetic amines like oxymetazoline (Afrin®) nasal spray or xylometazoline (Neo-Synephrine®) spray or drops which make them the drugs of choice for treating cold symptoms in the neurologically impaired individual.

The **fourth consideration** is to evaluate the *degree of specificity* of the medication. Whenever possible, it is desirable to use the drug which is the most specific or selective in acting on a target organ or receptor. An example of this consideration is the treatment of subacute or mild recurrent autonomic dysreflexia which is a problem limited to spinal cord-injured patients with lesions at or above T_6. It is characterized clinically by headaches and elevated blood pressure, accompanied by varying degrees of sweating, blotchy flushing, and goosebumps. The most common cause of this form of dysreflexia is bladder sphincter dyssynergia, which provokes a strong, unmodulated sympathetic discharge. When conservative management is unsuccessful, pharmacological treatment is usually directed at preventing endogenous norepinephrine from stimulating α-adrenergic receptors in the smooth muscles of peripheral arterioles and the urethra.

Four different types of medications have been used to control subacute dysreflexia: reserpine (Serpasil), mecamylamine (Inversine), guanethidine (Ismelin), and phenoxybenzamine (Dibenzyline). Within the nervous system, each works at different receptors and by a different mechanism of action. Reserpine acts by depleting stores of norepinephrine from portions of the brain and peripheral sympathetic neurons. Mecamylamine blocks sympathetic ganglia by preventing depolarization of the ganglionic postsynaptic membrane, which results in reducing the release of catecholamine from the peripheral sympathetic nerve endings. Both guanethidine and phenoxybenzamine act on the peripheral sympathetic nervous system. Guanethidine blocks the release of norepinephrine from the sympathetic nerve endings while phenoxybenzamine blocks the α-adrenergic receptors in the arterioles in a lasting noncompetitive manner. Although each of these medications could be fairly effective in treating this clinical problem, reserpine and mecamylamine are unacceptable because their effects are nonspecific and because they have a large number of adverse side effects. Guanethidine and phenoxybenzamine, by comparison, are relatively specific in preventing norepinephrine from stimulating peripheral α-adrenergic re-

Table 5.3
Neuroactive Drugs of Choice for Eight Clinical Problems

Clinical Problem	Generic Name	Trade Name	Primary Neuroactive Effect	Secondary Neuroactive Effect	Common Single Oral Dosages (mg)	Cost[a]
1. Allergic reactions	Chlorpheniramine[b]	Chlor-Trimeton	CNS inhibition	Muscarinic inhibition	4	$ 5.90
	Diphenhydramine	Benadryl	CNS inhibition	Muscarinic inhibition	25	6.00
	Hydroxyzine[c]	Vistaril	CNS inhibition	Muscarinic inhibition	25	22.00
	Promethazine	Phenergan	CNS inhibition	Muscarinic and α-adrenergic inhibition; occasional CNS stimulation	25	15.50
2. Anxiety	Chlordiazepoxide[b]	Librium	CNS inhibition	Muscarinic and spinal cord inhibition	10	13.00
	Diazepam[c]	Valium	Skeletal muscle and CNS inhibition	Muscarinic and spinal cord inhibition	10	25.00
3. Autonomic dysreflexia, subacute	Hydroxyzine[b]	Vistaril	CNS inhibition	Muscarinic inhibition	25	22.00
	Guanethidine[b]	Ismelin	α-Adrenergic inhibition	Muscarinic and β-adrenergic inhibition	10	15.00
	Mecamylamine	Inversine	α-Adrenergic inhibition	Muscarinic, β-adrenergic, CNS inhibition; CNS stimulation	2.5	6.00
	Phenoxybenzamine[c]	Dibenzyline	α-Adrenergic inhibition	β-adrenergic stimulation	10	6.50
	Reserpine	Serpasil	α-Adrenergic inhibition	Muscarinic, CNS stimulation; CNS inhibition	0.25	7.00
4. Bladder spasticity	Flavoxate	Urispas	Muscarinic inhibition	CNS inhibition	100	13.00
	Methantheline	Banthine	Muscarinic inhibition	Skeletal muscle inhibition	50	12.00
	Oxybutynin[c]	Ditropan	Muscarinic inhibition	CNS inhibition	5	13.00
	Propantheline[b]	Probanthine	Muscarinic inhibition	Skeletal muscle inhibition	15	13.00
5. Cold symptoms	Pseudoephedrine Triprolidine	Actifed	α-Adrenergic stimulation	Muscarinic and CNS inhibition; β- and CNS stimulation	Tablet	6.50
	Brompheniramine Phenylephrine Phenylpropanolamine	Dimetapp	α-Adrenergic stimulation	Muscarinic and CNS inhibition; CNS stimulation	Tablet	14.00

							Cost[a]
	Chlorpheniramine Isopropamide Phenylpropanolamine	Ornade spansule	α-Adrenergic stimulation	Muscarinic and CNS inhibition; CNS stimulation	Capsule		21.00
	Acetaminophen Phenylpropanolamine Phenyltoloxamine	Sinutab	α-Adrenergic stimulation	Muscarinic and CNS inhibition; CNS stimulation	Tablet		9.00
	Pseudoephedrine[c]	Sudafed	α-Adrenergic stimulation	β- and CNS stimulation		30	4.00
6. Insomnia	Chloral hydrate	Chloral hydrate	CNS inhibition	Muscarinic, CNS inhibition		500	5.50
	Diazepam	Valium	CNS and skeletal muscle inhibition			10	25.00
	Diphenhydramine[c]	Benadryl	CNS inhibition	Muscarinic inhibition		50	10.00
	Flurazepam[b]	Dalmane	CNS inhibition	Muscarinic inhibition		30	21.00
	Chlorpromazine[b]	Thorazine	CNS inhibition	Muscarinic and β-adrenergic inhibition; CNS stimulation		25	6.00
7. Nausea and vomiting	Dimenhydrinate	Dramamine	CNS inhibition	Muscarinic inhibition		50	13.00
	Hydroxyzine	Vistaril	CNS inhibition	Muscarinic inhibition		25	22.00
	Promethazine	Phenergan	CNS inhibition	Muscarinic and β-adrenergic inhibition; CNS stimulation		25	15.50
	Trimethobenzamide[c]	Tigan	CNS inhibition	Muscarinic inhibition adrenergic		250	14.00
8. Orthostatic hypotension	Ephedrine[c]	Ephedrine	α-Adrenergic stimulation	β- and CNS stimulation		25	3.00
	Phenylpropanolamine	Propadrine	α-Adrenergic stimulation	β-Adrenergic and CNS stimulation		25	6.00
	Sodium chloride[b]	Sodium chloride	α-Adrenergic stimulation			1000	1.50

[a] Cost per 100 tablets or capsules to outpatients at TIRR Pharmacy as of Spring 1980.
[b] Alternate choice.
[c] Drug of choice.
[d] See text for drug of choice.

ceptors, they have fewer side effects and are both acceptable forms of treatment. Recent data show that guanethidine is safer and more effective than phenoxybenzamine, even though in theory, phenoxybenzamine is more specific. Therefore, at this time, guanethidine is the drug of choice.

OTHER CLINICAL PROBLEMS

In addition to the clinical conditions described above to illustrate the four considerations used in the selection of the NAD, five other common clinical problems are listed in Table 5.3. The table lists the trade and generic names of medications frequently used to treat these problems, along with the primary and main side effects of the medications, the usual dosage for a single administration, and the cost for 100 tablets or capsules. Drugs of choice are indicated with two asterisks and alternate choices with a single asterisk. The drugs in this table are selected specifically with spinal cord-injured patients in mind, but in most cases apply to other neurologically impaired patients as well.

SUMMARY

The **following questions** should be answered as an aid in selecting the best possible treatment strategy and NAD in managing your patients.
● Is there a way of managing the clinical problem with no medication at all?
● If the answer is no, what are the primary and secondary effects of the NAD being considered?

● Is the patient taking other NAD, either on a regular or "as required" basis, prescribed by you or by another physician?
● If question 3 is answered yes, are there any potential adverse drug interactions between the new drug and other NAD the patient is receiving?
● If this is a compound medication, can I substitute a single drug instead, which will achieve the same therapeutic result with fewer side effects?
● Is the drug the most specific one available for treating the clinical symptoms?
● Can the problem be treated using an alternate route of administration of a drug with fewer side effects?
● Is this the least expensive medication to achieve the desired clinical effect?

References

1. Banerjee SP, Kung LS, Riggi SJ, Chanda SK: Development of beta-adrenergic receptor subsensitivity by antidepressants. *Nature* 268 (5619):455–456, 1977.
2. Goodman LS, Gilman A (eds): *The Pharmacological Basis of Therapeutics*, ed. 5. New York, MacMillan, 1975.
3. Halstead LS, Claus-Walker J: *Neuroactive Drugs of Choice in Spinal Cord Injury: A Guide for Using Neurologically Active Medications in Spinal Injured Patients.* New York, Raven Press, 1981.
4. Hansten PD: *Drug Interactions*, ed. 4. Philadelphia, Lea & Febiger, 1970.
5. Lefkowitz RJ: Beta-adrenergic receptors: Recognition and regulation. *N Engl J Med* 295 (6):323–328, 1976.
6. Woosley RL, Nies AS: Guanethidine. *N Engl J Med* 295:1053–1057, 1976.
7. Sommers DK: Paroxysmal neurogenic hypertension and its prevention in patients with cervical spinal cord lesions. *South Afr Med J*:14–18, 1979.

Nerve Blocks

A. A. KHALILI

Peripheral nerve blocks are used as diagnostic or therapeutic procedures in the rehabilitation management of patients with severe motor impairments or pain.

DIAGNOSTIC ASPECTS

Contractures vs. Spasticity

Restriction of range of motion (ROM) of a joint, among other causes, might be secondary to contracture and/or hypertonia (e.g., spasticity). Contracture which is a passive shortening of a muscle, tendon, capsule, ligament, or skin may require a surgical approach if prolonged and if sustained stretching does not relieve it significantly within a reasonable length of time. Spasticity, on the other hand, often is managed by oral pharmaceutical agents or by semipermanent nerve block or by nerve section. Therefore, accurate differentiation is important because of the difference in the means of management.

Clinically, contracture is diagnosed when normal ROM is restricted and comes to a rather abrupt halt, after which further brief stretching provides no significant gain. In spasticity the stretch reflex is increased; this is detected by exaggerated deep tendon reflexes and, sometimes, clonus. Alternatively, postural hypertonia may be detected. In spasticity, restriction in ROM is present and is usually more pronounced in one group of muscles than another, e.g., flexors vs. extensors. In spasticity, the restriction can usually be overcome in a few seconds or minutes by gentle sustained stretching.

A problem arises when there is a combination of spasticity and contracture or when spasticity is so severe that it mimics the combined form. In such a case, a temporary block of the related peripheral nerve relieves spasticity, and the remaining restriction will be related to contracture. Selective block of the obturator nerve is often used before obturator neurectomy and occasionally before phenol nerve block. After neurectomy, not only are all α and γ motor fibers sectioned, but also deprivation of sensory input takes place, and this will affect the outcome. More similarity exists in the outcome between selective lidocaine HCL block and phenol nerve block.

Voluntary Contraction vs. Spasticity

Normally, muscle fibers are contracted and relaxed volitionally. The number, rate, and distribution of the muscle fibers to be contracted depends on the work that is to be done and the result to be achieved. In spasticity, various trigger mechanisms cause contraction of the muscle fibers, although the degree of recruitment does not necessarily follow a normal pattern. Often, mass contraction occurs. Sustaining the desired level of contraction as a source of energy often is not possible. A spastic hemiplegic with no voluntary contraction in quadriceps may bear weight on the involved extremity with the knee locked in extension due to spastic contraction of quadriceps. Therefore, in the stance phase of ambulation, spasticity can be helpful. At the time of the swing phase, on the other hand, no relaxation often takes place in the quadriceps and, therefore, no shortening of the extremity occurs by normal flexion of the knee. To compensate, the patient has to circumduct the extremity.

When there is a *combination of spasticity and voluntary contraction* in the same muscle, prior to relief of spasticity, one should know the extent of each. Lidocaine HCL block (0.5%) has a rather selective effect on γ motor fibers and, therefore, temporarily relieves spasticity and is used clinically for this purpose (3).

Variation in Normal Innervation

Knowledge of variation in normal innervation becomes important in clinical neuromuscular diagnosis and management. For example, the median nerve usually innervates abductor pollicis brevis, opponens pollicis, superficial head of flexor pollicis brevis, and first and second lumbricals; the remaining intrinsic hand muscles are innervated by the ulnar nerve; various degrees of variation in innervation may take place, and two extremes are completely ulnar and very rarely completely median hand. In a completely ulnar hand, all motor fibers to the intrinsic hand muscles are routed through the ulnar carpal tunnel and, therefore, a total injury of the ulnar nerve above the wrist would cause complete paralysis of the intrinsic hand muscles. A complete lesion of the median nerve at the wrist or above the wrist in such a patient will not cause any paralysis of the intrinsic hand muscles. Therefore, a complete lesion of the median nerve in a completely ulnar hand mimics a partial median nerve lesion in an average patient. A 2% lidocaine HCL block of the ulnar above the wrist will confirm such an anomaly by causing complete paralysis of the intrinsic hand muscles.

Diagnosis of Pain

Clinically, symptomatic neuroma may occur following a nerve injury or surgical section of the nerve, e.g., in amputation of a lower extremity. In rehabilitation of patients with amputations of limbs, the diagnosis and management of neuroma may become a dilemma. A 2% lidocaine HCL block of the neuroma will confirm the diagnosis, and repeated lidocaine HCL blocks or block of the neuroma with a neurolytic agent (e.g., 5–7% phenol solution) may be the management procedure of choice. Similarly, selective nerve root or somatic temporary blocks may assist diagnostic localization, as may a differential epidural or spinal block. However, pain is a subjective phenomenon, and beneficial results may be a placebo response. Alternatively, the source of the pain may be at some distance, with the alleviated pain a mere epiphenomenon.

THERAPEUTIC ASPECTS

A nerve block may be therapeutic in the management of pain. For instance, in the shoulder-hand syndrome (sometimes called "reflex sympathetic dystrophy"), a temporary block of the stellate ganglion with lidocaine HCL not only assists in the diagnosis of subclinical cases but also has therapeutic value by permitting active mobilization of the upper limb. If repeated blocks are necessary, consideration may be given to the use of neurolytic agents (e.g., 5–7% phenol solution) or ganglionectomy.

Peripheral Nerve and Motor Point Phenol Nerve Blocks*

Here, the management of spasticity with phenol nerve block will be outlined. Generally, a neurolytic block should not be used unless more conservative measures have produced no desirable result. Furthermore, neurolytic blocks should be used cautiously, because a painful dysesthesia is a complication in a small but significant minority of such blocks.

A direct current stimulator is used with a manually operated rheostat to regulate the current. The active electrode is usually a 22-gauge spinal needle 2 or 3 inches in length whose entire shaft, except at the bevel, is insulated with Teflon coating (Fig. 5.1).

The nerve is approached with the active needle electrode using the usual technique employed for nerve blocking, and stimulated by turning the foot switch on briefly. As the tip of the coated needle

---

* This section has been adapted with permission from Current Therapy in Physiatry (5).

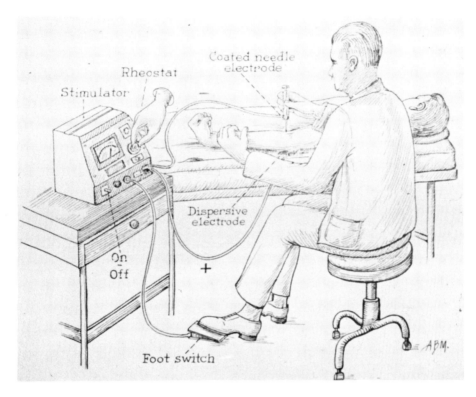

Figure 5.1.   Apparatus and procedure used for peripheral nerve and motor nerve phenol block.

approaches the nerve, less current is required to elicit the maximal contraction. The needle is in the desired location when the least intensity elicits the maximum contraction in the muscle fibers in which the spasticity is to be relieved or alleviated. In this manner, the entire nerve trunk or only the nerve fibers to a muscle or a portion of a muscle can be isolated and blocked. When isolation is perfect, the phenol solution is injected. If isolation of the nerve and injection of phenol are properly performed, there should be immediate relief of spasticity in the related muscles.

If a more localized blocking is desired, the nerve can be approached with a similar technique at a motor point. In such a case, the motor point is localized by percutaneous stimulation, after which a coated needle electrode is used for accurate isolation and injection of the blocking agent (1, 2, 4, 5).

CLINICAL PICTURES

Spasticity in finger and wrist flexors and in plantarflexors of the ankle and foot often causes problems in clinical rehabilitation and will be described, but specialized management of spasticity in the other areas requires advanced training (6).

Finger and Wrist Flexor Spasticity

Depending on the clinical status, there might be an indication for median and/or ulnar nerve block.

MEDIAN NERVE BLOCK

The median nerve is approached in the antecubital fossa at the level of the medial epicondyle where the nerve is medial to the brachial artery. Depending on the clinical picture, the primary goal might be to block flexor digitorum superficialis (sublimis) or related wrist flexors of flexor digitorum profundus (Fig. 5.2A and B).

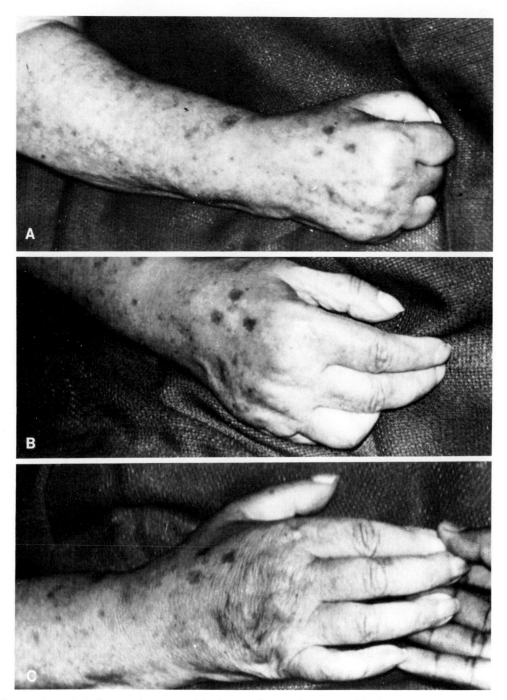

Figure 5.2. (A) Before median nerve block. (B) After median nerve block. (C) After ulnar nerve block.

The nerve fibers to pronator teres, which is a strong pronator, usually should not be blocked because, following the block, it is desirable for the hand to remain in semipronation, which is a more functional position for most patients with paresis and is more acceptable cosmetically. When there is spasticity in the elbow flexors, particularly the biceps brachii, relief of spasticity in the pronators would result in a semiflexed elbow, supinated forearm, and open hand—"beggar's hand"—which is very unsatisfactory cosmetically. When the nerve is approached at the medial epicondyle level, the fibers to pronator teres have usually already branched out from the median nerve.

ULNAR NERVE BLOCK

The ulnar nerve is approached about one digit proximal to the medial epicondyle, at the medial aspect of the distal part of the biceps, medial to the median nerve. Depending on the clinical picture, the fibers to flexor carpi ulnaris or flexor digitorum profundus to the fourth and fifth digits or to the interosseous muscles innervated by the ulnar nerve can be isolated and blocked (Fig. 5.2C). To prevent compression neuropathy or paresis, the solution must not be injected into the fibro-osseous canal which the nerve passes through at the medial aspect of the elbow.

In a severely spastic hand one usually plans a block of median and ulnar nerve. However, after the block of one nerve there is, in most cases, enough relief of spasticity in the territory of the other nerve to eliminate the need for a further block. Therefore, as a rule of thumb, the nerve with the maximum spastic territory is approached first, and generally about a week later a decision is made as to whether a further block is needed.

Plantarflexor Spasticity

Plantarflexor spasticity is the most commonly seen manifestation of central nervous system involvement with spasticity. The plantarflexors are gastrosoleus, plantaris, flexor digitorum longus, flexor hallucis longus, tibialis posterior, and peroneus longus and brevis. Spasticity in gastrosoleus causes the most problems. Prolonged spasticity in the muscles results in the development of contracture. Inappropriate stretching of the gastrosoleus may cause subluxation of Chopart's transverse tarsal joint.

Plantarflexor spasticity may cause plantarflexion during swing phase in an ambulatory patient. A patient usually is unable to compensate for this spasticity by flexing the knee or hip hiking, and the swing phase becomes cumbersome or impossible. In a wheelchair-bound patient, plantarflexor spasticity creates difficulty in transfer. Clonus of the ankle usually occurs while the patient is sitting in the wheelchair with the foot on the pedal. In a bed-bound patient, clonus of the plantar flexors may cause a friction sore at the dorsal aspect of the heel or heel cord. Plantarflexor spasticity may cause difficulty in putting shoes on or in keeping them on.

The spasticity can be managed either by motor point blocks or tibial (medial popliteal) nerve block (Fig. 5.3A and B). Motor point blocks require multiple nee-

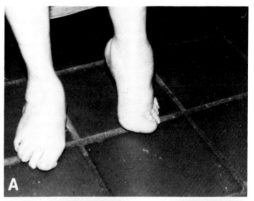
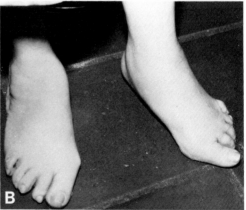

Figure 5.3. (A) Before tibial nerve block. (B) After tibial nerve block.

dling. For instance, gastrosoleus has six motor points and, frequently, besides reduction or relief of spasticity in the gastrosoleus, some reduction in spasticity in other flexors is also required. Therefore, a block of the tibial nerve is usually indicated, with fibers to gastrosoleus being the prime target.

After the popliteal artery is palpated, the nerve is approached lateral to the artery in the upper portion of the popliteal fossa, just distal to the bifurcation of the sciatic nerve, into the medial (tibial) and lateral popliteal (common peroneal) nerve—approximately four fingers above the popliteal crease.

INTRATHECAL PHENOL AND ALCOHOL BLOCK

In a paraplegic, quadriparetic, or quadriplegic patient with severe spasticity in the lower extremities, in whom the benefits of conversion of an upper motor neuron type of neurogenic bladder to the lower motor neuron type, changing a spastic anal sphincter to an atonic one, and possible loss or reduction of sensory appreciation outweigh the advantages of spasticity, intrathecal phenol or alcohol blocks are an alternative to surgical management.

References

1. Halpern D, Meelhuysen FE: Phenol motor point block in the management of muscular hypertonia. *Arch Phys Med Rehabil* 47:659–664, 1966.
2. Katz J, Knott L, Feldman DJ: Peripheral nerve injections with phenol in the management of spastic patients. *Arch Phys Med Rehabil* 48:97–99, 1967.
3. Khalili AA: Pathophysiology, clinical picture and management of spasticity. In: Harmel, MH: *Clinical Anesthesia. Neurologic Consideration.* Philadelphia, F. A. Davis, 1967.
4. Khalili AA: Peripheral phenol block for spasticity. In Ruge D: *Spinal Cord Injuries.* Springfield, Ill., Charles C Thomas, 1969, pp. 153–160.
5. Khalili AA: Physiatric management of spasticity by phenol nerve and motor point block. In Ruskin A: *Current Therapy in Physiatry.* Philadelphia, W.B. Saunders, 1983.
6. Khalili AA, Betts HB: *Management of Spasticity with Phenol Nerve Block.* Final Report RD-2529-M. Dec. 1970. Dept. of Health, Education and Welfare, Social and Rehabilitation Service.

CHAPTER SIX

Orthoses

J. B. REDFORD

An *orthosis* is defined as any device attached or applied to the external surface of the body to improve function, restrict or enforce motion, or support a body segment. Exclusively applied, the term "orthotics" refers to the development, manufacture, and application of orthoses. However, the field is often considered to include nonattached devices, such as environmental control systems and seating support systems, to improve functional disability.

In the past few decades, a large proportionate increase in the physically disabled population has spurred many advances in the field of orthotics. Cooperation between engineers, physicians, allied health personnel, orthotists, and manufacturers has enormously expanded the types and availability of orthotic devices.

Although *prescribing an orthosis* is a medical decision, close cooperation is mandatory between the prescribing physician, the therapist, the patient, and the orthotist. For the more complex biomechanical problems, orthotic prescription is best accomplished by this team which meets together with the patient. The prescription should include the medical diagnosis, including functional goals, and should outline special problems to be considered, such as skin anesthesia or vascular insufficiency. The patient ulti-

mately decides whether or not to use the orthosis, and the skill of the orthotist is indispensable if the device is to be custom made and fitted.

The physician's role is to determine the purpose of the orthosis, approve treatment plans, and describe any precautions necessary (Fig. 6.1). After the orthosis has been supplied, the physician must check as to whether it fulfills the need of the patient and must ensure that it is used effectively. If the patient requires special training with the device, the physician arranges this with the physical or occupational therapist.

Today's *orthotist* is a highly qualified specialist who knows how to select materials with an optimal balance between strength, flexibility, and weight. He recognizes the requirements of a useful orthosis as effectiveness, ease of application, cosmesis, comfort, durability, and minimal need for maintenance. Generally, the orthotist obtains the data required to construct orthoses, either by taking special measurements or tracings or by plaster wrappings which are later filled to produce a positive plaster mold. The almost yearly introduction of new materials and technology has added constant improvement to present techniques. Prefabricated components, for example, are replacing many items previously custom made, and

Summary of Functional Disability _____

_____

_____

_____

_____

_____

Treatment Objectives:

Prevent/Correct Deformity ☐   Improve Ambulation ☐
Reduce Axial Load   ☐   Fracture Treatment   ☐
Protect Joint   ☐   Other _____

ORTHOTIC RECOMMENDATION

LOWER LIMB		FLEX	EXT	ABD	ADD	ROTATION Int.	ROTATION Ext.	AXIAL LOAD
HKAO	Hip							
KAO	*Thigh*	▓	▓	▓		▓	▓	
	Knee							
AFO	*Leg*	▓	▓	▓	▓			
	Ankle	(Dorsi)	(Plantar)					
	Subtalar			▓	▓	(Inver.)	(Ever.)	
FO Foot	Midtarsal	—		▓	▓	▓	▓	
	Met.-phal.			▓	▓	▓	▓	

REMARKS:

_____   _____
Signature   Date

KEY: Use the following symbols to indicate desired control of designated function:

F = FREE   – *Free* motion.
A = ASSIST – Application of an external force for the purpose of increasing the range, velocity, or force of a motion.
R = RESIST – Application of an external force for the purpose of decreasing the velocity or force of a motion.
S = STOP   – Inclusion of a static unit to deter an undesired motion in one direction.
v = Variable – A unit that can be adjusted without making a structural change.
H = HOLD   – Elimination of all motion in prescribed plane (verify position).
L = LOCK   – Device includes an optional lock.

Figure 6.1. Summary and orthotic recommendation requisition (lower limb). (Reproduced with permission from: J. B. Redford. *Orthotics Etcetera*. Baltimore, Williams & Wilkins)

many thermoplastic orthoses can now be molded directly on the body, rather than over plaster molds (Fig. 6.2).

Physical and occupational therapists are often helpful in identifying functional problems and a patient's orthotic requirements. Later, they may teach the patient to use the orthosis and may help to evaluate its adequacy. A patient will readily discard an orthotic device if training in its use is lacking. Therapists may actually make orthoses in many situations, particularly fabricating upper limb orthotics from thermoplastics. Largely through the initiative of occupational therapists, a whole new scope for orthotics in hand rehabilitation has been developed (3).

Orthotics has suffered from a *lack of consistent terminology*. Some devices are described by their function, which has

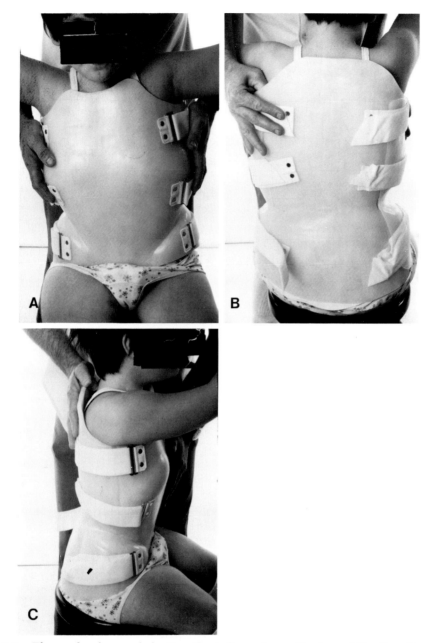

Figure 6.2. Thoracolumbosacral plastic orthosis for postoperative immobilization. (Reproduced with permission from: J. B. Redford. *Orthotics Etcetera*. Baltimore, Williams & Wilkins)

proved useful. On the other hand, some are simply described by eponyms using the name of the originator, such as the Williams brace: this has proved confusing (5). More anatomically descriptive terminology has now been widely accepted. This names orthoses according to the joints enclosed; for example, "knee-foot-ankle-orthosis," abbreviated "KAFO," much better describes the devices used to support the knee and ankle than "long leg brace." Details of this terminology, as well as a description of how orthotic prescription can include biomechanical and technical analysis, may be studied in the *Atlas of Orthotics* (1).

INDICATIONS FOR ORTHOSES

Indications for orthoses include one or more of the following:

(1) Relief of pain by reducing motion or weight bearing
(2) Protection of weak or healing musculoskeletal segments
(3) Prevention or correction of deformity
(4) Improvement of function.

Relief of pain may be accomplished by reducing the motion that contributes to the pain of inflammation or by reducing compression or traction on neural structures. A typical example is the use of a cervical collar in patients with cervical spondylosis and nerve root encroachment. A plastic splint to rest the hand and wrist (wrist-hand orthosis) in rheumatoid arthritis is another example. Pain in the lower back may be reduced by changing the line of weight bearing using wedges or elevation on shoes, or hip pain may be helped by a knee-ankle-foot-orthosis to unload the hip joint (as in aseptic necrosis of the hip).

Protection of weak or healing musculoskeletal segments which may also be painful is well illustrated by fracture bracing. In many centers, this orthotic technique has replaced traditional plaster casts. Fracture braces are lighter than casts and permit more mobility of the uninvolved joints, thus lessening the chances of joint stiffness following fracture healing. Perhaps the widest application of orthoses to support weakened or healing musculoskeletal segments arises in hand rehabilitation. Lightweight plastic orthoses are used to promote healing after hand surgery or burns and to support muscles weakened by neurologic diseases or nerve injury.

Orthotic prevention of deformity has its most common application in children. In a growing child, lack of balanced muscle forces or resistance to the pull of gravity can deform the limb or the spine. To prevent this occurrence, orthotic devices are often used as a counteracting force. Careful medical supervision and close cooperation of parents is essential for successful use of orthoses in children. A prime example of an orthosis of this type is the Milwaukee brace (cervicothoracicolumbosacral orthosis) to correct scoliosis (Fig. 6.3). Correction of deformities by orthoses is much more difficult than their prevention. This usually requires, for example, a static force such as serial application of a knee orthosis which gradually forces the flexed joint into extension. One also may use dynamic orthotic systems such as those applied after nerve injuries with springs or elastics counteracting the deforming forces.

Improvement of function is provided by virtually all orthoses through diminishing pain, relieving weight bearing, and preventing deformity. However, some devices have functional improvement as their primary purpose, e.g., the reciprocal wrist-extension finger-flexion orthosis which facilitates finger and thumb prehension by wrist extension in quadriplegic patients with function preserved above the sixth cervical segment (Fig. 6.4). As the wrist is flexed the hand opens; as it is extended the thumb is closed against the index and middle fingers. Many functional orthoses provide power to actively reinforce needed motions with springs, elastic, or even compressed gas, as in the artificial muscle powered by carbon dioxide (5).

LOWER EXTREMITY ORTHOTICS

Foot orthotics include shoes with inserts or modifications of heels, soles, and closures. For instance, heel shapes can be made to relieve ligamentous strain at the arch of the foot (e.g., Thomas heel) or to decrease the stress of heelstrike (e.g.,

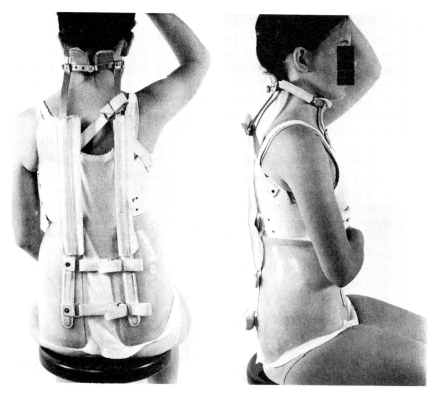

Figure 6.3. Views of the Milwaukee brace. (Reproduced with permission from: J. B. Redford. *Orthotics Etcetera.* Baltimore, Williams & Wilkins)

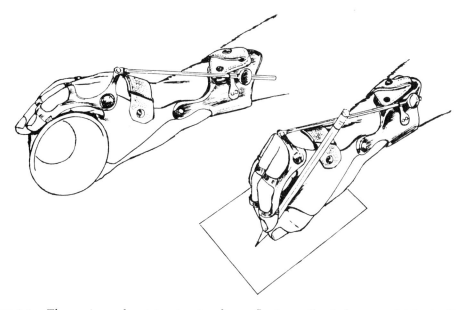

Figure 6.4. The reciprocal wrist extension finger flexion orthosis for a quadriplegic. (Reproduced with permission from: J. B. Redford. *Orthotics Etcetera.* Baltimore, Williams & Wilkins)

cushion heel). The height of the counter (firm back part of the shoe that grips the hindfoot) varies—generally being higher if everson or inversion of the hindfoot is to be controlled. Shoe closures with Velcro are much easier for patients with hand disabilities than traditional laceup shoes. Leather shoes are a necessity, and a firm shank is needed to support the arch and prevent the shoe from buckling under stress—a special problem when metal braces need to be attached. Internal shoe support or corrections can be provided such as longitudinal or transverse arch support pads individually sized (Fig. 6.5). Molded nonrigid or semirigid shoe inserts can be custom fitted to redistribute weight bearing loads on the sole of the foot or to correct mild degrees of valgus or varus ot the heel for such painful conditions as rheumatoid arthritis (2, 5).

Ankle-foot-orthoses (AFOs) used in ambulation are generally designed to control mediolateral ankle instability or provide dorsiflexion assistance. The older metal design with bilateral uprights attached to the outside of the shoe and held by a calf cuff proximally has been superceded in selected cases by plastic molded orthoses that fit inside the shoe (Fig. 6.6). The foot and ankle can be partly unloaded, or ro-

tational shear stresses on leg fractures can be minimized by molded AFOs designed to bear weight over the patellar tendon and condyles of the tibia (Fig. 6.7). Passive orthoses, either preformed or custom made, are widely used to prevent heel cord contracture or other limb deformity while the disabled patient is at rest.

Knee orthoses are mainly designed to control pain, prevent hyperextension, or control mediolateral instability. Some permit continued athletic participation within reasonable limits. Most have some elastic component to hold them in place, as the common difficulty in all designs is maintaining them securely above and below the joint.

The knee-ankle-foot orthosis (KAFO), because of its secure attachment to the foot, is a better choice than the knee orthosis for gross knee instability. Another use for the KAFO is to lock the knee in extension if there is so little muscle strength that the limb will not support body weight. Bilateral KAFOs, for example, are prescribed for patients with low level paraplegia. A quadrilateral ischial weight-bearing brim can be attached proximally to supply partial weight-bearing relief when there is otherwise unmanageable disease of the hip, such as after

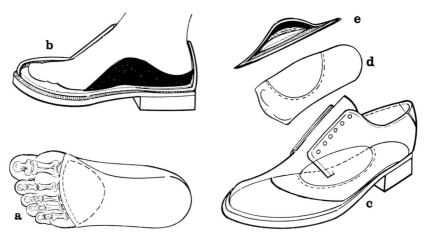

Figure 6.5.   Arch supports. (a) Fitting of arch support to the foot. (b) Arch support in shoe. (c) Wafer type arch support in shoe. (d) Dorsal view of wafer support. (e) Medial cutaway of wafer support. (Reproduced with permission from: J. B. Redford. *Orthotics Etcetera.* Baltimore, Williams & Wilkins)

example of a hip orthosis to correct deformity is a prewalking hip abduction and external rotation pillow inserted between the thighs in infants to correct congenital hip dislocation (Frejka pillow) (2, 5).

SPINAL ORTHOSES

Spinal orthoses can be classed among those that control pain (primarily by limiting anteroposterior mobility) and those that prevent lateral and rotational spinal deformity. The less rigid and more comfortable corsets or narrower belts that control the lower spine (lumbosacral orthoses or LSO) may act by augmenting the anterior pneumatic weight bearing system—the air- and fluid-filled abdominal cavity surrounded by strong abdominal muscles, or their orthotic supports. However, when severe instability occurs, a rigid thoracolumbosacral orthosis (TLSO) may be required (Fig. 6.9). Lately, because of the difficulty providing comfort in back orthoses made of metal and cloth such as

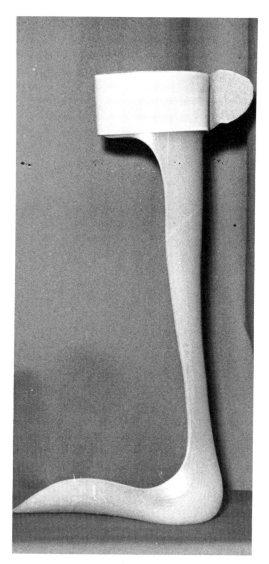

Figure 6.6. Plastic (polyurethane) molded "shoe-horn brace," or right-angle ankle orthosis. (Courtesy of Guy Martel, Department of Prosthetics & Orthotics, Chedoke Rehabilitation Centre.)

removal of an infected total hip replacement.

Some hip orthoses act by altering the position of the femoral head within the acetabulum. One such example is the ambulatory bilateral abduction orthosis (Toronto) for Legg-Perthes disease (Fig. 6.8) fitted with a universal midline joint to allow bipedal gait and ease in sitting. An

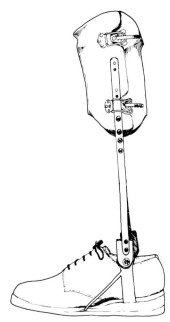

Figure 6.7. Patellar tendon-bearing ankle-foot-orthosis for limiting weight bearing. (Reproduced with permission from: J. B. Redford. *Orthotics Etcetera.* Baltimore, Williams & Wilkins)

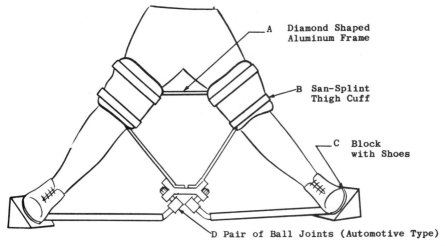

A   Diamond Shaped
     Aluminum Frame

B   San-Splint
     Thigh Cuff

C   Block
     with Shoes

D Pair of Ball Joints (Automotive Type)

Figure 6.8.   Hip orthosis to reduce weight bearing—the Toronto Legg-Perthes orthosis. (Reproduced with permission from: J. B. Redford. *Orthotics Etcetera*. Baltimore, Williams & Wilkins)

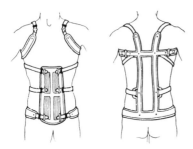

Figure 6.9.   A rigid thoracolumbar sacral orthosis (TLSO), the Taylor brace. (Reproduced with permission from: J. B. Redford. *Orthotics Etcetera*. Baltimore, Williams & Wilkins)

the Taylor brace, there has been a trend towards molded plastic TLSOs (Fig. 6.2). These are now available in preformed sizes or can be molded directly on the patient (1, 5).

The cervicothoracolumbosacral orthosis (CTLSO), used for controlling scoliosis (such as the Milwaukee brace), must be custom fitted to realign the head over the pelvis. This orthosis is used, not only to correct scoliosis but also the rotation and kyphotic or lordotic deformities accompanying it. Although an orthosis for scoliosis demands a high degree of skill in fitting with proper application and regular adjustment, the Milwaukee brace has spared many adolescents with idiopathic

scoliosis from spinal fusion (1, 5). It is a dynamic orthosis that requires the patient's musculature for optimal use, and is not indicated in patients with scoliosis secondary to neuromuscular disease.

Cervical orthoses range from very rigid ones attached to a shoulder harness with four uprights—two in front and two at the rear—to soft collars. Most are prefabricated and prescribed according to the degree of motion desired. Soft orthoses simply serve as a reminder to prevent unwanted neck motion; very rigid ones can control most motion during fracture healing. However, absolute rigidity in the neck or spine is only achieved by the *halo orthosis*. The head is held fixed by a metal halo through screws fastening it to the skull (Figs. 6.10 and 6.11). Vertical bars affix this halo to a molded body jacket and/or pelvic band gripping the upper part of the pelvis and thus preventing motion in any plane from occiput to sacrum (1).

STANDING AND SEATING DEVICES

Standing or seating devices constitute a special class of orthoses that are used primarily with the severely handicapped. Children born with paraplegia from neurologic defects accompanying meningo-

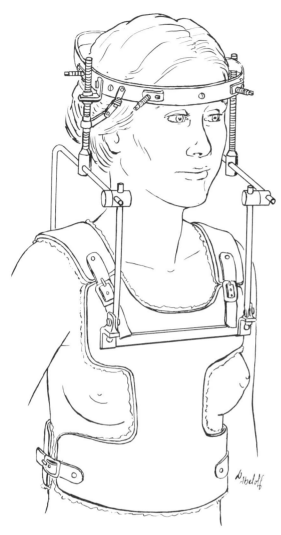

eases, and spinal cord injuries, seating clinics to prescribe and test such devices have become quite popular. For example, a modular plastic insert for patients with cerebral palsy has been designed to encourage better seating posture, inhibit abnormal reflexes, and allow better upper extremity function. Other special positioning seats have been used for patients with muscular dystrophy (who, if neglected, invariably develop scoliosis) and for those with desensitized skin such as children with meningomyelocele who need improvement in tolerance of tissue trauma and pressure (4). To permit the patient to sit at any location (e.g., in the car), these seats generally are detachable from the patient's wheelchair and so must be light and durable.

WHEELCHAIRS

Most such nonambulatory severely handicapped patients require specially designed or specially modified wheelchairs as well e.g., the reclining wheelchair (Fig. 6.13). For many handicapped persons, the type of chair used to a great extent determines their life-style and general mobility. It therefore is imperative that they receive the expert advice and team assessment found in rehabilitation centers when purchasing a permanent wheelchair.

Figure 6.10. Low profile halo with sheepskin-lined plastic jacket. (Reproduced with permission from: A. F. Brooker. *The Orthopaedic Traction Manual.* Baltimore, Williams & Wilkins)

UPPER EXTREMITY ORTHOTICS

Finger orthoses are mainly designed to prevent contractures of individual joints or specifically designed to preserve the thumb webspace. Some are molded from plastic, but others consist of spring wire and cloth-coverd metal and may feature built-in dynamic forces.

Wrist - hand - finger - orthoses (WHFO) consist of a forearm segment either attached or free from the hand and finger portion. There are many designs, but a typical example is the dynamic orthosis for radial palsy with loss of digital extension. This consists of a molded wrist and

myelocele can be stood upright early and some can later be trained to walk using special standing frames such as the *parapodium* (Fig. 6.12).

Adapted seating for those who cannot walk, often custom made, using various combinations of foam, wood, and plastic, has become a specialty of some orthotic programs. In rehabilitation facilities which treat large numbers of patients with cerebral palsy, neuromuscular dis-

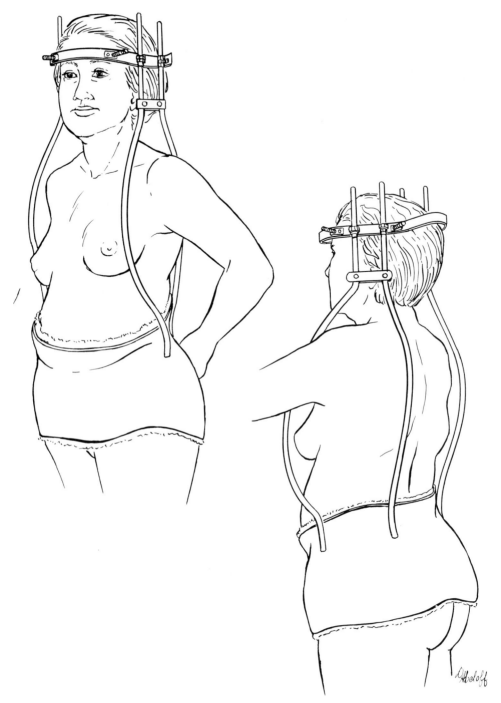

Figure 6.11. Halo ring in conjunction with pelvic girdle for thoracic and lumbar spinal deformity or injury. (Reproduced with permission from: A. F. Brooker. *The Orthopaedic Traction Manual*. Baltimore, Williams & Wilkins)

hand portion with an outrigger attached to the dorsal surface suspending elastics and leather cuffs looped around the prox-

imal phalanges (Fig. 6.14). This orthosis substitutes for lost metacarpophalangeal joint extension and prevents flexion con-

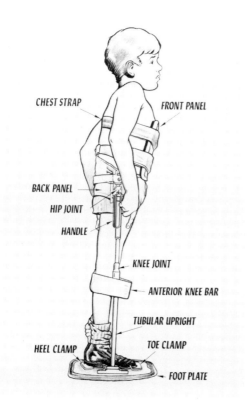

CHEST STRAP

FRONT PANEL

BACK PANEL

HIP JOINT

HANDLE

KNEE JOINT

ANTERIOR KNEE BAR

TUBULAR UPRIGHT

HEEL CLAMP

TOE CLAMP

FOOT PLATE

Figure 6.12. The parapodium. (Reproduced with permission from: J. B. Redford. *Orthotics Etcetera.* Baltimore, Williams & Wilkins)

tractures. Another typical wrist-hand-orthosis is the "cock-up splint," which immobilizes the wrist in a slightly extended position. It is usually custom molded on the patient's volar forearm and hand and is used in painful conditions about the wrist or to prevent flexion deformities in spastic hemiplegia (3, 5).

Elbow orthoses are mainly used to protect or immobilize unstable elbows following trauma. Some static orthoses are used, such as those with adjustable dial locks or adjustable turnbuckle bars to reduce elbow flexion contractures.

The shoulder is vital to reaching and hand placement, but its multiple axes of movement present very difficult problems to the orthotist, either to stabilize or restore even limited degrees of function. Generally, to control shoulder movement, the elbow must be supported so that the humeral head will be retained in anatomical relation to the glenoid.

The most common *shoulder orthoses* are the various types of slings used to support the paralyzed hemiplegic shoulder. As the scapula rotates away from the midline in the hemiplegic patient, the humeral head subluxes away from the glenoid, often causing severe pain and disability. Slings to support such a shoulder vary from the three-cornered first aid bandage to elaborate webbing and plastic devices that may be too complex for either the patient or his relation to learn to apply correctly. None has proved entirely satisfactory.

Static support with the shoulder in abduction following certain shoulder injuries or burns involving the axilla may be provided by the *airplane splint.* The patient's arm is held at about 90°, and the arm and forearm are held away from the side like the wing of an airplane.

Dynamic shoulder supports can be provided through "mobile arm supports," including *ball bearing balanced forearm orthoses* (Fig. 6.15), overhead sling suspensions, and "functional" arm braces with specially molded shoulder caps. These supports are all designed to replace lost motor function or assist shoulder mobilization by removing as much gravity effect from the weakened extremity as possible. Most are only used in patients who are confined to wheelchairs and are used more to retrain weakened muscles or mobilize stiff shoulders than to actively replace lost function.

ENVIRONMENTAL CONTROL SYSTEMS

When the upper extremities are so weakened that almost all useful function is lost, no externally applied orthotic device has really proved successful. Such a multiaxis orthosis requires extensive hardware, hours of fitting and training time, and an expensive external source of power. Those designed in the past have had really limited functional capability or portability and were cosmetically unap-

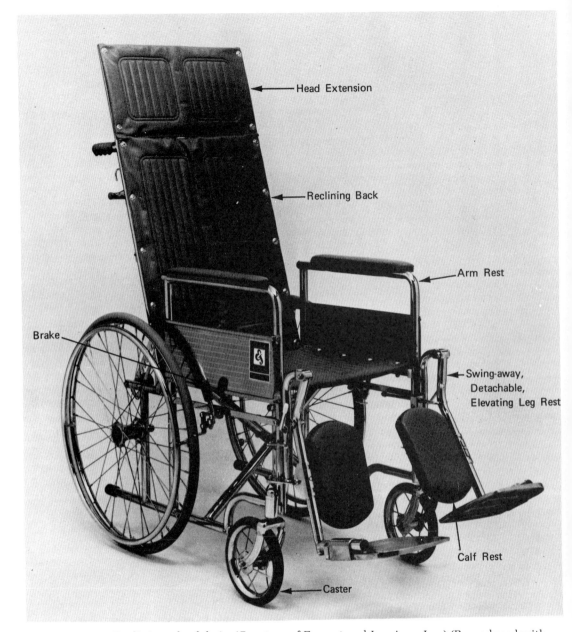

Figure 6.13. Reclining wheelchair. (Courtesy of Everest and Jennings, Inc.) (Reproduced with permission from: C. A. Trombly and A. D. Scott. *Occupational Therapy for Physical Therapists.* Baltimore, Williams & Wilkins)

pealing. The only purpose of a functional upper limb orthosis is to manipulate objects in the environment. If a simpler system not involving devices attached to limbs can serve this purpose, there is no need for further research into multiaxis types of orthoses.

Furthermore, if a patient has extensive paralysis, it is more important to be concerned with actual mobility in the wheelchair and ability to control environmental objects which pertain to ADL or comfort. Today, there are commercially available, reasonably priced, sophisticated environmental control systems that attach to the patient's wheelchair, van, or bed (Fig. 6.16). A patient with no function below the neck can drive into a dark room preceded by his headlights, switch on the room lights, activate his telephone, dial a number, speak and listen to the telephone, turn on a radio or television, set the station and volume, and then tape record and play back any part of the input received (5, 6).

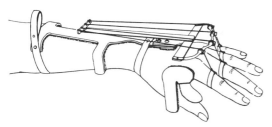

Figure 6.14. A wrist-hand-finger orthosis for radial nerve palsy. (Reproduced with permission from: J. B. Redford. *Orthotics Etcetera.* Baltimore, Williams & Wilkins)

SUMMARY

In summary, orthotics is an extensive field allied closely with rehabilitation medicine and under constant development. Prescription of more complex devices is best performed by a team composed of physician, orthotist, and therapist, but in the final analysis, the patient remains supreme—no one can make a patient use a device for which he or she does not perceive a specific need. In addition to utility, cost, portability, comfort, and cosmetic acceptance must be considered when ordering a device. Orthoses can never substitute for strengthening exercises, active joint mobilization, or corrective surgery. They can only serve as assistive devices in rehabilitation, but when properly prescribed and effectively used, they transform the life of a severely disabled person from one of dependence and misery to independence and relief from pain and discomfort.

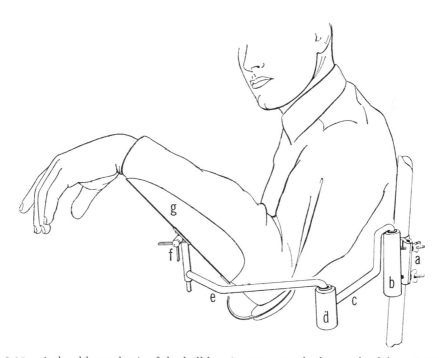

Figure 6.15. A shoulder orthosis of the ball bearing type attached to a wheelchair. (*a*) Bracket assembly. (*b*) Proximal ball bearing. (*c*) Proximal swivel arm. (*d*) Distal ball bearing. (*e*) Distal swivel arm. (*f*) Rocker arm assembly. (*g*) Trough. (Reproduced with permission from: J. B. Redford. *Orthotics Etcetera.* Baltimore, Williams & Wilkins)

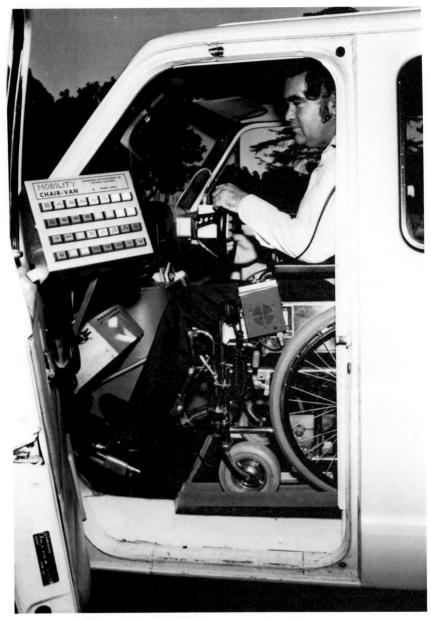

Figure 6.16.   Push button and servo controls in van (Scott). (Reproduced with permission from: J. B. Redford. *Orthotics Etcetera*. Baltimore, Williams & Wilkins)

References

1. American Academy of Orthopedic Surgeons: *Atlas of Orthotics*. St. Louis, C.V. Mosby, 1975.
2. D'Astous J (ed): *Orthotics and Prosthetics Digest*. Ottawa, Canada, Edahl Productions, 1981.
3. Fess EE, Gettle KS, Strickland JW: *Hand Splinting Principles and Methods*. St. Louis, C.V. Mosby, 1981.
4. Matlock WM: Seating and positioning for the physically impaired. *Orthot Prosthet* 31:11–21, 1977.
5. Redford JB: *Orthotics Etcetera*. Baltimore, Williams & Wilkins, 1980.
6. Sell GH, Stratford CD, Zimmerman ME, Youdin M, Milner D: Environmental and typewriter control systems for high level quadriplegic patients: evaluation and prescription. *Arch Phys Med Rehabil* 60:246–252, 1979.

CHAPTER SEVEN

Prostheses

L. F. BENDER

A prosthesis is a substitute for a missing body part, used for cosmetic or functional purposes. The physiatrist most frequently utilizes protheses designed to replace part of a leg or arm (as discussed in Chapter 11 by Dr. Banerjee), but protheses may replace a breast, an ear, an eye, or any other superficial body part. Surgeons implant protheses to replace various joints, bones, and tissues in the body.

Arms perform significantly different functions than legs, and the requirements for prosthetic function vary accordingly. The shoulder girdle is the most mobile of all joints in the body, and a hand has the most sophisticated function. The shoulder-elbow-wrist complex enables the hand to move to positions where it can perform intricate and delicate or powerful tasks. One- or two-handed manipulative ability, placement of the terminal device, and appearance are of prime importance.

The leg, through its hip-knee-ankle-foot complex, provides stability and mobility; it resembles a series of pendulums and levers and is most often covered by apparel. The leg prosthesis allows mobility that otherwise might be accomplished only with crutches or a wheelchair.

THE PROSTHETIC SOCKET

The interface requirements between the distal portion of an amputated limb and a prosthesis are similar in arms and legs. The socket of the prosthesis must fit snugly, yet comfortably, must provide a stable base for attachment of the rest of the prosthesis, and must be held securely on the stump. Leg sockets bear the full weight of the body during stance while arm sockets maximize placement of a terminal device through useful arcs of motion. Generally, one expects leg sockets to be sturdier and heavier than arm sockets, but both reflect the contour of the stump and must not damage the skin or constrict the stump proximally.

Sockets for above-knee stumps are approximately quadrilateral in internal contour with channels for the hamstrings and thigh adductors, a bulge over Scarpa's femoral triangle, and a broad seat for support of the ischium. The lateral wall is high to limit lateral bending during stance; the medial brim is low to avoid pressure on the pubis (Figs. 7.1 and 7.2).

Below-knee, below-elbow, and above-elbow sockets vary from triangular to oval in contour, depending on the site of amputation and the shape of the stump. Weight bearing on below-knee stumps is concentrated over pressure-tolerant areas along the proximal tibial flares and the patellar tendon.

Socket inner walls are usually constructed by vacuum molding epoxy resins and stockinette over a mold of the stump.

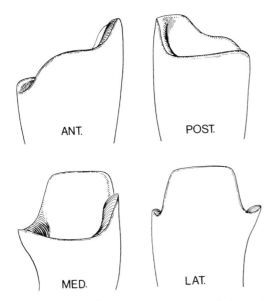

ANT.   POST.

MED.   LAT.

Figures 7.1 and 7.2.   Views of a quadrilateral socket as seen from each side (1) and from above (2) showing a high lateral wall, low medial brim, and a broad seat for the ischium.

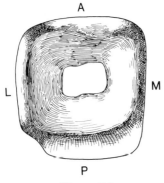

A

L   M

P

Figure 7.2.

Correct contour of the mold to distribute pressures from the prosthesis is crucial to satisfactory fit and ultimate function.

Thin liners of porous material or of silicone gel may be used between the stump and socket of a prosthesis to absorb some of the stresses that otherwise might be transmitted to the skin and subcutaneous tissues. A rigid socket provides a more intimate fit and fewer perspiration problems. Added pads inside the socket usually indicate a less than optimal fit of the socket and eventually point to the need for a new socket.

The outer wall of a prosthetic socket is shaped to resemble the body part it is to replace. At its distal end, it is built over a prefabricated joint which serves as the attachment point for the next segment of the prosthesis, *i.e.*, wrist, elbow, shoulder, ankle, knee, or hip.

LEG COMPONENTS

Ankle and Foot

The foot-ankle preferred for nearly all below-knee and most above-knee amputations is called a SACH (Solid Ankle, Cushioned Heel) foot. Varying durometers of rubber in the heel cushion the heel strike (Fig. 7.3). Modest mediolateral movement is available and is helpful on uneven surfaces. Active walkers prefer this foot and it can be obtained with simulated toes for use in sandals.

The most stable foot-ankle mechanism is the single-axis ankle with a soft poste-

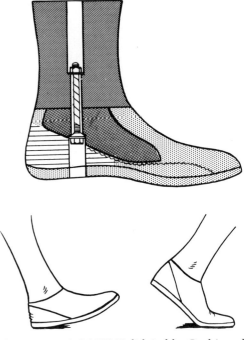

Figure 7.3.   A SACH (Solid Ankle, Cushioned Heel) foot bolted to a below-knee prosthesis. Rubber in the heel cushions heelstrike, a rigid internal keel provides stability, and the flexible toe break enhances push-off during walking.

rior and firm anterior rubber bumper; it allows easy plantar flexion at heel strike and provides a strong force through resistance to ankle dorsiflexion to prevent knee flexion during push-off.

A universal ankle held together with a flexible vertical cable and utilizing a circular rubber bumper is less stable but permits more motion than the single-axis or SACH.

Knees

Prosthetic knee movement must be controlled to prevent forceful terminal impact at the end of the swing phase of gait and to reduce excessive knee flexion after push-off. A constant friction knee accomplishes this; the degree of friction can be adjusted to meet individual needs. A constant friction knee is available with a locking mechanism that is activated either by the downward thrust exerted in stance (safety knee) or by a hand-operated lever, providing increased stability, particularly for the elderly.

A variable friction knee is available to accommodate a limited variation in an individual's walking speed. For maximum adaptation to varying walking speeds, a hydraulic swing-phase control unit may be used. Hydraulic knee units add several hundred dollars to the cost of the prosthesis but reduce the energy requirements of walking and should be considered for young, active walkers.

Hips

For persons with amputation at the hip disarticulation or hemipelvectomy level, the Canadian hip-disarticulation unit is the standard appliance. It has a flexion-extension hinge whose axis of motion is in front of the weight bearing line.

LEG SUSPENSION

Below-Knee

The standard patellar-tendon bearing prosthesis uses a supracondylar strap or a narrow cuff in most cases to hold the prosthesis on the stump (Fig. 7.4). Some

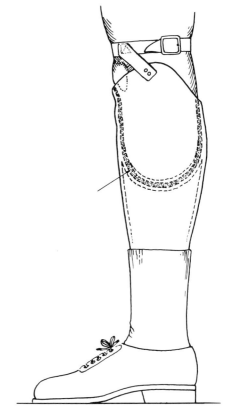

Figure 7.4. Double-wall, below-knee socket with suprapatellar strap suspension, patellar-tendon bearing design, and a removable liner (*arrow*).

users prefer a rubber sleeve that fits tightly over the upper area of the socket and is unrolled up the thigh to cover it as well as the knee. Additional suspension can be obtained through a thigh corset or a waist belt; corsets are needed only for very short, below-knee stumps or for unstable knees.

Above-Knee

A Silesian band provides minimal stability and enhanced mobility; it is a flexible strap attached to the anterior and posterior brims of the socket which runs around the opposite iliac crest (Fig. 7.5). A pelvic band with a metal hip joint increases stability and prevents rotation of the socket. It is most useful for short or flabby stumps or for the elderly who cannot manage to put on a suction socket.

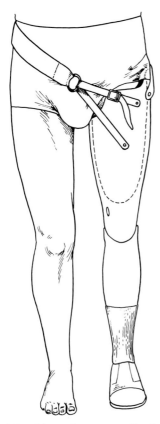

Figure 7.5. Above-knee prosthesis with a quadrilateral suction socket and a Silesian band.

Suction alone may be adequate to hold the prosthesis on the stump, especially if the stump is long and firm. A one-way valve is screwed into an air hole that enters the inner wall of the socket at its distal portion. The valve allows air to leave during stance, but not to reenter, thus maintaining suction.

ARM COMPONENTS

Terminal Devices

In contrast to lower extremity prostheses, terminal devices to replace the lost functions of the hand are numerous. A variety of hooks, hands, and special devices are available. Hooks are split so one side can be pulled away from or opposed to the other side. Tension devices such as rubber bands or springs are used to close

some hooks and hands called voluntary opening devices. Other devices are closed voluntarily and are opened by springs. Most devices are voluntary opening (Fig. 7.6).

The hooks are available in gradations of size and weight suitable for the newborn up to adulthood. Functional hands are not available for the newborn, infant, or toddler but are available for school age children and adults. Also available are special devices to hold tools, a bowling ball, a bowl, a rifle, and so forth. Electric motor-driven hands have been available for more than a decade in adult sizes, but electric motor-driven hooks are not available other than on an experimental basis.

Wrists

Throughout the world, terminal devices use a standard stud (½ inch, 20-thread) for attachment to a wrist unit of a prosthesis. All devices are therefore interchangeable. To enhance interchangeability, quick-disconnecting wrists are also available. The terminal device is screwed into an adaptor that plugs into a locking unit. In these wrists, the terminal device can be rotated by unlocking the adaptor and can be relocked in any position of rotation by pushing the terminal device proximally. In the simplest wrist units the terminal device screws into a threaded base, and rotation is controlled by a friction device of rubber or plastic.

Elbows

Persons with below-elbow amputations require some type of hinge at the elbow in the socket suspension harness. Both flexible and rigid hinges are available. Rigid hinges are preferred by some for short stumps to provide stability. There also are hinges which multiply the amount of flexion by utilizing a single wall socket over a short stump plus a forearm shell which is attached to the step-up hinges but not directly to the socket.

Above-elbow prostheses customarily

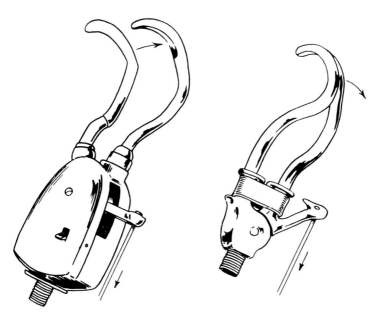

Figure 7.6. On the left is a voluntary closing hook developed by the Army Prosthetics Research Laboratory (APRL). Tension on the control cable causes the hook fingers to close; the force of prehension is proportional to the pull on the cable. On the right is a Dorrance No. 5 hook which is voluntary opening. Tension on the control cable pulls one side of the split hook away from the other; prehension force is dependent on the number of rubber bands used to close it when tension on the control cable is relaxed.

utilize a positive-locking elbow with fore-arm lift-assist. This unit can be locked in 11 different positions between 5 and 135° of flexion. Just above the elbow there is also a friction-plate turntable so the fore-arm shell can be positioned in "humeral" internal or external rotation. An adjustable spring mechanism mounted on the medial aspect of the unit assists elbow flexion by partially counterbalancing the weight of the forearm and the terminal device. Several electric elbow units are available, but they are extremely expensive.

For very long above-elbow and elbow-disarticulation stumps it is necessary to place the elbow hinges on the outside of the socket since there is no room for the positive-locking unit.

Shoulders

These units are needed for shoulder-disarticulation and for forequarter levels of amputation. A cosmetic unit may be all the patient desires rather than a functional upper extremity prosthesis. Such a unit can be constructed from polyethylene or from a block of polyfoam and can be held on with a chest strap. Patients who desire functional prostheses can be provided with one of several units which act as universal joints at the shoulder.

ARM SUSPENSION AND CONTROL

Below- and Above-Elbow

Various harnesses are available to hold the complete prosthesis on the stump and to provide an attachment for the control of the terminal device. The harness most commonly used is shaped like a figure eight. Instead of the straps being sewn in back where they cross, the O-ring harness utilizes at this point a circular ring which allows adjustment (Fig. 7.7). The anterior strap which lies in the deltoid-pectoral groove on the amputated side attaches directly to the socket of an above-elbow

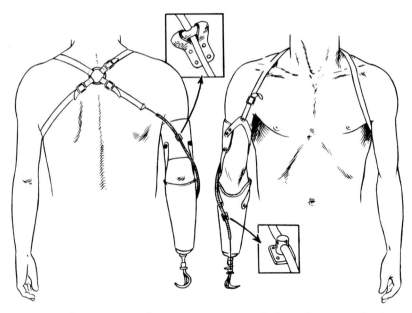

Figure 7.7. Front and rear views of a person wearing a below-elbow prosthesis with an "O" ring harness. The harness provides suspension of the prosthesis and anchors the cable which controls the hook. Insets show the method of attachment of the control cable housing to the triceps pad (above) and to the socket (below).

prosthesis or to a Y-strap and triceps pad for a below-elbow prosthesis. The posterior strap on the amputated side provides the attachment for the proximal end of the control cable.

For persons who do heavy work, a polyethylene shoulder saddle harness may be used. The shoulder saddle provides a larger weight-bearing area and permits the lifting of a heavy axial load with comfort (Figs. 7.8 and 7.9).

When the upper brim of the socket extends up over the tip of the acromion, a chest strap will usually provide adequate suspension and a proper attachment for a control strap. This type of harness is used with prostheses for amputations at the following levels: forequarter, shoulder disarticulation, humeral neck and, in some cases, short above-elbow.

Control Cables

Mechanical control of functional terminal devices and elbow units is achieved by metal cables. A cable housing is used to guide the cable from its point of origin on the harness to the point of attachment on a terminal device. The housing is composed of wire tightly wound to form a tube.

One cable may provide either single or dual control functions. In a system which provides two actions, the control cable slides through two separated pieces of housing. Force is transmitted to a terminal device, and force is applied to move the separated pieces of housing toward each other. Therefore, it can be used to bend the elbow as well as to operate the terminal device, depending on whether the elbow unit is locked or unlocked. A single cable thereby becomes a dual control system for above-elbow type prostheses.

Myoelectric Control

Electromyographic control has been utilized with proportional-type electronic switches to operate motor-driven hands and elbows. Surface electrodes are placed

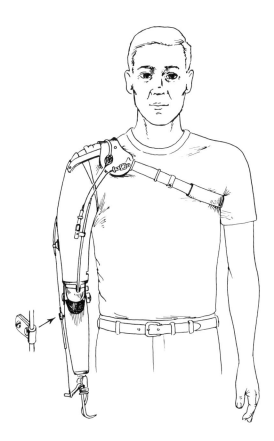

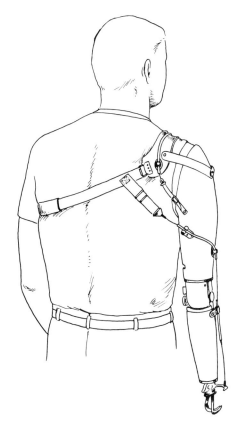

Figures 7.8 and 7.9. Front and rear views of a person wearing an above-elbow prosthesis with a shoulder-saddle harness. Suspension of the prosthesis is accomplished through a cable attached to the anterior and posterior aspects of the socket which transfers the weight to the saddle over the top of the shoulder. The dual control cable which operates the hook and elbow attaches to the chest strap posteriorly. The elbow lock is activated by the cable running anteriorly from the shoulder saddle to the elbow.

Figure 7.9.

inside the inner wall of the socket over appropriate muscles, the action of which was similar to that now to be performed by the prosthetic component. A tiny two-channel electromyograph is built into the prosthesis, and the electric activity generated in muscles beneath the electrodes is used to control the flow of stored electricity from a battery to the motor (Fig. 7.10).

EXOSKELETAL AND ENDOSKELETAL PROSTHESES

Below-elbow and below-knee prostheses are usually exoskeletal; the outer layer of the socket provides the strength and stability of the prosthesis and is attached to the ankle or wrist component. For amputations above the knee or elbow, an exoskeletal forearm or shin piece may be used to connect the wrist or ankle with the elbow or knee, or, a small-diameter, hollow tube of metal may be used, covered with a layer of plastic foam shaped to resemble the forearm or lower leg—an endoskeletal prosthesis. Endoskeletal prostheses are less durable and more expensive but lighter and more easily adjusted, and they provide enhanced cosmesis.

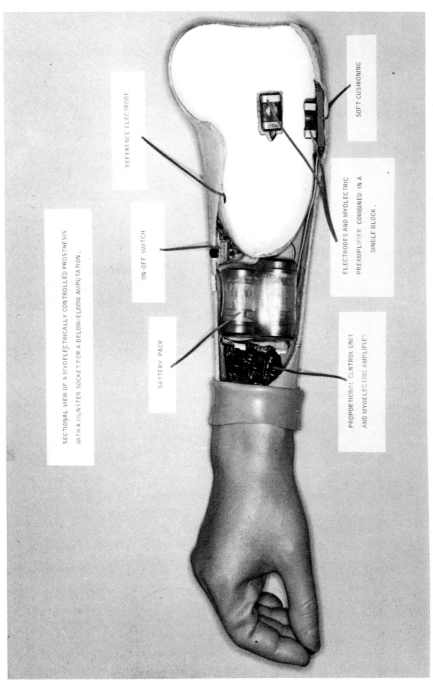

Figure 7.10.   Below-elbow myoelectric prosthesis with Muenster type socket cut away to show internal arrangements. (Reproduced with permission from C. A. Trombly and A. D. Scott, *Occupational Therapy for Physical Therapists.* Baltimore, Williams & Wilkins.)

NONFUNCTIONAL PROSTHESES

Prostheses designed purely for appearance are occasionally used to replace legs or, more often, arms. A person with weakness or paralysis coupled with leg amputation may want a leg prosthesis for a more normal appearance when sitting in a wheelchair. Similarly, a person with any level of arm amputation may not wish to cope with the complexity and weight of a functional prosthesis. In such cases, endoskeletal prostheses of light weight can be used to provide cosmesis and to simulate normal body contours under clothing.

PROSTHETIC TEAM

Adults and children with amputations are best served by attending an amputee clinic where a team of medical professionals listen, examine, and advise. Clinic teams usually include a physician with special interest and training in prosthetics, a physical and/or occupational therapist, a prosthetist, a social worker, and a vocational counselor. They may recommend specialized treatment to the stump, counseling and guidance, prevocational testing, or other procedures. They will decide if a prosthesis should be provided, and they will prescribe its components. After fabrication of the prosthesis, the team members will examine its fit and function and will provide instruction and training in its use. Any problems can be detected early and addressed quickly.

PRESCRIPTION DECISIONS

To write the prescription as accurately as possible, the prosthetic team must have adequate information about the patient. Such information, best obtained during a private interview, should include educational achievements, marital status, previous jobs, age, distance from home to the clinic or prosthetist, desire and aptitude for further educational or vocational training, motivation to wear a prosthesis, potential for continuing in a previous vocation or in a new one near home, and previous hobbies and diversional activities. Consulting together in the clinic, the prosthetic team decides when the stump is ready to be fitted with a prosthesis. Their considerations should include stump length, shape, muscle tone, stump circumferences at various levels, state of healing at amputation site and in other areas which will be in contact with the socket or harness, and motion and strength at the suspension and control sites. If there are deficiencies in any of these, the patient may require preliminary treatment. When the amputee and his stump are ready to be fitted with a prosthesis, the prescription should be written out, specifying each structural component.

THE PROSTHETIST

Artificial limbs have been constructed for centuries, but only in the past few decades have they been fabricated primarily by prosthetists, specialists trained to design, fabricate, and fit prostheses. In the United States prosthetists are certified by the American Board for Certification in Orthotics and Prosthetics, Inc. They must possess a bachelor's degree or an associate degree, and they must have successfully completed a specified number of approved courses in prosthetics to qualify for admission to the Certification Examination. In other industrialized countries, similar training and qualifying examinations are required.

IMMEDIATE POSTOPERATIVE FITTING

A temporary prosthesis may be constructed immediately after surgical amputation or within the next few days. Either plaster or a heat-moldable plastic is used to construct a temporary socket. Special attachment pieces are available for an elbow or a wrist on an upper limb or for a walking pylon on a lower limb. The socket must be reshaped or replaced every few days, but it offers the advantage of immediate standing and mobility or manipulative skills. Proponents of this management program describe decreased formation of edema in the stump, improved circulation to the skin, improved body metabolism through exercise, and enhanced healing. However, the cost of multiple temporary sockets is high, and the time from surgery to fitting of the final prosthesis may be approximately the same as when one uses a rigid dressing or elastic wraps postoperatively. A person who has experienced traumatic amputation of both hands is a candidate for immediate postoperative fitting with a temporary prosthesis, at least on one side, so that the most basic activities of daily living can be performed independently.

PROSTHETIC CHECKOUT AND TRAINING

After the prosthesis has been fabricated, the therapist and the physician check its fit and function. Specific checkout routines are available. The initial checkout of the finished prosthesis takes only a few minutes and involves primarily an inspection of the components and function of the prosthesis before the patient begins to wear it. After the patient dons the prosthesis, its position on the patient is observed, and its efficiency is checked. The checkout includes the conformance with prescription, dimensions, components, harness, cable system, socket, and workmanship.

Training in the control and use of the prosthesis begins as soon as it is delivered to the amputee. The length of the period of training varies from a few hours to a few weeks.

Follow-up

Prostheses remain effective therapeutic tools through continued monitoring of progress and problems by the prosthetic team. Advances made in prostheses and their components should be incorporated and used during periodic follow-up evaluations by the team.

CHAPTER EIGHT

Spectrum of Physical Treatment Measures*

B. J. de Lateur

This chapter deals with several major clinical applications of physical agents: modalities (especially heat and cold), traction, manipulation, therapeutic exercise, electrical stimulation, and massage.

MODALITIES

The "modalities" used in physical medicine include heat and cold, both deep and superficial.

Physiologic Effects of Heat

Since the diathermies and superficial heat have their therapeutic effect through the production or transfer of heat, it would be well to begin wih a statement of some of the general physiologic effects of heat which have therapeutic benefit as well as the general contraindications to heat. Heat alleviates pain by a direct effect on nerve and nerve endings as well as indirectly by alleviating painful conditions such as muscle spasms and joint stiffness. Subjectively, and by objective measurement, heat decreases the morning stiffness of rheumatoid arthritis. An

important effect of heat is that it alters the visco-elastic properties of collagen tissues, making joint contractures more amenable to stretching exercise. Heat increases blood flow and may assist in the resolution of chronic inflammatory processes (15).

It is often desirable to distinguish between vigorous heating and mild heating. In vigorous heating the highest temperature in the temperature distribution is applied at the site of pathology. Relatively high temperatures are achieved which are reached rapidly and maintained for relatively long periods of time. Vigorous heating is appropriate for chronic disorders. The therapeutic temperature range is 40–45°C. The effective duration of treatment is generally 5–30 minutes.

In acute disorders, particularly in acute inflammatory disorders, either heat should not be used at all or only mild heating should be used. In contrast to vigorous heating, with mild heating the highest temperature in the distribution is at some distance from the site of pathology (for example, superficial heat may be used over a deeply placed acutely inflamed joint); relatively low temperatures are achieved at the site of pathology.

General contra-indications to heat in-

* This chapter is in part based on research supported by Research Grant No. G008003029 from the National Institute of Handicapped Research, Department of Education, Washington, D.C. 20202.

clude malignancy or ischemia in the area to be treated, impairment of sensation or obtundation of consciousness, and hemorrhagic diathesis. In addition to these general contraindications there are some specific contraindictions with the specific diathermies.

DIATHERMY

The term diathermy, from the Greek "dia" meaning through and "thermos" meaning heat, implies that diathermy heats through tissues or at least deeply into tissues rather than just heating the surface. The three forms of diathermy are *shortwave, microwave,* and *ultrasound.* They, plus infrared radiation, are said to heat by conversion, because a different form of energy is converted into heat (15, 16).

Shortwave Diathermy

Shortwave diathermy (SWD) is the therapeutic application of high frequency electrical currents which are converted into heat as they pass through the tissues. This is perceived by the patient as warmth and not as a shock or the usual type of electrical stimulation. The types of equipment available for SWD vary, but all SWDs have in common the three basic components of the circuitry, which are the power supply, the oscillating circuit, and the patient's circuit. Tolerances for the oscillating circuit are specified by the Federal Communications Commission (FCC) in the U.S. (10). These machines operate at a frequency of 27.33 MHz, with a wavelength of 11 m. The patient circuit is part of the total circuitry and, therefore, the equipment must be tuned at a low output so that the frequency of the patient's circuit is made equal to the frequency of the oscillating circuit of the machine (resonance frequency). This is done at low output to avoid a surge of current which might result in a burn.

After the machine has been properly tuned to the patient's circuit, the output can be increased, depending on the vigor of heating desired. Accurate dosimetry is not available for shortwave diathermy, and therefore one must rely upon intact sensation of warmth and pain to effectively and safely use this modality.

Various types of applicators are available using either a condenser or an induction coil. Examples of the use of condenser plates are shown in Figures 8.1 and 8.2, and examples of the induction coil are shown in Figures 8.3–8.5. With condenser plates as shown in Figure 8.1, spacing is provided by the space plates which are part of the equipment. For the other types of application, spacing must be provided by several layers of terry cloth to avoid burns caused by too great a current density in the superficial tissues.

In general, with shortwave diathermy heating is greatest in deep subcutaneous tissue and superficial musculature, depending to some extent upon the technique of application and the thickness of subcutaneous fat. In addition, with SWD there are available internal vaginal and rectal electrodes which are used with an external belt and alcohol thermometer (see Fig. 8.6). This allows very accurate dosimetry because of the presence of the alcohol thermometer. This must be used with caution and may be contraindicated in borderline congestive heart failure because of the great increase in pelvic blood flow which may put a strain on a failing heart.

Caution: With SWD there is also the potential for hazardous interference with *cardiac pacemakers.* Shortwave diathermy should not be used on patients with implanted pacemakers and in particular should not be used to treat the area containing the device or electrode wires. Precaution should be used to avoid accumulation of sweat beads, as these may be selectively heated. The layers of terry cloth thus serve a dual function in that they not only provide spacing but also prevent accumulation of sweat beads. General contraindications to heat should

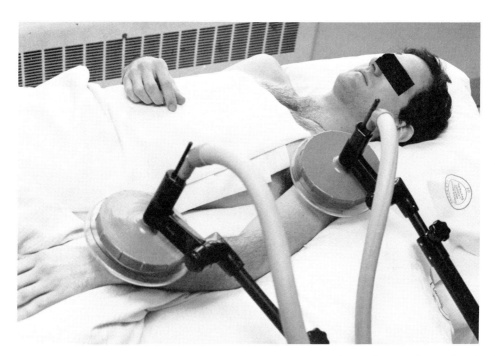

Figure 8.1. Shortwave diathermy application to the arm with condenser plates. Spacing is provided by space plates. (Reproduced with permission from: JF Lehmann *et al.* (16).)

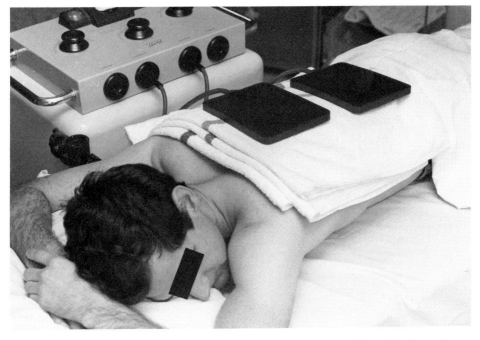

Figure 8.2. Shortwave diathermy application with condenser pads to back, with spacing between skin and electrodes provided by layers of terry cloth. (Reproduced with permission from: JF Lehmann (16).)

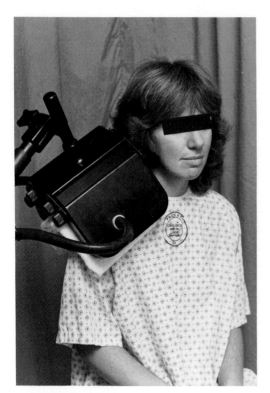

Figure 8.3. Shortwave diathermy application with induction coil (drum applicator). (Reproduced with permission from: JF Lehmann and BJ deLateur (16).)

be observed. In addition, shortwave diathermy should be avoided where there are *metal implants*.

Microwave Diathermy

Microwave diathermy (MWD) is the therapeutic application of electromagnetic radiation, identical to radar. It is propagated even in a vacuum and, thus, the patient is outside of the circuitry. As with light waves, microwaves can be reflected, scattered, refracted, or absorbed. The basic components of the apparatus for microwave consist of a power supply, a magnetron which produces the high frequency oscillation, and the applicator, which is an antenna. The applicators are often referred to as directors. The commercially available directors are called A, B, C, and E. The field pattern produced by these varies with the director.

Although there are some nonthermal effects of microwaves, all demonstrable therapeutic effects are due to heat. The pattern of relative heating varies with the frequency of the machine. Frequencies allowed by the FCC in the use of micro-

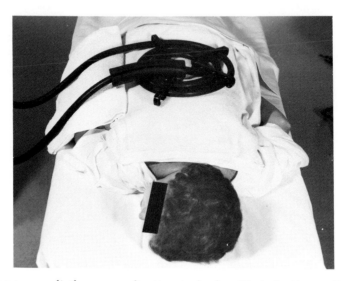

Figure 8.4. Shortwave diathermy application to back with induction coil (pancake coil). Spacing between coil and skin is provided by layers of terry cloth. (Reproduced with permission from: JF Lehmann and BJ deLateur (16).)

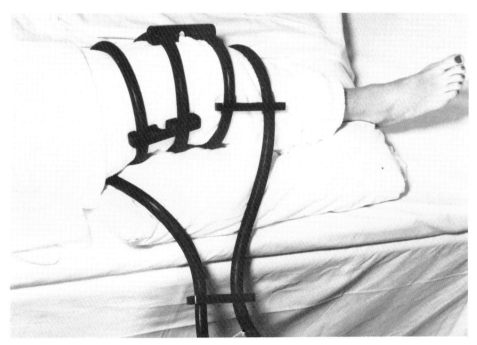

Figure 8.5. Induction coil application to knee, with spacing provided by layers of terry cloth. (Reproduced with permission from: JF Lehmann and BJ deLateur (16).)

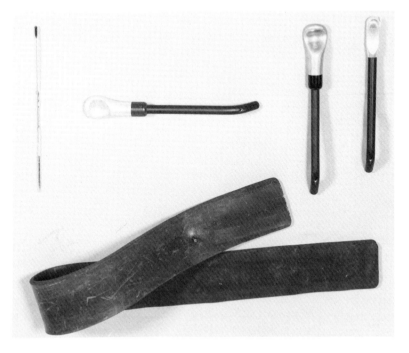

Figure 8.6. Internal vaginal and rectal electrodes with external belt and alcohol thermometer. (Reproduced with permission from: JF Lehmann and BJ deLateur (16).)

wave diathermy include 2456 MHz and 914 MHz. At this time, only machines operating at 2456 MHz are commercially available. Figure 8.7A and B shows the patterns of relative heating produced by microwaves operating at 2456 (A) and 915 MHz (B). From this it may be predicted that microwaves operating at 915 MHz have a greater depth of penetration, particularly in the muscle, which may be more desirable than merely heating the fat (8). Furthermore, the depth of penetration may be enhanced by using a contact applicator (instead of one of the standard

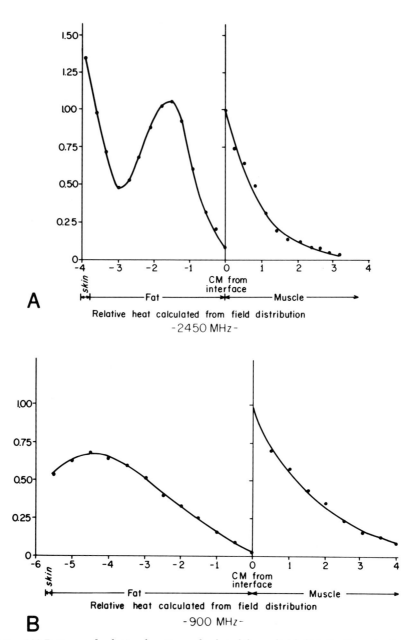

Figure 8.7. (A) Pattern of relative heating calculated from field distribution at a frequency of 2450 MHz. (B) Pattern of relative heating calculated from field distribution at a frequency of 900 MHz. (Reproduced with permission from: JF Lehmann et al. (18).)

directors) with preliminary superficial cooling. Figure 8.8 shows actual temperature measurements in the thigh of a live human who had 10 minutes of superficial cooling before turning on the power of the microwave. It can be seen that at minute 30 (20 minutes of microwave heating) uniform heating of muscle had been obtained.

Depth of penetration with microwave, then, depends upon the frequency at which the machine operates, the thickness of subcutaneous fat, the type of applicator, and the presence or absence of superficial cooling. The greatest depth of penetration and most uniform muscle heating occur with the contact applicator with previous superficial cooling. At this time, such applicators are not commercially available, but probably they will be soon.

As with shortwave diathermy, *caution* should be taken to avoid selective heating in *accumulations of fluid* and with *metal implants. Pacemaker inhibition* may also occur, and it should be avoided. Care should be taken to avoid exposure to the eye as cataracts may occur from long-term exposure. Experimentally, cataracts have not been shown to occur at intensities below 100 milliwatts/cm^2. Less stray radiation occurs with the contact applicator which will be an advantage when it becomes available commercially. An advantage for currently available directors is their great ease of application, which is roughly as easy as shining a light on a part to be heated.

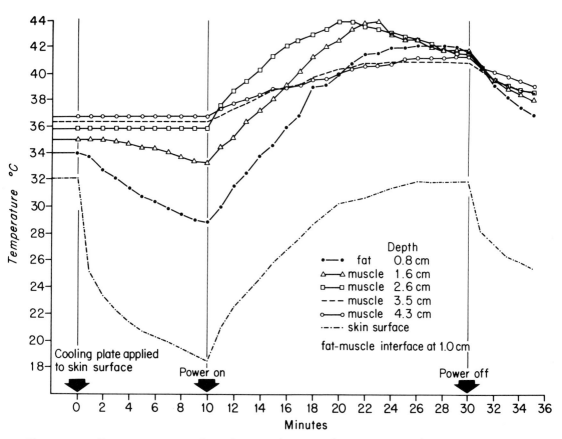

Figure 8.8. Temperatures resulting from application of microwave with a 915 MHz contact applicator in a typical experiment at various depths of tissue. (Reproduced with permission from: JF Lehmann et al. (8).)

Ultrasonic Diathermy

Ultrasound is an acoustic vibration characterized by compression and rarefaction of particles in a medium. It is similar to audible sound in all respects, except for its frequency. Somewhat arbitrarily, frequencies below 17,000 Hz are referred to as sound, and higher frequencies are referred to as ultrasound.

The propagation of ultrasound depends upon a medium; ultrasound cannot be propagated in a vacuum (in contrast to microwave). Since wavelength is inversely proportional to frequency it follows that the wavelength of ultrasound is very much shorter than that of sound. Thus, anatomic structures in the body are large relative to the wavelength; bones and joints represent a barrier to ultrasound. For this reason multiple aspects (fields) of joints like the shoulder must be treated.

For therapeutic purposes it is desirable to have an ultrasonic applicator with good beaming properties. Other things being equal there will be less divergence with applicators of large diameter. However, when applicators are too large, contact with tissues, which is essential for propagation, may be lost. Therefore, the applicator size chosen is a compromise between these two considerations. An applicator with a radiating surface of 7–13 cm^2 is a useful range.

Ultrasonic diathermy (USD) is a very effective deep heating agent and has the deepest penetration of the three diathermy modalities. Figure 8.9 shows the temperature inside the hip joint of a pig in response to ultrasound, shortwave, and microwave. USD easily brings the temperature of the hip joint into the therapeutic range whereas shortwave and microwave have little or no effect. USD can also be used safely in the presence of metal implants in the area to be treated, but the available data suggest that it should not be used in the presence of methyl methacrylate, the "bone cement" widely used in joint replacements.

Accurate dosimetry is available for USD. Therapeutic intensities range from 1 to 4 watts/cm^2. The appropriate amount depends on the vigor of heating required as well as the volume (area times thickness) of tissue to be treated. If a deeply placed joint capsule is to be heated, it is desirable that an intensity be chosen which would produce pain in approximately 11 or 12 minutes. In the actual treatment, which would be, for example, 10 minutes, the patient will not experience pain because the treatment stops short of this time. If it is possible to treat an area for 20 minutes or more without ever producing pain, it is likely that the intensity used is too low and that the structures intended to be heated will not be brought into the therapeutic temperature range.

In general, the benefits from ultrasound relate to its heating effect, but streaming of fluids may also result in a stirring effect which may be beneficial in accelerating diffusion of injected medications. There is no evidence to support the use of "pulsed" over continuous SWD. General contraindications to heat should be observed, although it is possible under carefully controlled conditions to heat an area of impaired sensation if the ultrasonic dosage is first standardized on the unaffected side and then, for safety, the wattage is cut back slightly. So, for example, a stiff shoulder in a hemiplegic patient might safely be treated if the dosage were standardized in this way on the unaffected side. Gaseous cavitation can occur in fluids of low cell density but does not occur clinically as long as proper equipment with full wave rectification and filtering is used along with adequate pressure of the applicator on the tissue and a stroking technique.

Because the ultrasonic beam, even with good equipment, is not perfectly uniform in the so-called "near field," stroking technique must be used to mix or "average" the maxima and minima of intensity. A good coupling medium must be used be-

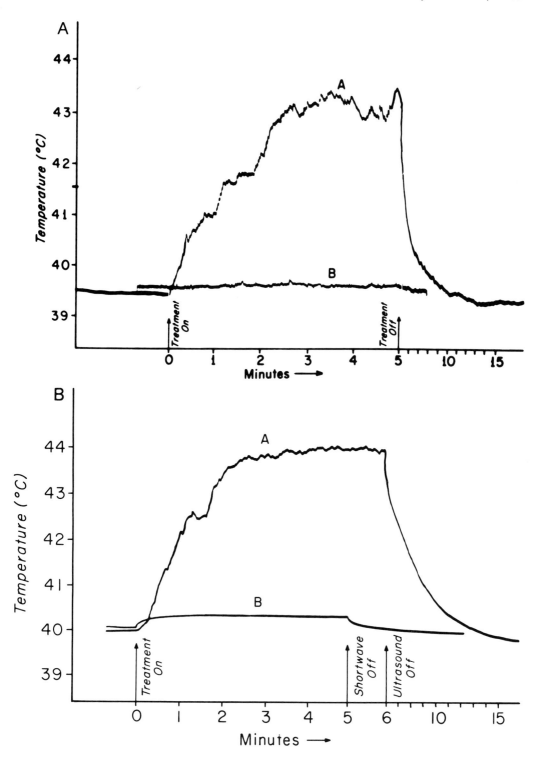

Figure 8.9. (A) Change in temperature inside hip during exposure to "A" (ultrasound) and "B" (microwave). B, change in temperature inside hip joint during exposure to "A" (ultrasound) and "B" (shortwave). (Reproduced with permission from: JF Lehmann *et al.* (17).)

cause of the mismatch of acoustic impedance between the applicator and air. Ultrasound is reflected at interfaces; this contributes to its utility for heating deeply placed structures such as joint capsule. However, nerve may be heated selectively so that care must be taken to avoid inadvertent heating of nerves, although a low intensity application to nerves may be desirable and helpful in pain control in an area supplied by the nerve, or in the case of an amputation neuroma.

Ultrasound is most useful when combined wih a therapeutic exercise program of stretching and active exercises of a contracted joint such as the shoulder or hip. For maximum effectiveness the stretching should be applied with low loads for relatively prolonged periods (20 minutes or more) during the application of the ultrasound or immediately thereafter if it is not possible to stretch during the application. A *typical prescription* for a patient with a flexion contracture of the right hip might be as follows: "Place patient in Thomas position with prolonged low load static stretch to the right hip flexors. Apply ultrasound to the anterior aspect of the hip joint; 2–2.5 watts/cm^2 with stroking technique for 10 minutes."

SUPERFICIAL HEAT

Superficial heat can be applied with a wide variety of techniques and equipment. Virtually all methods of superficial heat application have the same depth penetration, i.e., a few millimeters and, therefore, the modality chosen is due to factors other than penetration. For example, with hydrotherapy, the other factors include buoyancy and cleansing. Figure 8.10 shows a Hubbard tank. The shape

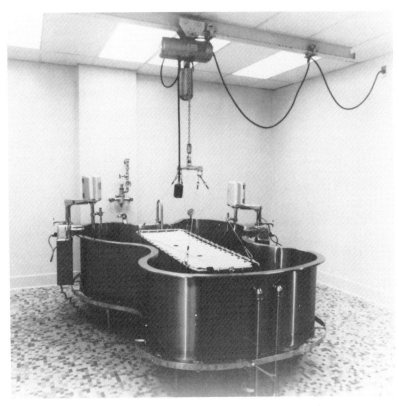

Figure 8.10.   Hubbard tank. (Courtesy of J.A. Preston Corp., 1982.) The patient is supported on the canvas plinth.

of the tank allows the patient to exercise upper and lower extremities in the tank while utilizing a minimum of water and also permitting the therapist access to the patient to assist in range of motion or dressing changes at the point at which the Hubbard tank narrows. Deeper walk-in tanks are available in some facilities. This allows the patient to walk with less stress on the joints and with some support provided from the water, although if the patient is unstable, additional external support from an overhead harness may be needed.

Hydrotherapy is very useful in the management of burns and pressure sores where the cleansing effect is desired. It is also useful in rheumatoid arthritis where many joints are affected and a mild heating effect may be desired. The temperature of various forms of hydrotherapy baths depends on the amount of the body to be heated. For the Hubbard tank, 102° (39°C), would be the upper limit, although the author personnally does not go beyond 100°F (38°C); 105°F (41°C) may be used for the extremities, although if one is treating an ischemic ulcer, the temperature should be kept in a more neutral range of 95° to 98°F (35°–37°C) so that only the cleansing effect of the agitated water is used without additional heating.

Superficial heat is also conveniently applied in the form of hot water bottles, which are inexpensive and readily available. Also available are pads with circulating water which are thermostatically controlled at a safe level; heating pads which (if of good quality) prevent exceeding a safe level; and Hydrocollator® packs which are commercially available and contain a silica gel that retains the heat of the water bath in which the packs are heated to a temperature of 140–160°F (60–71°C). Prevention of burn is assured by applying several layers of terrycloth towels between the Hydrocollator® pack and the skin.

Noncontact dry heat may be applied by various types of heat lamps, either the powerful lamps available in a physical therapy department or by the relatively inexpensive heat lamps (such as the Mazda® lamp) available in most drug and hardware stores. Care should be taken that the patient does not inadvertently obtain a sun lamp which emits ultraviolet radiation when only heat is desired. In addition to the benefit of the heat from infrared lamps, drying may be useful in some stages of pressure sores.

THERAPEUTIC COLD

Application of cold has some things in common with therapeutic heat. Both alleviate pain and muscle spasm, although some patients will have a definite preference for one over the other. Cold is more appropriate in acute processes, particularly in acute inflammatory processes which might be aggravated by the addition of heat. Superficial cold may paradoxically raise the temperature slightly in a deeply placed underlying joint. In acute trauma (such as sprains and strains), application of cold plus compression immediately following the injury may lessen the extent of swelling and hemorrhage. In contrast to heat, cold increases joint stiffness—although many patients with rheumatoid arthritis find relief of the pain and stiffness (1) by alternating heat and cold in the so-called contrast baths.

TRACTION

Traction of the cervical and lumbar spine is used to provide an axial distracting force (2–5). Prolonged low-force traction may be applied with tongs in the distraction and realignment of cervical fractures. In the physical therapy department and, occasionally, in the home, however, shorter-duration relatively high-force traction, often with the patient in a seated position, is applied to the cervical spine to alleviate pressure on nerve roots. It is important that the traction pull the neck toward slight flexion to obtain the desired effect. Flexion alone will increase the vertical diameter of the intervertebral foramina. Traction added to the slightly flexed position will further increase this diameter and alleviate pressure on the nerve roots.

After a series of treatments, the benefit obtained often far outlasts the treatment time. Although the mechanism of this effect is unclear, one hypothesis is that of interstitial fluid returning into the intervertebral discs.

It is also possible to produce demonstrable distraction in the lumbar spine, but special equipment with the application of relatively high forces is required. It is important here that traction be applied to the pelvis and not to the legs, as the latter will increase the lumbar lordosis, an undesired effect in patients with low back pain or an acutely herniated disc. Bed rest with application of 10–30 lbs (4.5–13.3 kg) pelvic traction is simply a form of enforced bed rest with no additional benefit of this low level of traction.

Muscle and Tendon Stretching

Physical therapists are often called upon to stretch tight musculotendinous units or periarticular connective tissue (Fig. 8.11). The rule is to use low loads for long durations, i.e., at least 1 minute and preferably as long as 20 minutes. Ballistic stretch and bouncing stretch should be avoided, since residual length increases will not be produced and damage may occur.

MANIPULATION

Manipulation is a treatment modality for which efficacy has been difficult to confirm scientifically, but which has its advocates, among them many patients who have obtained prompt and long-lasting relief. Theories differ regarding what is actually done by manipulation and how it produces its relief. Perhaps the foremost proponent of manipulation in the United States is John Mennell (19, 20). He theorizes that the most important effect of manipulation as he describes it is restoration of "joint play." By joint play he refers to the nonvoluntary range of motion of a joint. An example of Mennell's manipulations would be long axis extension of the interphalangeal joints of the finger or a distracting force pulling the humerus away from the body in the long axis of the arm (Fig. 8.12). These movements should be short and sharp, not prolonged. These movements are referred to as nonvoluntary, because none of the patient's own muscles can produce them.

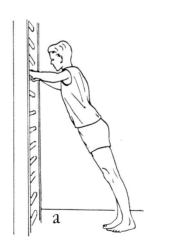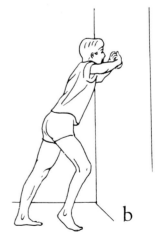

Figure 8.11. Stretching the heel cords (a) bilaterally and (b) one at a time. (Reproduced with permission from: J. Rogoff (ed): *Manipulation, Traction and Massage*, ed 2. Baltimore, Williams & Wilkins.)

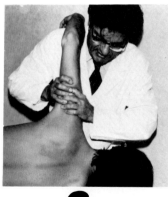

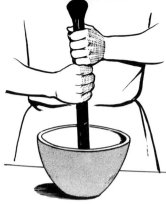

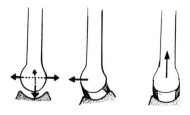

Figure 8.12. Mobilization of the glenohumeral joint is compared to a mortar-and-pestle. (Reproduced with permission from: J. Rogoff (ed): *Manipulation, Traction and Massage,* ed 2. Baltimore, Williams & Wilkins.)

They must be done passively by specially trained therapists or physicians.

THERAPEUTIC EXERCISE

Purposes and Definitions

STRENGTH

Even an apparently simple concept such as "strength" must be defined in view of the various capabilities that muscle has (6). Muscle can shorten actively.

This is called a concentric contraction. Muscle can lengthen actively; this is called an eccentric contraction. Muscle can maintain an overall length against resistance. This is called an isometric or setting contraction. The kinesiologic functions of each of these types of contractions are, respectively, acceleration, deceleration (shock absorption), and stabilization. Strength, then, may be defined either as the maximal force one can exert either concentrically, eccentrically, or isometrically.

The measured values for each of these will differ in any one individual. The highest value will be seen with a fast lengthening contraction; lower values with slow lengthening contractions; lower still with isometric; lower with slow shortening contractions; and the lowest force or tension in the muscle with fast shortening contractions. These are referred to as the classic force-velocity relationships first described by A. V. Hill (13, 14). In addition, owing to length-tension relationships and variations in leverage related to the angle of insertion of the muscle tendon, the torque which a muscle can exert even at a constant velocity of contraction varies throughout the joint range. All of these considerations are important to the question of angle-specific and rate-specific effects of muscle training. Strength is determined by the physiologic cross-sectional area of the muscle plus certain neural or skill elements such as the ability to synchronize.

ENDURANCE

Endurance is defined as the ability to continue a specified task. This can be specified in time or repetitions. Endurance is one factor in work capacity which is a product of force times distance times number of repetitions. Endurance is the converse of fatigue, which may be defined operationally as the inability or unwillingness of the subject to continue the prescribed task.

AEROBIC CAPACITY

This is the maximal ability of the subject to consume oxygen despite increasing performance of external work.

ENDURANCE EXERCISE

This is a term used by exercise physiologists to describe an activity which requires the prolonged and reciprocal use of multiple groups of muscles.

Other Anatomical Aspects

Muscle is under neural control in its anatomic as well as physiologic aspects. Motor units, including the nerve and muscle fibers it innervates, fall into two basic types and follow the size principle as described by Henneman (12). The smaller units described as type I have slow twitch characteristics, are recruited early (at low forces) in a voluntary contraction, fire regularly, exert low tensions, have high oxidative ability, and are fatigue-resistant. Type II units have fast twitch characteristics, are larger, are recruited at high thresholds, fatigue rapidly, fire irregularly, and are low in oxidative ability. There is a subtype of the Type II which has an intermediate fatigue resistance and oxidative ability but retains the fast-twitch characteristics. The twitch characteristics of a motor unit are highly stable and change only with cross innervation. Type I are also referred to as slow oxidative (SO). The two subtypes of the type II are referred to as fast-glycolytic (FG) and fast-oxidative glycolytic (FOG), respectively.

Using histochemical techniques the three types of fibers can be distinguished by staining for myosin ATPase preincubated at pH 9.4 or 10.2. Adjacent serial sections can then be identified, and stained for other metabolic properties such as NADH-diaphorase, reflecting oxidative ability, and phosphofructokinase, reflecting glycolytic ability.

Response to Training

Muscle may respond to training by improvement of skill (neural factor), which generally includes efficiency of contraction (lower metabolic demand for a given task). It may also respond by an increase in strength (increase in physiologic cross-sectional area plus certain neural factors such as the ability to synchronize); and by enhancement of metabolic capability, either the aerobic or the anaerobic capacity or both. Endurance at a given task is related to strength and metabolic capacity, which in turn are related to the metabolic apparatus (such as the cytochrome oxidase system) and the amount of glycogen contained in the muscle. Within rather wide limits of the actual strength of contraction, endurance is mathematically related to strength. These limits may be as wide as 20 to 100% of maximal voluntary contraction (MVC) capacity.

The higher the force of contraction, the more closely is endurance related to strength. As one moves further and further down in force, the more important metabolic capacity becomes. When one gets down to an intensity that may be maintained for 1 to 2 hours or more, the endurance will be limited by the glycogen contained in the muscle, assuming an adequate metabolic apparatus.

What type of exercise produces such training effects? Within wide limits, i.e., between 40 and 100% of MVC (and perhaps as low as 20%), there is a high degree of positive transference from low intensity training to high intensity performance and high intensity training to low intensity performance as long as the subjects go to fatigue in training. However, for extreme quantitative differences as well as for qualitative differences (e.g., isometric vs. isotonic—i.e., static vs. dynamic) in exercise there will be little positive transference, and there is even some evidence, albeit limited, that there may be such a thing as negative transference, i.e., interference. It may be safely said that the best type of training for a given task is that task itself.

Programs and Equipment

A wide variety of programs and equipment exist. Only a few can be mentioned here. Perhaps the most well-known strengthening program is that described by DeLorme (9) and modified by Zinovieff (21). The latter is referred to as the "Oxford" technique. In either of these, the 10-repetition maximum (RM), i.e., the highest weight which can be lifted by the subject 10 times, is determined once per week for each muscle group to be trained. At each treatment session, then, 10 repetitions each are done at 50% of the 10 RM, 75% of the 10 RM, and 100% of the 10 RM. In the DeLorme technique it is done by adding weights; in the Oxford technique it is done by removing weights. Although the Oxford technique is more widely used today, in the author's opinion the DeLorme technique is probably the superior of the two because contracting initially at the lower force provides a warm-up, and working gradually to the higher forces results in fatigue which has a long-term beneficial effect in training.

In addition to strengthening by increasing the load, strengthening may be done by increasing the rate of contraction at a constant weight, as described by Hellebrandt (11). This is referred to as progressive rate training. It is not widely used but has as an advantage the fact that it is relatively economical in time.

Brief isometric exercises have been advocated. Their advantage is that they are very effective and efficient in developing isometric strength. However, because most activities require some dynamic strength and because transferability from isometric to dynamic contractions is limited, training for dynamic tasks should not be confined to isometric exercises.

Two of the newer types of equipment which are available deserve mention. Isokinetic apparatus (e.g., the Cybex II® al-lows one to preset a rate of contraction which cannot be exceeded no matter how hard the subject pushes against the resistance arm (Fig. 8.13). It provides accommodating resistance to the concentric contractions throughout the range of motion and thus, it is suggested, provides rate-specific and angle-specific training. It has a write-out device which gives immediate feedback to the subject regarding his contraction ability. Another set of devices is available in the Nautilus® equipment which, through its nautilus-shaped cam, provides variable concentric and eccentric resistance to approximate the torque curves of the muscle as previously described. Because the resistance varies to match the torque curves, it subjectively feels *uniform* throughout the range and provides uniform muscle training throughout the range.

Rate of Increase and Loss With Immobilization

The most rapid increases of strength with training and the most rapid losses of strength with immobilization occur early in the course, and therefore reported average figures will vary, depending on the length of the training or immobilization. A good average figure for 6 weeks of immobilization is 8% loss per week and for a 6-month training program 5% gain per week. These figures must be taken as a rough rule of thumb only. Both figures will be higher for shorter training programs and shorter immobilization periods.

ELECTRICAL STIMULATION

It is the property of innervated muscle that it is able to respond to short duration stimuli, as can nerve. Denervated muscles can respond to stimuli only of long duration. With a relatively long duration of 300 msec, denervated muscles may be even more sensitive to stimuli, i.e., may respond at a lower intensity in milliamps, than innervated muscles. However, as

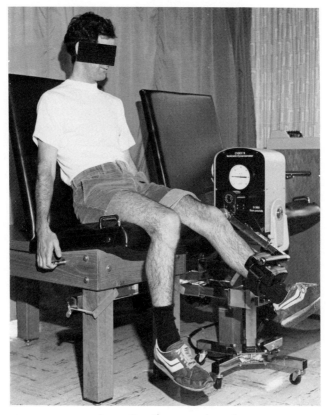

Figure 8.13.   Cybex II® isokinetic strengthening apparatus.

one proceeds to relatively shorter durations the intensity required to produce a contraction becomes for practical purposes "infinite." So-called faradic current is of necessity short duration current; galvanic (direct) current may be of long or short duration. Innervated muscle may be stimulated by either type of current.

Denervated muscle must be stimulated by long duration current; the optimal is said to be direct current made into a slow sinusoidal curve, with the frequency of the sine wave being 1/sec. Innervated muscle might be stimulated, for example, as a re-education technique in someone who has temporarily lost central control, as in stroke patients. Denervated muscle may be stimulated to maintain muscle bulk until expected re-innervation occurs. In order to have any significant effect this stimulation of denervated muscle must be carried out several times a day with multiple contractions each session.

TRANSCUTANEOUS ELECTRICAL NERVE STIMULATION

TNS, or TENS (as it is popularly abbreviated), is now widely applied to many types of pain syndromes, both in acute surgery and medicine and in medical rehabilitation, growing out of theories of pain conduction and modulation in the CNS. Widely divergent techniques of electrode placements, currents and voltages, stimulus frequencies, etc. have been advocated, but consensus has not yet been reached on when and how this therapeutic technique should be used.

MASSAGE

Massage has both reflex and mechanical effects. The most important of the reflex effects include relaxation. The mechanical effects include improvement of circulation and intramuscular movements which may assist in the removal of

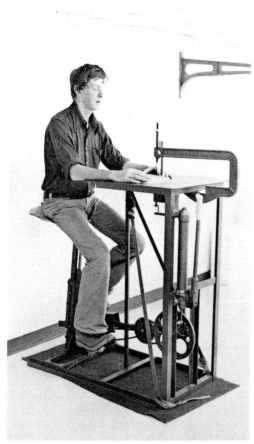

Figure 8.14. Bicycle jigsaw trains muscles, coordination, and endurance. (Reproduced with permission from: CA Trombly and AD Scott: *Occupational Therapy for Physical Therapists*. Baltimore, Williams & Wilkins.)

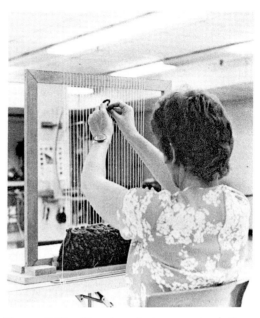

Figure 8.15. Weaving trains manipulative functions in particular, but many other functions are involved. (Reproduced with permission from: CA Trombly and AD Scott: *Occupational Therapy for Physical Therapists*. Baltimore, Williams & Wilkins.)

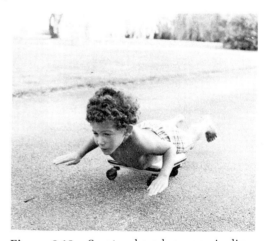

Figure 8.16. Scooter board on an incline. (Reproduced with permission from: CA Trombly and AD Scott: *Occupational Therapy for Physical Therapists*. Baltimore, Williams & Wilkins.)

adhesions. The general types of massage are stroking (effleurage), compression (petrissage), and percussion (tapotement). The subtypes of compression (*i.e.*, kneading, squeezing, and friction) are useful in mobilizing adhesions. Stroking and well done percussion are relaxing. Stroking is also useful in assisting the circulation and must always be done in the direction that will assist the venous circulation, *i.e.*, toward the heart. Massage is contraindicated in infection, malignancy, deep-vein thrombosis, and hemorrhagic diathesis. Massage does not provide muscle strengthening and is not a substitute for active exercise.

OCCUPATIONAL THERAPY

A wide variety of quite specialized procedures are carried out by the occupa-

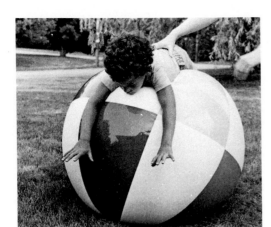

Figure 8.17. Large beach ball elicits equilibrium reactions (Reproduced with permission from: CA Trombly and AD Scott: *Occupational Therapy for Physical Therapists.* Baltimore, Williams & Wilkins.)

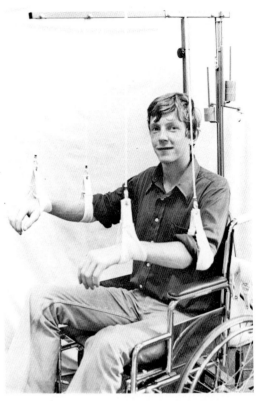

Figure 8.19. The Deltoid Aid® counterbalancing sling permits easier antigravity motions of the weak upper-limb—"progressive assistance exercise." (Reproduced with permission from: CA Trombly and AD Scott: *Occupational Therapy for Physical Therapists.* Baltimore, Williams & Wilkins.)

provide purposeful and pleasant ways of restoring functions in the activities of daily living (Figs. 8.14–8.19).

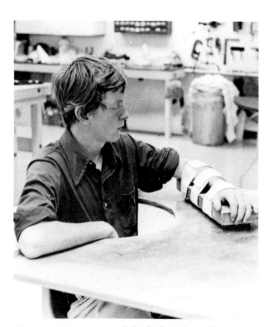

Figure 8.18. A modified skateboard permits easier shoulder and elbow joint movements. (Reproduced with permission from: CA Trombly and AD Scott. *Occupational Therapy for Physical Therapists.* Baltimore, Williams & Wilkins.)

tional therapist members of the rehabilitation team to accelerate the recovery of mobility in both neuromuscular and musculoskeletal problems. The basic aim is to

References

1. Backlund L, Tiselius P: Objective measurement of joint stiffness in rheumatoid arthritis. *Acta Rheum Scand* 13:275–288, 1967.
2. Colachis SC Jr, Strohm BR: A study of tractive forces and angle of pull on vertebral interspaces in the cervical spine. *Arch Phys Med Rehabil* 46:820–830, 1965.
3. Colachis SC Jr, Strohm BR: Cervical traction: relationship of traction time to varied tractive force with constant angle of pull. *Arch Phys Med Rehabil* 46:815–819, 1965.
4. Colachis SC Jr, Strohm BR: Effect of duration of intermittent cervical traction on vertebral separation. *Arch Phys Med Rehabil* 47:353–359, 1966.

5. Colachis SC Jr, Strohm BR: Radiographic studies of cervical spine motion in normal subjects: flexion and hyperextension. *Arch Phys Med Rehabil* 46:753–760, 1965.

6. de Lateur BJ: Exercise for strength and endurance. In Basmajian JV: *Therapeutic Exercise.* ed 3, chap 3. Baltimore, Williams & Wilkins, 1978, pp 85–92.

7. de Lateur BJ: The role of physical medicine in problems of pain. *Adv Neurol* 4:495–497, 1974.

8. de Lateur BJ, Lehmann JF, Stonebridge JB, Warren CG, Guy AW: Muscle heating in human subjects with 915 MHz microwave contact applicator. *Arch Phys Med Rehabil* 51:147–151, 1970.

9. DeLorme TL: Restoration of muscle power by heavy resistance exercises. *J Bone Joint Surg* 27:645–667, 1945.

10. Federal Communications Commission: *Rules and Regulations*, vol 2, subpart A, section 18.13. Washington, D.C., US Government Printing Office, 1964.

11. Hellebrandt FA, Houtz SJ: Methods of muscle training: the influence of pacing. *Phys Ther Rev* 38:319–322, 1958.

12. Henneman E: Peripheral mechanisms involved in the control of muscle. In Mountcastle VB: *Medical Physiology*, ed 13. St. Louis, CV Mosby, 1974.

13. Hill AV: Dynamic constants of human muscle. *Proc R Soc (Lond) Ser B* 128:263–274, 1940.

14. Hill AV: The heat of shortening and dynamic constants of muscle. *Proc Roy Soc (Lond)* 126:136–195, 1938.

15. Lehmann JF (ed): *Therapeutic Heat and Cold*, ed 3. Baltimore, Williams & Wilkins, 1982.

16. Lehmann JF, de Lateur BJ: Diathermy, superficial heat and cold therapy. In Kottke FJ, Lehmann JF (eds): *Handbook of Physical Medicine and Rehabilitation*, ed 3, 1983.

17. Lehmann JF, McMillan JA, Brunner GD, Blumberg JB: Comparative study of the efficiency of shortwave, microwave and ultrasonic diathermy in heating the hip joint. *Arch Phys Med Rehabil* 40:510–512, 1959.

18. Lehmann JF, Guy AW, Johnston VC, Brunner GD, Bell JW: Comparison of relative heating patterns produced in tissues by exposure to microwave energy at frequencies of 2450 and 900 megacycles. *Arch Phys Med Rehabil* 43:69–76, 1962.

19. Mennell JM: *Back Pain*. Boston, Little, Brown, 1960.

20. Mennell JM: *Joint Pain*. Boston, Little, Brown, 1964.

21. Zinovieff AN: Heavy-resistance exercises; the "Oxford technique." *Br J Phys Med* 14:129–132, 1951.

CHAPTER NINE

Rehabilitation Management and the Rehabilitation Team

T. P. Anderson

A recent survey (13) showed that many medical students who choose Physical Medicine and Rehabilitation (PM&R) as a specialty do so because of special attributes of its style of patient management, namely, the humanistic approach to the patient, the regard for the whole patient (holistic health care), and the team approach. One of the aims of this chapter will be to delineate how and why PM&R has earned this reputation.

The editors deliberately chose the wording "Rehabilitation Management" for this chapter, rather than "Rehabilitation Treatment." The term "treatment" implies activities directed toward the disease whereas the term "management" is much broader in scope. It involves the whole patient, along with his or her nonmedical problems as well as the medical ones. "Physical medicine" deals more with assessment and treatment of disease or impairment; however, rehabilitation is concerned with the control or reversal of the consequent disability and handicap in the performance of daily living (14). Perhaps the French word, "readaptation," better conveys what happens to the patient as a result of rehabilitation (1).

FRAME OF REFERENCE

In order to better understand rehabilitation management, it is helpful to con-sider its frame of reference, as contrasted with those of the more traditional medical-surgical aspects with which most readers are familiar (Table 9.1) (adapted from a conceptual framework by Halstead and Halstead (9)). The objective of both traditional medicine-surgery and rehabilitation is diagnosis and treatment, but the latter also deals with the patient's ability to perform a variety of functions and to readapt. Halstead and Halstead (9) stated: "Although a person in any specialty in the health professions can practice a blend of humanistic and scientific medicine, rehabilitation as a field is uniquely suited to achieving this balance. From its inception, the philosophy of rehabilitation has been strongly oriented toward the humanistic approach while developing an ever expanding scientific base."

Rehabilitation uses a problem-oriented approach to the entire patient, particularly the patient's ability to perform activities of daily living (Fig. 9.1). Emphasis is on helping the patient become as independent as possible, and achieving with the patient and family an optimal level of health and quality of life.

The focus of traditional management is on immediate problem(s), which is also true of rehabilitation, but also included in rehabilitation are a problem-oriented approach to the entire patient (true holistic

Table 9.1
Management Frames of Reference (1, 9)[a]

Element of Health Care	Traditional	Rehabilitation
1. Orientation	Disease	Patient
2. Objective	Diagnosis and treatment	Diagnosis and treatment plus patient's ability to perform and readapt
3. Scientific vs. humanistic	Scientific medicine tends to predominate.	Conscious attempt to maintain balance between scientific and humanistic medicine
4. Focus	Immediate problems	Immediate problems plus wider issues including: Problem-oriented approach to whole patient; Ability to perform; Potential for independence; Patient and family education; Quality of life
5. Approach	Empirical; Rational; Quantitative	Empirical and subjective; Rational and intuitive; Quantitative and qualitative
6. Role of patient	Passive; Little responsibility; Inconsistently compliant	Active; Trained to become responsible; More consistent in compliance
7. Evaluation, planning, delegation, and review	Physician	Physician with team
8. Role of Physician	Active, knowing, directive	Learner, evaluator, educator, trainer, advisor, counselor, encourager, enabler in problem solving, coordinator of team approach
9. Physician's relationship to:		
Patient	Episodic; Reserved; Cautious involvement	Continuing; Personal; Involved
Health team	Directive, dominant, authoritarian	Facilitative, coordinative
Other physicians	Competitive	Collaborative
Patient's disability	"All or none"	Balance between disability and residual ability
10. Education of patient and family:		
Process	By chance and/or by nursing	Planned, organized, and presented by rehab team
Materials	Presentation fulfills the educational function	Interaction and evaluation
11. Evaluation	None, or possibly peer	Management outcome assessed at discharge and follow-up
12. Setting	Isolated individual rooms	Therapeutic community of patients with similar problems learning from one another
13. Psychosocial-vocational (PSV) factors	Concern about PSV effects on disease process	Concern about disease process's effect on patient's quality of life
14. Problem-solving	Physician takes responsibility	Responsibility shared with, and gradually shifted to, the patient

[a] Note: Readers will recognize that extremes on the spectrum between traditional and rehabilitation approaches are presented and that the more desirable dimensions are achievable by all physicians, regardless of their special interests.

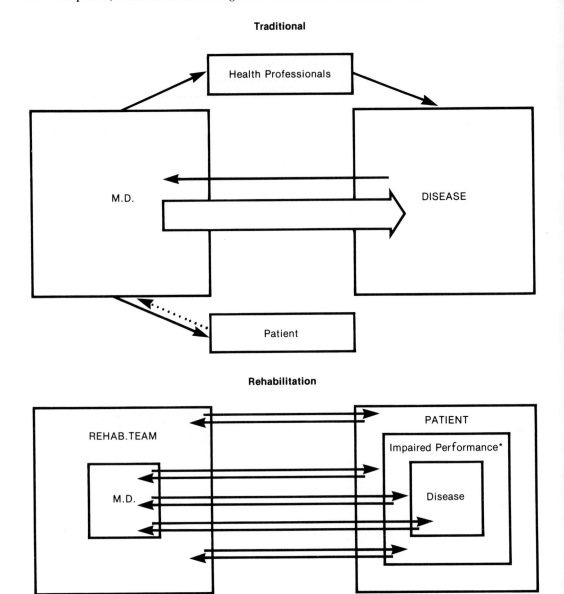

* Impaired physical, physiologic, and psychologic performance in readapting.

Figure 9.1.   Relationships: traditional compared to the rehabilitation approach.

health care), the patient's ability to perform common functions such as activities of daily living (Fig. 9.1), the potential for the patient again becoming as independent as possible, the education of the patient and family in understanding the patient's condition and learning the optimal way of maintaining as high a level of health as possible, and the patient's qual-ity of life. While the traditional approach is empirical, rational, and quantitative, the rehabilitation approach in addition is subjective, intuitive, and qualitative, with concern for the patient's quality of life.

Many in medicine and surgery feel that the timing for beginning rehabilitation is after the acute care is completed, whereas in rehabilitation management it is believed these principles should be instituted early in the acute phase in order to avoid potential but preventable complications. Traditional services are organized so that the physician writes orders for the involved allied health professionals to carry out, whereas in rehabilitation the rehabilitation team (which is coordinated by the physician) actively assists in the evaluation and formulation of plans for many of the patient's problems.

Other features which distinguish the rehabilitation team are that it includes the patient and the family (6) and it sets goals of management. Traditionally, the role of patients is to remain passive. Rehabilitation patients are urged to become more and more active and are trained to become responsible and hence tend to have more consistency in their compliance to recommendations. The physician in rehabilitation management is a fellow-learner, reports evaluations to the patient, serves as an educator and trainer, advises the patient on courses of action, serves as a counselor and encourager and in problem solving is an enabler to the patient. In all of this, the physician is helping to serve as a coordinator of the team approach.

A consideration of the physician's relationships provides interesting contrasts. In his relationship to the patient, traditionally it is episodic, while in rehabilitation it is continuing, personal, and not fearful of becoming involved. Traditionally, physicians appear dominant, directive, and competitive, but those in rehabilitation tend to be collaborative. This may be due in part to the fact that most of the patients on rehabilitation wards are referred from other services.

The attitudes toward the patient's disability are different. Traditionally the patient is viewed as being able or disabled—an all-or-none situation, but in rehabilitation the concept of partial disability prevails, with the emphasis on minimizing the effects of the patient's disease.

Traditionally, education of the patient and the family, if it occurs, is by chance or performed only by nurses; in rehabilitation (3), it is planned, organized, and presented by the full rehabilitation team. The topics covered in traditional education are usually only the current disease process; in rehabilitation the patient is taught avoidance of potential problems by enlightened self-care. Educational materials such as printed handouts, videotapes, and motion pictures are used in both frames of reference, not just the educational function. In rehabilitation the presentation of the materials is followed by discussions to see if the patient and the family truly understand what was presented. Often, there are required classes held, and then the patient, before graduating from rehabilitation training, is required to perform both written and practical tests, and actual outcomes that were affected by the rehabilitation are assessed at follow-up as well as at discharge.

It seems optimal to have pateints in private or semiprivate rooms in medicine and surgery, but this is not true in rehabilitation; there, patients with similar problems are placed in 4- or 6-bed wards on a special rehabilitation station so that a therapeutic community is promoted for the patients to learn from each other. Although it is true that more and more people in traditional medicine and surgery are giving attention to psychological, social, and vocational aspects of the patient, usually only the effects that these have on the disease process are considered; in rehabilitation, consideration is given to the effect of these on the patient's entire quality of life.

For some of the psychological and social problems of the patient, a behavioral type of approach is taken by the rehabilitation team. This is particularly true if various therapies have delineated frequently and easily attained goals so that the patient can see that he can become less dependent on others through further rehabilitation training. The pharmacologic approach is often not necessary in rehabilitation management of depression and is utilized only when counseling and patient achievement have not been effective.

The approach to problem solving provides interesting contrasts also. In rehabilitation (2) this responsibility is shared with and then gradually shifted to the patient as he is trained and helped to grow in taking on the responsibility of his own problem solving.

THE REHABILITATION TEAM

Team Concepts

Over the past two decades there has been an increasing emphasis on the team approach to health care. Rothberg (12) believes this emphasis on the team concept "arose from a need to deal with the increasingly complicated delivery of health services that resulted from the knowledge explosion in the basic sciences and medical technology." She has pointed out that, as time passed, each new specialty group narrowed its focus, increased its depth of knowledge, and became more expert regarding a smaller portion of the patient's problems, needs, and life-styles. The frequent result was little communication among the several types of professional and even less coherent communication with the patient. Hence, the team concept of health care delivery evolved as a compromise between the benefits of specialization and the need for continuity and comprehensive integrated care. The team approach was considered a solution by which evaluation, management, and care could be provided to a patient in a coordinated nonfragmented way by specialists representing several disciplines.

Rehabilitation Team Characteristics

The health care team in rehabilitation is composed of two or more representatives of disciplines involved in the patient's evaluation, management, and training. Flexibility is one of its most significant characteristics. Its flexible membership depends on the particular needs

and problems of the individual patient and family.

All health teams are multidisciplinary in composition, but rehabilitation teams pride themselves on being truly interdisciplinary in function. Melvin (11) has pointed out that the multidisciplinary team involves the efforts of individuals from a number of different disciplines. Their efforts are discipline oriented, and although they may impinge upon clients or activities dealt with by other disciplines, they approach them primarily through each discipline relating to its own activities. Through their efforts the results represent, at best, the sum of each discipline's unique achievements.

In contrast, in an interdisciplinary team the activities of individuals from different disciplines are complementary and symbiotic and are directed toward shared goals. This requires group interaction skills and the knowledge of how to translate integrated group activities into a result which is greater than the simple sum of individual accomplishments. They share the responsibility for the group activity.

Each team member needs to have knowledge regarding the general principles, and specific technical awareness, of the activities of the others.

Many rehabilitation teams aspire to the ideal of interaction stated by Given and Simmons (7): "Patient care should be approached by team members on the basis of joint problem formulation, data collection, problem evaluation, goal setting, problem solution, outcome prediction, and determination of activities to achieve this outcome. ... Collaborators must have strong common values, confidence, and trust in each other's abilities and certainty about members' interest in contributing to the common goal."

Although the team approach has demonstrated broad achievements, research on its efficacy is also in progress (4, 5). A critical review by Halstead (8) of the literature of the past 25 years on the rehabilitation team revealed 10 studies which were not just descriptive or anecdotal but actually tried to compare results with control groups. Six studies concluded that coordinated, comprehensive care was more effective; in two studies, more effective in some areas but not in others; and in two studies, no more effective than care provided in the control groups. Hence, of the 10 studies (most of which used serious research efforts to investigate the effectiveness of team care in various settings) the majority demonstrated better outcomes in one or more areas for patients receiving coordinated team care, when compared to control groups.

Task-oriented patient care favors the learning of team skills, especially when all levels of administration support and participate in the processes (10). Interdisciplinary team training for students seems most timely during the clinical phase of their education as students appear to be unable to participate effectively as team members until they have learned the basic skills of their own disciplines.

MEMBERS OF THE REHABILITATION TEAM

Roles of the various members of the rehabilitation team often overlap and vary somewhat from patient to patient. Variations are also found among institutions.

Patients and Family

Becker et al. (6) have made the following observations regarding written goal setting by the rehabilitation team (including patient and family) for severely disabled patients: early identification of conflicts among any combinations of patient-staff-family goals; truly individualizing treatment programs; enhancing family-patient-staff interaction through negotiation and the setting of treatment priorities; including the patient and his family as active and responsible team members; teaching the staff how to achieve longer-

lasting rehabilitation goals through intermediate and compromise goals; and reducing sabbotage of treatment goals by the patient or family.

Physician

The role of the physician (family physician or specialist) on the rehabilitation team has been adequately described elsewhere in this chapter. Not all teams will include all the persons named below, nor are they all needed together. However, their inputs can help to change the handicapped person's life.

Rehabilitation Nursing

In addition to the usual nursing responsibilities, the rehabilitation nurse works with the team to aid the patient in the transition from being sick and hospitalized to being well and disabled, toward attaining maximal independence. The nurse is often called the "general practitioner of rehabilitation," helping the patient apply during everyday activities on the ward what has been learned in various therapies. More independent functions of rehabilitation nursing are the management, treatment, and education of patient and family in programs for care of bowel, bladder, and skin.

Psychologist

Psychologists explore their client's history for vocationally significant facts and add data from tests, inventories, and work evaluation to this information. They integrate all information with medical prognoses to help clients select appropriate goals. With the psychologist's support, most clients arrive at a more optimum level of adjustment than without this counseling effort. The psychologist may also guide rehabilitation teams in behavior modification programs.

Social Service

The social worker counsels individual patients and families centering around coping, adjustment, and future planning and may focus on family, marital, or parent-child relationships; patient or family adjustment to disability; social skills development training; sex education; or sexual adjustment. The social worker is the liaison person with community agencies such as welfare departments, public health nursing, schools, and nursing homes—often using these resources in doing discharge planning. Social workers also discuss and help with finances, arranging transportation, helping with equipment, and initiating and coordinating both post-discharge arrangements and family conferences.

Occupational Therapy

The occupational therapist is concerned with the total life role of the individual, including the ability to function at work, at play, at school, or in the community. OT goals include the remediation of physical and emotional deficits, minimizing the disabling effects of a handicap, and the development of attitudes and skills basic to the pursuit of independent functioning. Through participation in an activity, an individual explores his or her interests, needs, capacities, and limitations, and then develops skills and learns the range of interpersonal and social attitudes and behaviors.

Physical Therapy

The physical therapist focuses primarily on the neuromusculoskeletal, pulmory, and cardiovascular systems, assisting in evaluating the functions of these systems; and on the selection and application of appropriate therapeutic procedures to maintain, improve, or restore these functions. Assessments are made of muscle strength, motor development, functional capacity, or respiratory efficiency. Therapeutic procedures include exercises for increasing strength, endurance, coordination, or range of motion; stimulation to facilitate motor activity

and learning; and instruction in activities of daily living.

Speech Pathology

The speech pathologist on the rehabilitation team determines the nature and significance of communication disorders, and what kinds of treatments, if any, are appropriate. These might include: impaired hearing, language comprehension, or expression deficits (either developmental or as a result of brain injury), articulation disorders, voice disorders, problems of fluency, and difficulties related to oral functioning. The speech pathologist also guides the team on how to communicate with the patient.

Vocational Counselor

In general, the vocational counselor is responsible for initiating and directing the evaluation, planning, and treatment procedures that relate to the patient's vocational functioning. The counselor is responsible for knowing what vocational services are available in the community, for referring patients to appropriate vocational agencies after discharge from the hospital, and for maintaining liaison with these agencies. The counselor is also usually the only member of the rehabilitation team who has any responsibility for job placement.

Work Evaluation

Clients are referred to Work Evaluation to determine their eligibility and/or readiness for vocational training or employment, their eligibility to meet referral resource requirements, and whether their level of employability is competitive, sheltered, or work activity. Clients are given actual job samples, and based on the client's interests, behavior, and test results, recommendations are made to the appropriate agency. Some work evaluation units are a source of information for handicapped driving controls, lifts, ramps, and other assistive devices and equipment.

Recreational Therapy

Through the utilization of play and social interaction in purposeful and leisure time activities, the recreational therapist guides the disabled, the aged, or the retarded individual toward self-help in achieving the fullest physical, mental, social, and economic life possible, individually and in the family or community. The staff helps the person in returning to the community by structuring activities involving him in the community, such as outings to shopping centers and sports activities out of the hospital. In recreational therapy, a person can test out in a supporting group experience the skills learned in other therapy areas.

Dietician

The dietician assists in the evaluation of the patient's nutritional status, in the development of modified diets or feeding patterns, and in the necessary education of the patient and family to ensure compliance with recommendations.

Prosthetist and Orthotist

The roles of the prosthetist and orthotist are elaborated in earlier chapters.

Conclusion

Medical rehabilitation of the disabled or handicapped person presents many nonmedical as well as medical problems. During the various periods of recovery and return to a full life, the patient (and family) require experts and teams of experts to help.

References

1. American Medical Association Criteria Development Project. Sample Criteria for Short-Stay Hospital Review. Chicago, American Medical Association, 1976.
2. Anderson TP: An alternate frame of reference for rehabilitation: the helping process versus the medical model. Arch Phys Med Rehabil 56:101–104, 1975.
3. Anderson TP: Educational frame of reference: an additional model for rehabilitation medicine. Arch Phys Med Rehabil 59:203–206, 1978.
4. Anderson TP et al: Stroke rehabilitation: evaluation of quality of assessing patient outcomes. Arch Phys Med Rehabil 59:170–175, 1978.
5. Anderson TP, Baldridge M, Ettinger MG: Quality of care for completed stroke without rehabilitation: evaluation by assessing patient outcomes. Arch Phys Med Rehabil 60:103–107, 1979.
6. Becker MC, Abrams KS, Onder J: Goal setting: a joint patient-staff method. Arch Phys Med Rehabil 55:87–89, 1974.
7. Given B, Simmons S: Interdisciplinary health care team: fact or fiction? Nurs Forum 15:166–184, 1977.
8. Halstead LS: Team care in chronic illness: a critical review of the literature of the past 25 years. Arch Phys Med Rehabil 57:507–511, 1976.
9. Halstead LS, Halstead MD: Chronic illness and humanism: rehabilitation as a model for teaching humanistic and scientific health care. Arch Phys Med Rehabil 59:53–57, 1978.
10. Masur H, Beeston JJ, Yerxa EJ: Clinical interdisciplinary health care: an educational experiment. J Med Educ 54:703–713, 1979.
11. Melvin JL: Interdisciplinary and multidisciplinary activities and the ACRM. Arch Phys Med Rehabil 61:379–380, 1980.
12. Rothberg JS: The rehabilitation team: future direction (abstr). Arch Phys Med Rehabil 62:407–410, 1981.
13. Scheer S: Rehabilitation medicine as a specialty choice: qualities which recruit residents (abstr). Arch Phys Med Rehabil 62:533, 1981.
14. Spencer WA: Changes in methods and relationships necessary within rehabilitation. Arch Phys Med Rehabil 50:566–580, 1969.

PART THREE

Rehabilitation Problems

CHAPTER TEN

Neurological Problems

Neurological Weakness

D. D. MURRAY

Many problems of the neurologically impaired patient require attention from all members of the health-related professions. The eight subchapters of Chapter 10 (of which this is the first) review the most significant ones that the student must be familiar with before graduation.

For this section, neurological weakness may be defined as that weakness of muscle which results from interference with upper or lower motor neuronal control. This is distinct from muscle weakness due to myopathies (e.g., those associated with metabolic disease or endocrine disorders), familial dystrophies, disuse, or aging, and from weakness due to disorders of the neuromuscular junction (e.g., myasthenia gravis).

Muscle weakness of neurological origin can have its etiology either centrally (motor cortex, motor pathways, brainstem, spinal cord, and conus medullaris) or peripherally (cauda equina, roots, and peripheral nerves). There is a broad clinical spectrum of the presentation of neurological weakness. With upper motor neuron weakness, probably the most common presentation is that of weakness, with increased tone, hyperreflexia, and resultant poor fine motor control. At the other end of the spectrum is the patient with spasticity and either no voluntary function, or movement only in synergy patterns without the ability to isolate single movements. The initial weakness in stroke may be flaccid and hypotonic, even though spasticity may (or may not) develop with time.

Lesions of the cauda equina or nerve root present classically as a lower motor neuron picture with weakness, wasting, hypotonicity, and areflexia. Such a lesion with Wallerian degeneration shows clinical evidence of denervation with fasciculations and atrophy. Secondarily, deformities resulting from muscle imbalance in the involved limbs may be seen.

The extent of weakness can be reduced by a specific exercise program, and the effects of the weakness can be minimized by orthotic assistance or aids.

MUSCLE TONE AND SPASTICITY

Muscle tone is involuntary in origin and is reflexly maintained and adjusted. Stretching a muscle stimulates the muscle spindles and thereby adjusts the sensitivity of the primary endings appropriate to the new muscle lengths. Muscle spindles lie in parallel with extrafusal fibers and thus are influenced by changes in muscle length. Within the spindle are small intrafusal muscle fibers which are innervated by the axons of small γ motor neurons of the γ anterior horn cells. These fibers actually sensitize the stretch reflex arc and, thus, the gamma efferent system becomes important in the regulation of muscle tone (Fig. 10.1). Besides the system of setting or detecting length changes in extrafusal muscle fibers, there is also a protective reflex which damps muscle contraction following excessive stretch and is mediated by the Golgi tendon organs.

Internuncial neurons are present diffusely in the anterior horn of the spinal cord. The interconnections between these cells, and the anterior motor neurons are responsible for many integrative functions of the cord. Incoming sensory signals can be modified, as can outgoing motor responses. Thus, the γ-loop (α-γ linkage) refers to the reflex system which registers disparity between the intra- and extrafusal systems and acts to reduce this difference. Supraspinal controls may facilitate or inhibit this γ system.

In lesions interrupting the pyramidal tracts, besides weakness and paralysis, there is an increase in muscle tone due to loss of supraspinal damping of the γ efferent system. Clinically, this causes muscle spasticity and is thought of as a lack of suprasegmental inhibition or a release phenomenon. Such spasticity can be influenced by a number of medications, although in many patients spasticity is either not a limiting factor, or its positive effects (e.g., on bone mass and on improving some forms of transfers by the patient) outweigh its disadvantages. Dantrolene acts directly on the contractile mechanism without action on the reflex pathways. Its mechanism of action is to reduce the depolarization-induced calcium efflux into the sacroplasm. Baclofen (Lioresal®) seems to have a site of action at the spinal cord level and to work best in the paraplegic or quadriplegic patient. Diazepam, a benzodiazepine, enhances or potentiates the postsynaptic effects of γ-aminobutyric acid (13). Problematic spasticity also may be managed by nerve blocks or neurolytic surgery (e.g., Bischoff's frontal myelotomy or radiofrequency rhizotomy). The long-term effects of these procedures tend to be disappointing.

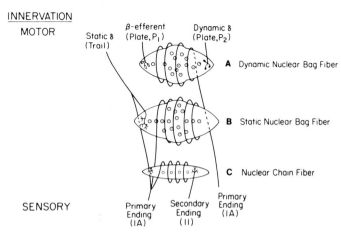

Figure 10.1. Alpha-gamma (α-γ) linkage. The group II and Ia afferents are sensory from the nuclear bag and chain of the muscle spindle. They connect to the fusimotor nerves (γ) and to the extrafusal fibers to complete the cord level reflex arc. The supraspinal centers descend the cord to connect to the (γ) motor neurones to innervate the spindle. (Reproduced with permission from JV Basmajian (ed): *Therapeutic Exercise, ed 4.* Baltimore, Williams & Wilkins.)

HEMIPLEGIA

This term refers to the clinical picture of upper motor neuron paralysis or paresis of the hemibody with increased tendon reflexes, spasticity, and an extensor plantar response. Strokes from occluded cerebral blood flow are the most common; infarction in the territory of the middle cerebral artery is a common cause. The deficit occurs on the side opposite the lesion (Fig. 10.2), and in addition to paralysis of the hemibody, sensory changes and visual field defects often occur. Spatial disorientation and neglect often complicate the rehabilitation of the left hemiplegic patient. Speech may be involved (see *Aphasia*, later in this chapter). Occasionally, a patient will not recover from the initial flaccid stage and is spoken of as having a flaccid stroke.

The weakness due to middle cerebral artery occlusion is characteristic. Usually, after a week or two, tone returns to both upper and lower limbs, but more function returns to the lower limb. The leg recovers more function because of a different (anterior *vs.* middle cerebral) blood supply and possibly because of its larger musculature and cruder function.

Upper Limb

Proximally in the arm, patients often retain shoulder shrug. They may retain elbow flexion and hand closure "in pattern," which essentially means a mass action which incorporates the motion of elbow flexion, hand closure, and adduction of the arm, as well as some internal rotation. If hand closure can be isolated from this pattern, it is clumsy with loss of fine motor control such as individual finger motion or use of the intrinsic hand musculature. Opening the hand and extending the wrist and elbow all require adequate neurological recovery to isolate these extensor movements. The arm is usually carried in the typical posture of shoulder adduction, flexion, and internal rotation, with the elbow semiflexed and the wrist in flexion and pronation.

Lower Limb

In the leg the proximal groups recover tone and function first and usually best. Good knee control without recurvatum usually requires training. Dorsiflexion weakness gives a foot drop gait, plantarflexor spasticity results in equinovarus during the swing phase of gait, and difficult flexion of the hip and knee requires circumduction for toe clearance. A patient is often unable to dorsiflex as an isolated movement, but in concert with hip and knee flexion in synergy pattern, is able to do so, even against resistance. In the lower limb the presence of extensor spasticity with weakness in the leg can be useful. In the absence of adequate voluntary contractions, some hemiplegics can use spasticity in the leg extensors to stand, transfer, and walk (usually with auxiliary aids).

Muscle Testing (Stages)

Muscle testing for power grading in the hemiplegic is not the same as with the lower motor neuron lesion or other causes of muscle weakness. Perhaps the most widely known classification is that of Brunnstrom (4), which is based on motor recovery. *Stage 1* is the postinsult period of flaccidity. As spasticity appears with some primitive limb synergies or patterns, *Stage 2* is reached. With recovery of some voluntary control over movement patterns and increase of spasticity, *Stage 3* is present. *Stage 4* recognizes the patient's ability to isolate movements from patterns. Often, there is a decrease in spasticity. More sophisticated movement, isolation, and combinations of movements mark *Stage 5*.

Treatment Principles in Hemiplegia

The treatment program can begin as soon as the patient is medically stable. The aims are to encourage neurological recovery by control of cerebral edema and arterial hypertension, as well as to augment any remaining strength. In the flaccid stage, support and the maintenance of

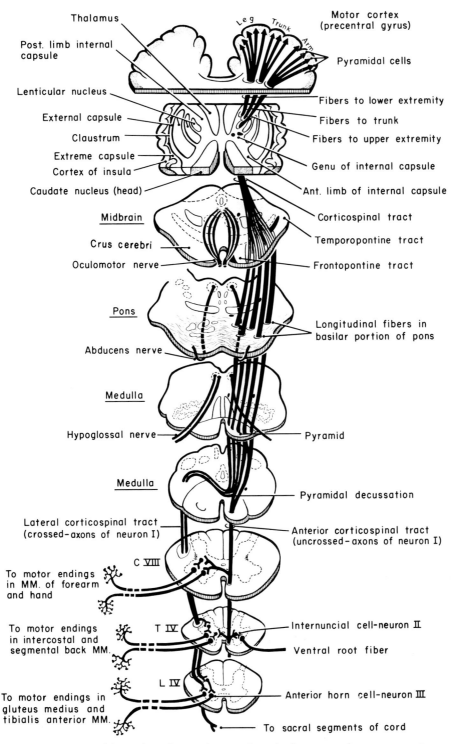

Figure 10.2.   Diagram of lateral and anterior corticospinal tracts—the upper motor neuron pathways to the anterior horn cells. (Reproduced with permission from RC Truex and MB Carpenter: *Strong and Elwyn's Human Neuroanatomy.* Baltimore, Williams & Wilkins.)

range of motion prevents contracture and, especially in the upper limb, prevents subluxation or a painful restricted shoulder.

With the return of tone, the program shifts its emphasis towards the restoration of function, including power and active range. Several treatment programs apply such principles as reflex inhibition of unwanted patterns or proprioceptive neuromuscular facilitation techniques. These put the patient in positions and postures which discourage certain patterns and thus allow the emergence of more isolated voluntary movements (3, 7).

A painful shoulder is best dealt with by the use of heat, support, and a gradual restoration of range of motion. Spasticity is dealt with by both the exercise program and various medications. Residual weakness can be augmented by bracing or external assistive devices such as a cane to improve locomotion. The overall aims of therapy are to make the patient independent for the activities of daily living and to help the patient and family to deal with the psychosocial impact of such a catastrophic event.

Implications for Functional Independence

The expectations for the patient with a stroke include major recovery and function in the leg; in the arm and hand recovery is usually rudimentary. The shoulder in the hemiplegic often becomes restricted in range but remains functional and free of pain. Subluxations in the flaccid upper limb remain a problem for which supportive orthoses are often used (including variations on the theme of sling). Most times, the patient wisely discards such devices as the shoulder settles into its final level of function or range.

As the leg progresses from Stage 3 to 5, the observer can begin to estimate whether ambulation will be possible and whether aids will be necessary. Often, the spastic gait pattern allows enough foot clearance in the swing phase to obviate the need for an ankle-foot orthosis (AFO)

for mediolateral support, dorsiflexion assistance, or prevention of plantarflexion. A cane on the sound side may act as both an outrigger for balance and an adjunct to weak hip abductors, often imparting a sense of confidence to the patient.

Prognosis

As far as prognosis is concerned, figures vary, but from 42 to 90% of patients regain independent self-care and unaided ambulation following hemiplegia. These figures depend on the selection process for rehabilitation, as well as on the severity of the stroke. We can expect some 65% of patients to be restored to independent activities of daily living and ambulation and, perhaps, 25% of these to be able to return to work (1, 10). Negative predictive factors include a prolonged period of unconsciousness, disorientation, aphasia, and perceptual problems. Incontinence of bladder and bowel is also a poor prognostic sign. Rehabilitation programs are able to achieve significant gains that could not otherwise be accounted for on the basis of spontaneous recovery alone (2, 8, 9).

PARAPLEGIA

This term refers to a paralysis which affects the lower limbs, with sensory loss and neurogenic bladder and bowel. The usual cause is trauma, although other etiologies include inflammatory processes, vascular lesions, and compressive lesions from central disc extrusion or neoplasm.

Lesions between T_2 and L_1 produce a picture of spastic paralysis which may involve chest, trunk, and leg musculature, as well as impaired sensation and impaired bladder and bowel function.

The spinal cord ends at the conus medullaris at the L1-L2 bony vertebral level. At this vertebral level conus medullaris syndrome is produced with injuries to the S2-S3-S4 roots (Fig. 10.3). Clinically, this syndrome is characterized by paralytic incontinence, bladder distention, impotence, and saddle anesthesia with normal

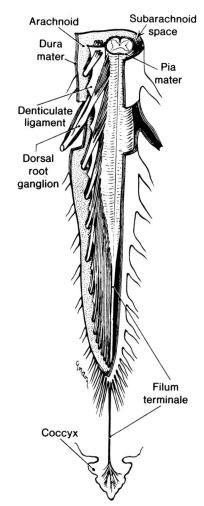

Arachnoid

Subarachnoid space

Dura mater

Pia mater

Denticulate ligament

Dorsal root ganglion

Filum terminale

Coccyx

Figure 10.3. Spinal cord ends as conus medullaris, below which the filum terminale and lower spinal nerve roots make up the cauda equina. (Reproduced with permission from: JV Basmajian: *Primary Anatomy*, ed 8, Baltimore, Williams & Wilkins.)

sensory and motor function of the lower limbs (11).

Below the conus is the cauda equina which, when injured, produces lower motor neuron lesions with sensory and motor involvement in the legs and a neurogenic bladder and bowel. In patients with incomplete lesions, weakened lower motor neuron muscles can be retrained, and by hypertrophy of the remaining functioning motor units, often progress to useful power for ambulation. The story for the flaccid bladder and sexual function in

these cases is much less heartening. With partial injuries to the cauda equina, because it is the beginning of a peripheral nerve, there is the possibility of some proximal muscle recovery with regeneration of the axon. Lower motor neuron wasting and lack of spasticity promote more accentuated osteoporosis, rendering such long bones more susceptible to fracture.

Paraplegia is either spastic or flaccid, depending on the level of injury, and complete or incomplete, depending on the degree of injury.

Treatment Principles for Paraplegia

During the flaccid stage of the disease, the emphasis of the therapy program is on prevention of deformity and the complications of bed rest. For instance, the patient's involved limbs are put through full range of motion at least twice a day. Equally, attention is paid to arrangement of bed clothing and foot boards in order to discourage a foot drop deformity. With the return of tone, the program's emphasis shifts to augment and capitalize on remaining or returning strength. Further exercises are designed to increase upper limb strength to aid in the activities of daily living and transfers, as well as locomotion by either wheelchair or braces and crutches.

Implications for Functional Independence

Functionally, the healthy paraplegic at any level can be taught to be independent for the activities of daily living and ambulation. Lesions below the cervical spinal cord supply to the hands (C8-T1) allow bimanual power and skill. The more the thoracic cord is spared, the better the ventilatory capacity and trunk balance. Between T3 and T12 the wheelchair is the recommended and preferred mode of transport, with independence coming through super arm strength and skill to allow car, bed, toilet, and bath transfers. Although technically possible, most paraplegics do not elect to walk as a primary mode of travel unless they have some motor power at or below the hips, providing proximal stability of the pelvis when on long leg braces and crutches or walker. With the addition of knee extensors (L2-3-4), the braces may be reduced to support below the knees, primarily for the ankles and feet. With lower lesion (L5-S1), the practical major problem is often that of hip abductor weakness, resulting in a waddling type of gait requiring crutches or canes, as well as plantarflexion and hip extensor weakness, and bladder, bowel, and sexual disruption (S2-3-4) (5).

QUADRIPLEGIA

Lesions above and including the spinal supply to the hands (C8-T1) results in quadriplegia, which is to say paralysis of all four limbs. Lesions above C3-4, because of the nerve supply to the diaphragm, may produce a so-called pentaplegia with respiratory dependency. In the quadriplegic patient the intercostal muscles of respiration will be lost, and respiratory work is performed by the diaphragm and accessory muscles of respiration (the upper part of the trapezius and the sternocleidomastoid). This fine balance can be disturbed by a respiratory infection, by an intraabdominal problem (e.g., distension, ileus) or by spinal bracing which may limit diaphragmatic excursion.

The usual traumatic cervical spinal cord injury results from spinal column damage at C5-6. This is understandable, as the major amount of flexion and extension occurs here, and at the same time, there is both a bulge in the cord for the origin of the brachial plexus and a critical spinal column canal space for the cord.

With partial quadriplegia, the neuroanatomy of the cord dictates several patterns of injury which are classical (Fig. 10.4). In the acute *central cord syndrome*, central damage affects the arms more than the legs and the hands more than

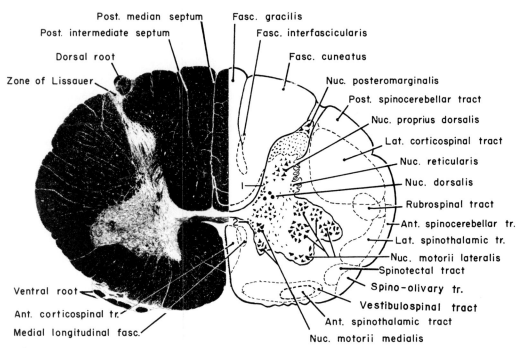

Figure 10.4.   Cross-section of the spinal cord at C8 level (Weigert's stain on *left*). (Reproduced with permission from RC Truex and MB Carpenter: *Strong and Elwyn's Human Neuroanatomy.* Baltimore, Williams & Wilkins.)

the arms. If a neurogenic bladder is present initially, it often recovers. The fibers to the hands and arms lie centrally, and the more peripherally placed fibers serve the lumbar and sacral segments supplying the legs and bladder. Moreover, in the peripheral area, perforating radicular arteries assist in the cord blood supply. This fact explains the occasional finding of sacral sensory sparing in an otherwise complete quadriplegic.

Anterior spinal artery involvement of the cervical cord (the *anterior cord syndrome*) gives rise to a picture similar to that in the quadriplegic, with involvement of all four limbs. In these patients, there is motor paralysis but preservation of proprioception and deep pain because of posterior column sparing. This assists the patient in balance and in skin care.

Damage of just the posterior columns with preservation of the lateral corticospinal tract is much more unusual because of the arterial supply of the cord. Incomplete lesions, especially in the thoracic cord, often lead to a high degree of spasticity, sometimes to the point where it interferes with the activities of daily living (ADL) by throwing the patient from bed or chair.

A *Brown Sequard lesion* of the spinal cord is one-sided, resulting in weakness on the same side due to interruption of the corticospinal tract, with loss of pain, temperature, and some touching on the opposite side due to interruption of the crossing lateral spinothalamic tracts. Thus, the limb with the best power has the poorest sensation.

Treatment Principles—Quadriplegia

The program after the initial insult is similar in principle to that for paraplegia. In the C5-C6 type of quadriplegia it may take up to a year to get adequate power and skill in the upper limbs to allow most of the ADL and transfers, as well as pushing a wheelchair successfully. In the quadriplegic lower limb, orthoses are not used but for the upper limb may occasionally augment hand function, such as in the handling of tableware, pencils, or typewriters.

Implications for Functional Independence

The functional prognosis is almost wholly determined by the level of the injury—given a healthy and well-motivated patient. Above C4, the patient will be respirator dependent unless some type of diaphragmatic pacing procedure can be done. Such a patient is completely dependent for self-care but may operate an electric wheelchair and environmental control system. With C5 preserved, shoulder power is present, and elbow flexors are active; this means the ability is present to feed, do some grooming, and type and use externally powered assistive devices. The powerful will be able to use a manual wheelchair, but independent transferring is very difficult without elbow extensors. With wrist extensors at C6 available, the tenodesis grip becomes possible; this is a functional hand grip performed by wrist extension with the somewhat shortened finger flexors passively producing a fist as the wrist is cocked. Such a grip is a major addition to functional independence. The patient can dress, do buttons, transfer more efficiently, and write.

At the C7-8 level, the presence of triceps makes the transfers much easier and more practical. Hand activities are more refined with finger flexors and extensors present. All aspects of self-care become more practical, such as self-catheterization and bowel treatments.

At the T1 level, control of the small hand muscles is present and, really, the patient does as well as a high paraplegic. Balance will be poor, being mainly dependent on the latissimus dorsi (6, 12). Besides the level of physical disability, the ultimate level of independence will depend on the patient's desire to maximize the remaining functional abilities and to rejoin the working world.

References

1. Adams GF: Prognosis and survival in the aftermath of hemiplegia. *Br Med J*, 5222:309–314, 1961.
2. Anderson TP, Bourestom N, Greenberg FR, Hilyard VG: Predictive factors in stroke rehabilitation. *Arch Phys Med Rehabil* 55:545–553, 1974.
3. Bobath B: The treatment of motor disorders of pyramidal and extrapyramidal origin by reflex inhibition and by facilitation of movements. *Physiotherapy* 41:146, 1955.
4. Brunnstrom S: *Movement Therapy in Hemiplegia.* New York, Harper & Row, 1970.
5. Burke DC, Murray DD: *The Handbook of Spinal Cord Medicine.* New York, Macmillan, 1975.
6. Ford JR, Duckwork B: *Physical Management for the Quadriplegic Patient.* Philadelphia, F.A. Davis, 1974.
7. Knott M, Voss DE: *Proprioceptive Neuromuscular Facilitation,* ed 2. New York, Harper & Row, 1968.
8. Lehmann JF, DeLateur BJ, Fowler RS, Warren CG, Arnheld R: Stroke: Does rehabilitation affect outcome? *Arch Phys Med Rehabil* 56:375–382, 1975.
9. Lehmann JF, DeLateur BJ, Fowler RS: Stroke rehabilitation: outcome and prediction. *Arch Phys Med Rehabil* 56:383–389, 1975.
10. Moskowitz E, Lightbody FEH, Freitag NS: Long-term follow-up of the poststroke patient. *Arch Phys Med Rehabil* 53:167–172, 1972.
11. Truex RC, Carpenter MB (eds): *Strong and Elwyn's Human Neuroanatomy,* ed 5. Baltimore, Williams & Wilkins, 1964, p 235.
12. Trombly CA, Scott AD: *Occupational Therapy for Physical Dysfunction.* Baltimore, Williams & Wilkins, 1977.
13. Young RR, Delwaide PJ: Spasticity. Parts 1 and 2. *N Engl J Med* 304:28–33, 96–99, 1981.

Movement Disorders

G. H. KRAFT

This section deals with motor dysfunction which is not due to disease of the pyramidal tract. These disorders are due to dysfunction in other portions of the central nervous system which are required for normal motor function. The deficit is not loss of strength; it is loss of intact motor function resulting in impairment due to ataxia, dystonia, or tremor.

Ataxia, or *dyssynergia*, is the incoordination during voluntary effort seen with a variety of neurological conditions. There are many types of ataxia, both congenital and acquired, which disturb purposeful movement from minor to devastating degrees. Most arise from either cerebellar or spinal cord lesions.

Chorea means irregular, spasmodic, involuntary movements of the limbs, trunk, neck, and face. It, too, has many types and causes (both congenital and acquired), with most due to lesions in the cerebral hemispheres and central ganglia of the brain. *Ballismus* (wild jerking or shaking movements) is related to chorea.

Athetosis, alone or combined with chorea—hence, *choreoathetosis*—describes constant slow writhing and involuntary movements of the wrists, hands, and fingers, in particular. It, too, has its cause in subcortical disturbances of the cerebral hemispheres.

Dystonia and dyskinesia literally mean any state of abnormal tone and movement. There are a number of rare childhood diseases (e.g., dystonia musculorum deformans) which lead to severe torsion deformities of the torso and limb-girdles because of alternating bouts of hypo- and hypertonicity of large muscle groups. Dystonia as a sign (hyper- or hypotonia) is seen in most neurological diseases and injuries. Spasmodic torticollis is an example of a dyskinetic wry neck.

Bradykinesia, literally, extreme "slowness in movements," becomes a diagnostic category in neurology as an accompaniment of other signs and symptoms of conditions such as parkinsonism.

MOVEMENT DISORDERS OF CHILDHOOD

The most common of these disorders is dyskinetic cerebral palsy. Cerebral palsy (CP) refers to a condition characterized by paralysis, weakness, and incoordination or some other motor functional aberration due to pathology in the brain. The diagnosis of cerebral palsy implies a nonprogressive disturbance of brain function due to an occurrence prior to birth, at the time of birth, or in the first few years of a child's development—generally before age 7. Ninety percent of cerebral palsy occurs prior to or at the time of birth. The incidence is approximately 1 in 250 live births.

There are two common types of cerebral palsy.

Spastic Diplegia

This type is typically due to prenatal disease, and is often thought to be due to hemorrhage in the central sulcus, affecting the motor cortical strips of the leg homunculus. Prenatal bleeding into this area produces damage to the lower extremity motor strips bilaterally and a nonspecific healing response of brain tissue which results in retarded development of those motor cells.

The clinical picture is a child with inadequately developed motor strips bilaterally. The child is hypotonic at birth, but subsequently develops spastic paresis of both legs classically, with especially marked adductor spasticity and consequent "scissors" gait. The upper limbs are also involved, but to a minor degree. This form of the disorder makes up two-thirds of all cerebral palsy. Spastic hemiplegia is also seen, with involvement of one side of the body and greater upper than lower limb involvement.

Dyskinesia

This category includes *athetoid CP*, *dystonic CP*, and other movement disorders. The pathology in these patients is thought to be *in utero* hypoxia to the brain, frequently associated with a variety of conditions, including icterus. Decreased oxygen affects the more rapidly growing structures of the brain, i.e., the basal ganglia, most severely.

The *athetoid* form of cerebral palsy consists of a child with constant, purposeless involuntary movements of the face, trunk, and extremities. This motor tone tends to involve the antagonists to antigravity muscles most severely. There tends to be a relatively greater control of the hands and feet than of the more proximal portions of the body. These patients are invariably slender due to their constant motor activity and often show facial grimacing which is most pronounced during periods of stress, such as attempts at purposeful motor activity. Speech is extremely difficult in many cases due to the poor motor control of muscles required for phonation.

ADULT MOVEMENT DISORDERS

There are several relatively common diseases which produce movement disorders in adults. Motor strength may not be diminished in these disorders, but the motor function which is present will be abnormal. Normally, the cerebellum is responsible for the smooth, accurate coordinated execution of movements. This portion of the brain receives information from the periphery regarding the actual position and rate of movement of the limbs, plus visual and auditory cues. It also samples information from the motor cortex regarding motor commands. Lesions of the cerebellum result in decreased tone and loss of the ability to move in a smooth and coordinated manner.

Parkinson's Syndrome

Parkinson's syndrome characteristically consists of rigidity, akinesia, tremor at rest, and a festinating gait. In contrast to spasticity, in which the resistance to passive movement is position- and rate-dependent and may reach a peak and suddenly decline, there is rigidity, in which the examiner perceives a constant resistance throughout the entire range of passive movement of affected joints. The patient with Parkinson's syndrome has an expressionless or mask-like face, soft monotonous speech, flexion posturing of limbs and trunk, and a resting tremor of about 3/second. Intention tremor is not present in this disorder.

Friedreich's Ataxia

This disorder is an hereditary spinocerebrellar degeneration. Striking clinical features seen in this disorder include intention tremor and ataxia of the lower extremities. Movements are not carried out smoothly, and as a patient approaches the conclusion of a purposeful movement with any muscle of the body—including the hands or feet—the feedback loops correcting the terminal phase of motor control do not function properly. As a result, there is a flailing movement which occurs with increasing rate of excursion as the hand or foot approaches the targeted position. Consequently, the patient may have serious problems in carrying out functional upper extremity activities and can be severely disabled. For example, satisfactory eating may be very difficult. As the patient's spoon nears his mouth, his arm may flail through progressively greater arcs, ineffectively reaching his mouth. The similar phenomenon in the lower extremities prevents accurate foot placement and makes safe walking difficult or impossible. Another condition in which intention tremors may frequently occur is multiple sclerosis.

TREATMENT OF MOVEMENT DISORDERS

These disorders are among the most difficult to treat, although neurosurgeons increasingly advocate surgical CNS ablations and implanted electrostimulation, etc., and other clinicians search for adequate chemical controllers. A discussion of these approaches is beyond the scope of this chapter. There are, however, two physical strategies which can claim some degree of success.

Use of the Mass Principle

In any rhythmic or pendular movement a given force on a constant mass will produce a given excursion. If the force producing the movement is held constant, increasing the mass of the object being moved will reduce the excursion. This can be shown in the following formula:

$$\text{Excursion} \propto \frac{\text{Force}}{\text{Mass}}$$

This principle can be applied to the treatment of patients with intention tremor in the following manner. Patients may have difficulty using a walker because when they pick up the walker and place it in front of them it may not be in a good stable position because of flailing movements. Weighting the walker will reduce the flailing movements and ensure more accurate placement safely in front of the patient. In a similar way, a patient with intention tremor who uses crutches may have poor accuracy in floor placement of the crutches during the gait cycle. However, weights on the tips of the crutches will reduce crutch excursion and ensure that they are more accurately placed. Similarly, weighted cuffs can be placed on the wrists for other tasks.

Training

A second treatment strategy consists of teaching a patient coordination exercises based on Frenkel's exercises; the patient practices repeated placement of the feet in adjacent squares on the floor. This is a retraining type of exercise to enhance the patient's ability for accurate foot placement during the gait cycle. A similar approach can be used for any necessary task.

Aids

If a movement disorder interferes with the accuracy of a task, the equipment with which the task is performed can sometimes be modified. For instance, a protective cover is commercially available which will prevent the wrong keys of an electric typewriter from being inadvertently depressed. Other examples include electronic scanning devices controlling typewriters or environmental control units with switches placed widely apart rather than the usual microswitches. For similar reasons, the control stick of an electric wheelchair should be of the "all-or-none" type, rather than a proportional control.

Neurogenic Bladder

S. L. STOVER

The neurogenic bladder is one of the most frequent problems encountered in patients with neuromuscular disorders. The ultimate goal of management is maintaining bladder drainage in a socially acceptable manner while preventing medical complications of the urinary tract.

Bladder dysfunction is usually a result of neurological impairment. Primary neurological impairment may occur from trauma, infection, or degenerative, vascular, or neoplastic processes. It may involve the peripheral nerves or the central nervous system at the spinal or supraspinal level. Bladder dysfunction may be congenital or acquired, acute or insidious. Whatever the cause of the nervous system involvement, the end result depends more on *how* bladder emptying is affected, rather than on the specific etiology.

ANATOMY AND PHYSIOLOGY

The bladder has both sensory and motor innervation from three sources (1, 8). The *somatic* pudendal nerve carries both sensory and motor fibers between the muscles of the external sphincter and pelvic floor to and from the micturition center in sacral spinal segments S2–S4. The parasympathetic pelvic nerves carry sensory and motor stimuli between the bladder wall and the micturition center. The hypogastric nerves carry *sympathetic* fibers from T10–L2 and provide both sensory and motor fibers to and from the bladder and urethra (Fig. 10.5). Sacrobulbar and reticulospinal tracts connect and integrate the spinal cord with a complex reflex system higher in the central nervous system.

Thus, initiating, inhibiting, sustaining, or interrupting bladder emptying consists of a highly coordinated set of reflexes controlled by all levels of the neuraxis (1). Although the upper urinary tract (e.g., the renal pelvis and ureter) has innervation, it is mostly passive and reflects the function of the lower urinary tract.

Voiding is initiated by bladder fullness (intravesical volume and/or pressure), providing stimuli for relaxation of the pelvic floor and external sphincter skeletal muscle and onset of reflex detrusor activ-

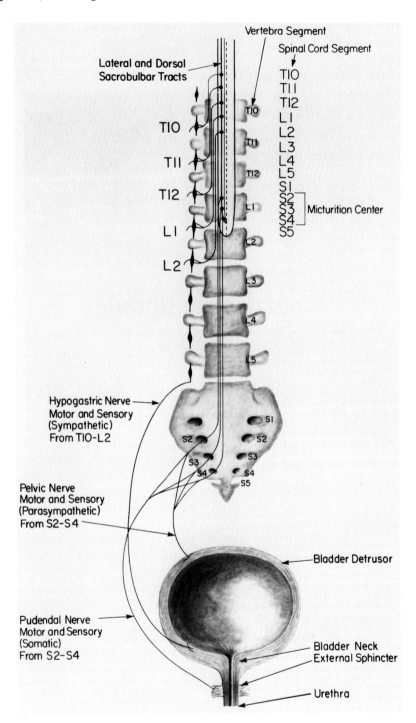

Figure 10.5.   Neural control of the bladder.

ity (1, 2). While the normal detrusor contracts, the bladder neck and sphincter relax by reciprocal inhibition. These synergistic actions are coordinated in the
brainstem and result in complete bladder
emptying (Fig. 10.6A). Neurologic lesions
may disrupt this coordinated synergistic
function, causing detrusor-sphincter dys-

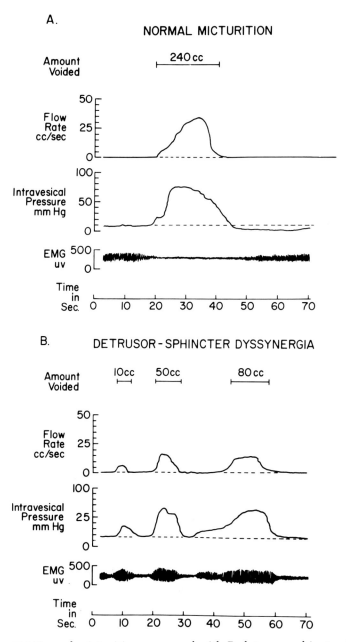

Figure 10.6.   (A) Normal micturition compared with B, detrusor-sphincter dyssynergia.

synergia that may lead to incomplete bladder emptying (Fig. 10.6B). Innervation of the bladder may be partially or completely disrupted. Neurological impairment of the cord at S1 or above usually leads to a reflex bladder (upper motor neuron) while pathology of S2 to S4 or below (either conus medullaris or cauda equina) leads to a flaccid areflexic bladder (lower motor neuron) (4).

CLASSIFICATION

The simple classification advocated by Comarr (4) is recommended (Table 10.1). This classification is based on a neurolog-

Table 10.1
Classification of Neurogenic Bladder

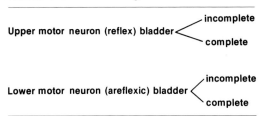

ical examination and is confirmed by urodynamic evaluation which includes a cystometrogram, sphincter electromyography, and urethral pressure profile.

The neurological examination includes sensory testing of the sacral segments, observation of volitional anal sphincter control, and reflex testing. In patients with an incomplete neurogenic bladder, pinprick sensation seems to correlate better than light touch sensation with a preserved desire to void and maintenance of volitional control. Reflex testing includes evaluation of anal sphincter tone, the anocutaneous (anal wink) reflex to perianal stimulation, and the bulbocavernosal reflex which is elicited by squeezing the glans penis of the male or the clitoris of the female, resulting in contraction of the external anal sphincter.

In most cases, these tests also provide accurate information about reflex activity of the autonomic pathways (4). An upper motor neuron bladder will usually empty automatically with reflexes. However, with a lower motor neuron bladder, voiding will take place only by overflow or by extrinsic pressure on the bladder through abdominal straining or the Credé maneuver (manual suprapubic pressure).

FUNCTIONAL PROBLEMS OF THE NEUROGENIC BLADDER

Incomplete bladder emptying is the common denominator in the neurogenic bladder, regardless of the neurological impairment. This may lead to infection and back pressure which are ultimately responsible for most complications associ-

ated with the neurogenic bladder (7). Whether infection or increased intravesical pressure is more harmful to the upper urinary tract remains unknown. Both are important factors and often coexist. Bacteria are normally cleared from the urinary tract by the combined effect of bladder washout and tissue defenses. Therefore, bladder volume, emptying intervals, intravesical pressure, and mural tension are important variables. Just having a low residual urine volume should not lead to a false sense of security, since detrusorsphincter dyssynergia may lead to increased sphincter resistance, increased intravesical pressure, reflux, and hydronephrosis even in a small capacity bladder (5). Incomplete bladder emptying, recurrent infection, and increased pressure are all interdependent.

COMPLICATIONS

Table 10.2 lists the most common complications seen in patients with neurogenic bladder dysfunction, most of which occur with any method of bladder management. In some cases, however, time after onset and method of management can also predispose to specific complications. For example, the penoscrotal abscess and its possible sequelae usually occur soon after onset in patients managed with an indwelling urethral catheter (1). Many times it is difficult to determine the relationship of one complication to another, e.g., are renal calculi caused by renal infection, or are calculi responsible

Table 10.2
Complications of Neurogenic Bladder
Management

Infection
   Cystitis and/or pyelonephritis
   Penoscrotal abscess and/or diverticulum, stricture, fistula
   Epididymitis and/or orchitis
   Prostatitis
   Septicemia

Vesicoureteral reflux

Hydronephrosis

Calculi

Autonomic hyperreflexia

Renal failure

for secondary infection? In neurogenic bladder patients, renal calculi are usually infection-associated or infection-induced. The combination of infection and recurrent calculi predispose to deterioration of renal function (3, 11). Increased professional interest in the overall care of patients with neurogenic bladder, irrespective of the bladder management method selected, appears to have reduced the incidence of complications.

Those who manage patients with neurogenic bladder should be familiar with autonomic hyperreflexia. This can occur in patients with upper motor neuron impairment at or above the T6 spinal segment which interferes with reflex control over the sympathetic nervous system (1). Many types of stimuli can trigger sympathetic reflexes, but bladder distention by obstruction or detrusor-sphincter dyssynergia seem to be the most common cause. Catheterization or other urological procedures may also precipitate hyperreflexia. Signs and symptoms include severe headaches, hypertension, sweating, flushing of the skin above the level of injury, nasal congestion, respiratory distress, and bradycardia. Recognition of the problem and alleviation of the stimulus, or treatment with medications which inhibit the autonomic nervous system, are important.

MANAGEMENT OF THE NEUROGENIC BLADDER

Optimal neurogenic bladder management employs whatever residual function remains. Adequate bladder emptying at regular intervals is probably the most important key to preservation of renal function (2). Selection of the method of bladder management must be individualized and based on the neurologic and urodynamic examination (classification), and existing pathology of the urinary tract must be determined by appropriate laboratory tests and x-rays. In addition, it may be influenced by social, educational, psychological, and vocational considerations.

The list of current methods of neurogenic bladder management in Table 10.3 suggests that the ideal and proven method has not yet been identified. With the onset of an illness or injury, an indwelling catheter or intermittent catheterization are now most frequently used for bladder drainage. During the acute period, intermittent catheterization has decreased the incidence of penoscrotal abscess and epididymitis (6, 9). Intermittent catheterization is often continued until the bladder empties by reflexes, stimulation, or voluntary pressure and can serve as a voiding trial. A majority of males with upper motor neuron bladders become catheter free using external condom drainage because reflex emptying remains involuntary and usually unpredictable (12). Without a suitable external collecting device for females with reflex bladders, voiding trials may be undertaken with intermittent catheterization, although an indwelling urethral catheter will most likely be the best method available. Fortunately, females tend to tolerate a urethral catheter better than the male population (5). In lower motor neuron bladders, the flaccid bladder must be voluntarily emptied on a regular basis by abdominal straining, Credé, intermittent catheterization, or an indwelling urethral catheter.

The term "bladder training" is frequently associated with neurogenic blad-

Table 10.3
Methods of Neurogenic Bladder Management

1. **Indwelling urethral catheter**
2. **Suprapubic catheter**
3. **Intermittent catheterization**
4. **External condom**
5. **Conduits - Ileal, colonic, etc.**
6. **Cutaneous vesicostomy**
7. **Bladder neck prosthetics**
8. **Bladder stimulators**
9. **Spinal posterior column stimulators**
10. **Selective sacral rhizotomy**
11. **Sacral nerve grafts**

ders, but the ability to train bladder reflexes is questionable. A reflex bladder emptying variable quantities of urine at regular intervals does not signify a "trained bladder." Selecting the most appropriate method of management and good medical follow-up, coupled with training of the patient in caring for the urinary tract, are most important to a successful outcome.

Drugs have limited value in modifying neurogenic bladder dysfunction. Proof of effectiveness is often lacking in drugs reported to have a physiologic basis for altering neurogenic bladder dysfunction. Hyperactive bladder reflexes which lead to urgency, frequency, and incontinence may be partially controlled by drugs which block the parasympathetic nervous system. By comparison, parasympathomimetic drugs have little value in improving bladder emptying. Drugs which block skeletal muscle spasticity are suggested to have some value in detrusor-sphincter dyssynergia, but these drugs are often unpredictable and can decrease detrusor function as well as sphincter spasticity. The value of urinary acidification, bladder irrigation, and prophylactic antimicrobial treatment is still debated.

In some patients, efforts to obtain a catheter-free state and a sterile urine are unsuccessful. Recurrent bacteriuria continues to be a problem with most current methods of management, and the long-term effects of asymptomatic bacteriuria are still uncertain. There are, as yet, no readily available and reliable clinical methods to determine if the source of bacteriuria is from the lower or upper urinary tract.

In patients with upper motor neuron bladders who are catheter-free, increased intravesical pressure over prolonged periods of time may be just as detrimental to the urinary tract as persistent infection. An external sphincterotomy may be quite beneficial in patients with detrusor-sphincter dyssynergia to decrease the residual bladder volume and pressure (10).

The indwelling urethral catheter can still be one of the better methods of management for certain patients. If an indwelling urethral catheter is used, penoscrotal abscesses can usually be prevented by taping the catheter to the abdomen. In the female, taping the catheter to the thigh can also prevent traction on the bladder neck which leads to bladder neck dilatation and leakage around the catheter. Urinary diversion, such as by connecting both ureters to an isolated loop of ileum which drains to a bag on the abdominal wall, is rarely required.

Increased interest and improved care in the management of the neurogenic bladder and total care of the patient have led to advances in preventing renal failure without necessarily crediting the improvement to any one specific method of bladder management.

References

1. Bors E, Comarr AE: Neurological Urology. Physiology of Micturition, Its Neurological Disorders and Sequelae. Basel, S. Karger, 1971.
2. Boyarsky S, Weinberg S: Urodynamic concepts. In W Lutzeyer and H Melchior: Urodynamics—Upper and Lower Urinary Tract. New York, Springer-Verlag, 1973, pp 1–13.
3. Coe FL: Clinical and laboratory assessment. In FL Coe: Nephrolithiasis: Pathogenesis and Treatment. Chicago, Year Book Medical Publishers, 1978, pp 1–26.
4. Comarr AE: Urinary bladder disorders from spinal cord injury. Comp Ther 5 (9):1979.
5. Graham SD: Present urological treatment of spinal cord injury patients. J Urol 126:1–4, 1981.
6. Guttman L, Frankel H: The value of intermittent catheterization in the early management of traumatic paraplegia and tetraplegia. Paraplegia 4:63–84, 1966.
7. Hinman F: Hydrodynamic aspects of urinary tract infection. In Lutzeyer W, Melchior H: Urodynamics, Upper and Lower Urinary Tract. New York, Springer-Verlag, 1973, pp 14–22.
8. Mason RC, Downey JA: Urogenital physiology. In Downey JA, Darling RC: Physiological Basis of Rehabilitation Medicine. Philadelphia, WB Saunders, 1971, pp 245–264.
9. Pearman JW, England EJ: Urological follow-up of 99 spinal cord injured patients initially managed by intermittent catheterization. Br J Urol 48:297–310, 1976.
10. Perkash I: An attempt to understand and to treat voiding dysfunctions during rehabilitation of the bladder in spinal cord injury patients. J Urol 115:36–40, 1976.
11. Price M, Kottke FJ, Olsen ME: Renal function in

patients with spinal cord injury: the eighth year of a ten year continuing study. *Arch Phys Med Rehabil* 56 (2):76–79, 1975.

12. Stover SL, Lloyd LK, Nepomuceno CS, Gale LL: Intermittent catheterisation: follow-up studies. *Paraplegia* 15:38–46, 1977 and 1978.

The Neurogenic Bowel

S. BERROL

A neurogenic bowel may result from disease or injury to the lower motor neuron or upper motor neuron. It may result from spinal cord injury, multiple sclerosis, cauda equina injury, diabetes mellitus, spina bifida, head injury, stroke, etc. The psychologic effects of bowel incontinence may be devastating. Regardless of etiologic disorder, effective control of fecal incontinence is possible and is essential for adequate integration of the individual into the mainstream of society.

MECHANISMS OF DEFECATION

The process of defecation is usually initiated following a meal when a strong peristaltic wave occurs in the colon as a result of food entering the stomach (gastrocolic reflex) and its contents spilling into the duodenum (duodenocolic reflex). The smooth muscle of the intestinal tract has an inherent "pacemaker" activity and cells that respond to extrinsic autonomic nerve supply and others that function from intrinsic nerves of the intestines independently.

Stretch receptors in the wall of the rectum are stimulated by the entrance of the fecal mass; the nerve impulses in the inferior hypogastric plexus pass to the parasympathetic fibers in the sacral cord as S2, S3, and S4. A spinal reflex may be initiated to evacuate the rectum or may travel up the cord to cerebral awareness, and the urge to defecate is appreciated. If defecation proceeds under voluntary control, it is initiated by closure of the glottis, voluntary descent of the diaphragm, and contraction of abdominal and pelvic muscles, resulting in increased intraabdominal and intrathoracic pressures (Valsalva maneuver); this forces the fecal material into the rectum. As feces enter the rectum, the ascending colon contracts (rectocolic reflex). The distention of the rectum further results in reflex relaxation of the internal anal sphincter (smooth muscle). Early entrance of fecal contents into the rectum causes reflex contraction of the (striated) external sphincter initially, followed by inhibition of sphincter tone.

MAINTENANCE OF CONTINENCE

Mechanical aids to continence include the acute anterior and posterior angulations of the sigmoid colon and its lateral curves. In addition, there exist several spiral folds containing circular muscle fibers (valves of Houston) that restrict fecal movements. The angulation of the colon at the entrance to the anal canal is increased with high intraabdominal pressure, producing a "flap-valve" effect.

The internal anal sphincter is comprised of smooth muscle and remains in a state of constant tonic contraction. The pelvic diaphragm (chiefly, levator ani) forms a U-shaped sling which produces a strong sphincter-like action to control fecal loss. The external anal sphincter consists of striated muscle and surrounds the internal sphincter; it is almost constantly contracting and is chiefly responsible for retaining solid feces. The internal sphincter is not under voluntary control, and its high resting tone controls the passage of liquid and gas.

UPPER MOTOR NEURON LESION

Upper motor neuron (UMN) lesions, such as spinal cord injury, may be complete (both motor and sensory loss) or varying degrees of incompleteness. UMN lesions are associated with spasticity of the extremities. Saddle anesthesia may be present if sensory tracts have been involved. The bulbocavernosus reflex is positive (reflex contraction of the rectal sphincter when the head of the penis or the clitoris is squeezed). An "anal wink" reflex is present. The anal sphincter contracts reflexly when a pin prick is applied peripherally to the skin around the anus. If these reflexes are absent in a spinal cord-injured individual, then the sacral centers (S2, S3, S4) have been injured.

LOWER MOTOR NEURON INJURY

When S2, S3, and S4 nerve fibers are damaged, flaccidity of lower extremities is found, as well as a negative bulbocavernosus reflex, a negative anal wink, and impaired or absent saddle area sensation. The defecation reflex is impaired, and external rectal sphincter tone is absent or decreased, so physical stress may be sufficient to cause loss of rectal contents.

BOWEL PROGRAMS

The purpose of a good bowel program for patients with a neurogenic bowel is to produce regular complete evacuations at a planned time, with minimal or no bowel accidents. The program must be individualized for the patient, taking into account emotional, cultural, and family needs. Active participation must be encouraged from the onset. The program must be adjusted as the individual's situation changes. Maintenance of bowel program records are essential to the comprehensive management in eliminating a trial-and-error approach.

Exercise

Prolonged bed rest and inactivity predispose the patient to constipation. The individual should be encouraged to participate as fully as possible in all ADLs, including dressing, transfers, wheelchair ambulation, and exercise. A bathroom or bedside commode should be used rather than a bedpan.

Fluids

Adequate fluid intake is required to adjust the consistency of the fecal mass. A daily intake of 2000–3000 ml is desirable. Patients on intermittent catheterization programs may be on restricted fluid intake and, therefore, may require the use of stool softeners to prevent a constipated stool. Large quantities of milk should be avoided.

Diet

A habit pattern of three regular meals a day should be established. It should consist of a well-balanced diet high in fiber-containing foods, such as whole grain cereals, bran, green vegetables, nuts, and fruits with skins and seeds. Gas-producing foods such as cabbage and beans should be avoided. Large quantities of natural laxatives such as prune juice should be avoided. Juices, however, may be a very effective natural means of correcting constipation.

Timing

The bowel program should be established at a time consistent with the premorbid pattern. It should be performed within an hour after the morning or evening meal, and a glass of hot or warm liquid should accompany the meal. This will take advantage of the residual gastrocolic and duodenocolic reflexes. Privacy during the bowel program has a positive effect.

Upper Motor Neuron Program

In the patient with an UMN lesion, evacuation results from stimulation or stretch to produce a reflex. The program is planned following a meal, and a commode or commode chair is used. The defecation reflex may be stimulated using a suppository (e.g., Bisacodyl®) inserted well into the rectum and against the rectal mucosa. The program is conducted usually every other day, but individual patterns prevail. Some patients may have their bowel program every 3 or 4 days without harmful effect. Eventually, the suppository may be replaced by the use of digital stimulation. This is performed by inserting a gloved lubricated finger into the rectum and moving it in a slow, gentle, circular, dilating pattern, until the external anal sphincter relaxes. Patients with inadequate hand strength or control may still achieve independence with the use of an orthosis or aid. Enemas should not be used, except in exceptional circumstances.

Lower Motor Neuron Program

Patients with a LMN lesion must use the Valsalva maneuver. This is accomplished most efficiently on a commode, attempting to increase intra-abdominal pressure to expel the feces through the flaccid sphincter. Not uncommonly, manual evacuation is required. If fecal contents are not present in the rectum, a Bisacodyl® suppository may be inserted as high as possible within the rectum to stimulate the colon to expel its contents.

Medications

Some patients appear to do better when mild, stimulating laxatives are given 12 hours before bowel evacuation. A change in bowel pattern frequently occurs with the use of concomitant medications. Constipating drugs include anticholinergics, narcotics, antihistamines, antacids, etc.

SUMMARY

Restoration of bowel continence establishes an increased level of independence for the disabled. Assessment and intervention to re-establish a more normal bowel evacuation pattern should begin with the initial diagnosis. To be effective, the program must be individualized, and the patient must take responsibility for maintenance of the program as early as possible. Medical responsibility requires that we develop strong and intensified learning programs for our patients.

Pressure Sores

F. NOWROOZI

Pressure sores are localized areas of tissue necrosis which tend to occur between underlying bony prominences and overlying compressing surfaces such as a bed, chair, or orthotic device. Prolonged local pressure is the most important factor causing these ulcers.

ETIOLOGY AND PATHOGENESIS

Neurotropic factors, in the past, were frequently claimed to play the most important role in causing pressure sores, but there is little to substantiate this hypothesis. It is the current belief that the most important etiologic factor is localized ischemia secondary to excessive pressure. Normally, pressure on the arterial side of the capillary loop is 32 mm Hg. This pressure increases up to a maximum of 60 mm Hg during hyperemia (7).

Kosiak (8) has shown that external pressure of as little as 60 mm Hg for 1 hour would produce microscopic degenerative changes of all tissues from skin to bone in dogs, and that there were no detectable microscopic differences between normal or denervated muscle following the application of either constant or alternating pressure. He found that external pressures of 35 mm Hg for up to 4 hours would not produce such microscopic changes.

In contrast, Daniel et al. (4) produced pressure sores over the femoral greater trochanter of both normal and paraplegic swine by applying continuous pressure. Their results indicate that primary ischemia occurs in the muscle and that skin destruction will follow as pressure and/or duration increase. Compromised circulation can be compensated for, and adequate tissue nutrition can be restored through the mechanism of reactive hyperemia. This phenomenon will permit the subjected area to be flooded with blood if the pressure is removed before the critical period of between 1 and 2 hours. Reactive hyperemia would be insufficient if pressure persisted longer than that critical period.

The "H" substance resembling histamine released from traumatized cells, and accumulation of metabolites such as potassium, ADP, hydrogen, and lactic acids, have been suggested as factors which, individually or in combination, dilate the blood vessels. In addition to external pressure, there are other contributing factors which produce pressure sores (Table 10.4).

CLINICAL PRESENTATION AND DIAGNOSIS

More than 90% of pressure ulcers are located in the lower part of the body. The ischial tuberosities (30%), greater trochanters (20%), and the sacrum (15%) are the most commonly involved. Other areas less frequently involved are the malleolus, the heel, and the fibular head. It is

Table 10.4
Etiological Factors in Pressure Sores (11)

1. Localized ischemia secondary to excessive wound pressure (the single most important factor)
2. Malnutrition and hypoproteinemia
3. Anemia
4. Circulatory impairment
5. Infection
6. Sensory loss
7. Paralysis
8. Joint limitation and contractures
9. Edema
10. Poor hygiene of skin
11. Mental status
12. Spasticity
13. Incontinence of bowel and bladder

174

important to distinguish between the superficial manifestations of pressure and those due to abrasion or local trauma (e.g., bumping the buttock on the wheelchair tire during a side transfer).

Clinical symptomatology of pressure sores may also be classified in four stages as follows (5, 8, 10).

Stage I

This stage is manifested by the redness of the skin that blanches when light finger pressure is applied. This stage represents a circulatory disturbance. The ulcer is limited to the superficial epidermal and dermal layer. An acute inflammatory response involving soft tissue layers is characteristic of the earliest stage of injury of Grade I pressure sores. A normally innervated patient may complain of pain in the involved area. The diagnosis of Stage I is very important because the process is reversible simply by the relief of the pressure. A complete healing may occur within 5–10 days.

Stage II

In contrast to Stage I, the reddening and congestion of the affected area do not disappear on decompression. Excoriation of the skin and blisters are among other findings. Superficial necrosis may be developed in more advanced Stage II cases. This stage is characterized by the extension of the acute inflammatory response, leading to a fibroblastic response in the previously mentioned tissue layers and also the adipose tissue. Microscopic examination will show both the acute and chronic inflammatory processes. The Stage II pressure sore is also a reversible lesion.

Stage III

This is essentially a full-thickness skin defect. The ulcer extends into the subcutaneous fat. There is no direct involvement of the muscle; however, it is distorted by swelling, inflammation, and infection, along with some loss of fibrillar structures. The ulcer margin is irregular and is outlined by a dark and light hyper- and hypopigmentation. Histologically, the ulcer margins are thickened and rolled with extensive epidermal reaction. Chronic inflammation reactive fibrosis and tissue necrosis now have extended peripherally and produced undermining. Systemic infection, including fever, leukocytosis, dehydration, and sometimes anemia may also be present.

Stage IV

A Stage IV lesion is characterized by extension of the ulcer into the deep fascia with involvement of the muscle and bone. There is an extensive undermining with profuse necrosis. This stage is characterized by the communication of the ulcer with the bone or joint structure (Fig. 10.7). One may find the pathological picture of septic arthritis or osteomyelitis during this phase. Exposure of the bone is common. Anemia and dehydration commonly occur.

In some situations, such as the later stages of paraplegia (i.e., ambulatory stage), prolonged pressure with or without repeated trauma may cause an ischemic necrosis in the subcutaneous fat. A small ulcer measuring a few millimeters in diameter normally over the ischial tuberosities or trochanters with associated tissue swelling is the only physical finding. An x-ray following contrast filling reveals a bursa-like cavity whtch is filled with necrotic tissue. These closed pressure sores are frequently overlooked unless they become infected and connected with joints when the signs of systemic infection may be evidenced with minimal external skin involvement. The ulcer base should be judged by palpation since a very small ulcer may overlie a large undermining defect below. Occasionally, other pathological processes such as vasculitis, deep mycotic infection, necrotic malignancy, and early ischial-rectal abscess may mimic a pressure sore.

Laboratory tests, such as wound and tissue culture, complete blood count,

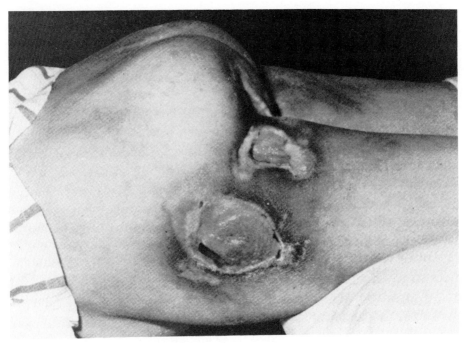

Figure 10.7.   Grade IV pressure sores. (Reproduced with permission from Guttmann: *Spinal Cord Injuries: Comprehensive Management and Research.* Oxford, Blackwell Scientific Publications, and Philadelphia, FA Davis, 1973.)

erythrocyte sedimentation rate, serum electrolyte, and albumin, may help to provide more comprehensive management. Diagnostic imaging studies, such as x-ray, bone scan, computerized tomography, sinography, and thermography, may lead to the early diagnosis of life-threatening complications such as osteomyelitis, infectious arthritis, and the formation of sinuses, cysts, and fistulae.

Complications

Complications are commonly seen in Grades III, IV, and closed pressure sores. Infection is, as a rule, part of the local clinical picture of Grades III and IV pressure sores. It is also common in more superficial ulcers, however. Infection is frequently multimicrobial. This microbial flora includes both aerobic and anaerobic bacteria. In a recent study (3) on geriatric patients, these organisms were *Staphylococcus aureus, Proteus mirabilis, Pseudomonas aeruginosa, Bacteroides fragilis,* and *Bacteroides asaccharolyticus.* Some infections are associated with necrotic and enlarging lesions. Involvement of deeper tissues and bone causes periostitis, osteitis, sinus formation, and osteomyelitis. Septic arthritis of the hip and joints with destruction of the femoral head and acetabulum is still reported (6). Septicemia may also follow if the necessary therapeutic steps are not taken in the early stage. Anemia is not only known as an etiological cofactor in the development of the pressure sore, but it can also be caused by chronically infected ulcers. The type of anemia is one which is associated with chronic infection. The septic condition caused by the chronic infected ulcer has at times disastrous effects on the nitrogen balance of the patient. Hypoalbuminemia and loss of protein may also be caused by draining pressure sores. Extreme states of malnutrition in some paraplegics are still occasionally reported (6). Secondary amyloidosis has been reported in chronically infected pressure ulcers.

PREVENTION

The most common neurological disorder associated with the pressure sore is paraplegia secondary to spinal cord injury (SCI). Prevention of pressure sores in SCI should begin at the scene of the accident. This includes removing hard objects from the patient's pockets, padding bony prominences, and early admission of the patient to a spinal cord center. Quality nursing care is critical. Frequent change of posture, at least every 2 hours day and night, is the cardinal prophylaxis.

Preventive devices are of three broad types (2). First are those designed to aid in turning or moving a patient. The Foster frame, the Stryker frame, the Circoelectric® bed, and the tilt table are among devices used. Of these devices, only the tilt table and the Circolectic® bed allow the patient to be placed in a head-up position. Second are those designed to support specific pressure areas of the body, such as the heels, sacrum, and buttock. Gel flotation pads and sheepskin have been widely used for the purpose of partial supports. Devices designed to support the entire body surface to change, minimize, or equalize pressure distribution are the third group.

There are various types of beds and mattresses employed in the prevention and treatment of pressure sores. The rationale for their construction is to alter points of pressure against the body surface at regular intervals, and also to allow the weight of the body to spread out over a sufficiently wide area. Several alternating pressure mattresses and molding devices are commercially available. For instance, recently air-fluidized sand or glass beads covered with a closely woven monofilament polyester sheet have been introduced (9) (Fig. 10.8). The depth of the fluidized material is approximately 12

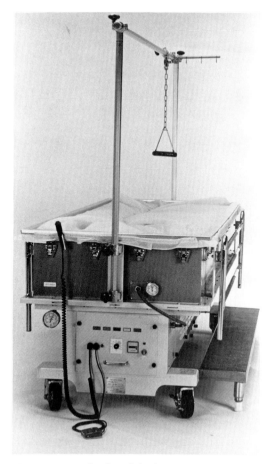

Figure 10.8. Fluidized bed. An air compressor forces warmed air through a thick bed of silicon-coated soda-lime glass microspheres which are thus converted to a thick "fluid" that looks rather like boiling milk. Over this bed is stretched a monofilament polyester filter sheet that permits the passage of air while it supports the patient with minimal pressure on various vulnerable pressure points. (Courtesy of "Clinitron" Manufacturers (9).)

inches (30 cm), and the normal penetration of the patient's body into this layer is 4 inches (10 cm).

No device is sufficiently good to eliminate the need for frequent careful position changes. Patient and family education regarding the continued necessity of preventive measures (e.g., wheelchair pushups) is mandatory.

TREATMENT

General supportive measures, including diet, correction of anemia, dehydration, control of spasticity, diabetes, and hygiene of the perineal area, especially in the case of the incontinent patient, are important parts of the management.

In Grade I and II pressure sores, relief of pressure by frequent change of posture and local cleansing of the skin to control bacterial contamination are all that should be done. Gentle soap and a soft cloth or sponge are needed to keep the skin clean. If the skin is sweaty, a lotion with an alcohol base may be used. If the skin is abnormally dry, a petroleum jelly may be applied. Adequate exposure of the skin to air can help avoid buildup of heat and perspiration.

Many topical agents being used are purported to speed up the healing process in Grades III and IV ulcers. For instance, a high molecular weight dextran polymer, in the form of beads which can be packed in the wound, has been used. This material not only absorbs fluid but also larger molecules and bacteria. However, studies so far do not support the advantage of using these agents over debridement of the ulcer and wet to dry dressing 3 and 4 times per day.

Many Grade III and IV pressure sores require surgical intervention. Surgical repair should be contemplated only when local or systemic infection is irradicated and healthy granulation tissue begins to appear. Anemia, protein depletion, and electrolyte imbalance should be treated prior to surgery. Systemic antibiotics beginning 36 hours before the operation to cover the operative phase are advocated by some physicians.

The objectives of such surgery include debridement of necrotic tissues and early closure of ulcers. Primary closure is possible in small ulcers with soft adjacent skin. Closure of large ulcers, however, is usually done by skin and muscle (or myocutaneous) flaps (1). Excision of femoral trochanters, ischial tuberosities, and head of the femur may become necessary in certain cases, especially if osteomyelitis has involved the bone.

CONCLUSION

Pressure sores constitute a common problem of disabled, chronically ill, debilitated patients. They delay rehabilitation. It is estimated that each pressure sore costs $5000 in care. Despite significant improvement in better understanding of pressure sores, this preventable complication remains a source of frustration to the patient, and a real challenge to the medical care team.

References

1. Antypas PG: The patient with spinal cord injury: Management of pressure sores. *Curr Prob Surg* 17:229–244, 1980.
2. Berecek KH: Treatment of decubitus ulcers. *Nursing Clin North Am* 10:171–209, 1975.
3. Daltrey DC, Rhodes B, Chatterood JG: Investigation into the microbial flora of healing and non-healing decubitus ulcers. *J Clin Pathol* 34:701–705, 1981.
4. Daniel RK, Priest DL, Wheatley DC: Etiologic factors in pressure sores: an experimental model. *Arch Phys Med Rehabil* 62:492–498, 1981.
5. Guttman L: The problem of treatment of pressure sores in patients with spinal paraplegia. *Br J Plast Surg* 8:1966, 1955.
6. Guttman L: Spinal cord injuries. In *Comprehensive Management and Research*, ed 2. London, Blackwell Scientific Publications, 1976, pp 512–542.
7. Kosiak M: Etiology and pathology of ischemic ulcers. *Arch Phys Med Rehabil* 40:62–69, 1959.
8. Kosiak M: Etiology of decubitus ulcers. *Arch Phys Med Rehabil* 42:19–29, 1961.
9. Parish LC, Witkowski JA: Clinitron therapy and the decubitus ulcer: preliminary dermatologic studies. *Int J Dermatol* 19:517–518, 1980.
10. Shea JD: Pressure sores: classification and management. *Clin Orthop Related Res* 112:89–100, 1975.
11. Tepperman PS, DeZwirek DCS, Chiarcossi AL, Jimenez J: Pressure sores. *Postgrad Med* 62:83–89, 1977.

Emergencies Related to Neurological Impairment

F. NASO

The patient who sustains acute major neurologic disease, such as stroke or spinal cord injury, may develop acute medical problems that can affect the course and prognosis of a restorative program. The risk of urinary tract infection, thromboembolism, and cardiac problems, to mention a few, may be considered a part of the total disability and will require aggressive intervention whenever they appear. Because of the frequency of these complications, the physician must be familiar with the diagnosis, initial treatment, and prevention. He must also be able to decide when a medical consultant should be involved. What follows is a survey of some of the more common problems.

GENITOURINARY EMERGENCIES

The neurogenic bladder that occurs after neurologic insult predisposes to urinary tract infection that plagues the patient during inpatient rehabilitation and frequently after discharge. Altered bladder and host resistance, and instrumentation in addition to inadequate drainage, are predisposing factors. Optimal management requires adequate emptying by an appropriate bladder program with either continuous or intermittent catheterization (see p. 169).

Careful screening for urinary tract infection is critical, particularly during the acute rehabilitation period. When a positive culture appears, controversy exists about treatment. In the presence of an indwelling catheter, treatment is not necessary without systemic signs of infection (fever, leukocytosis). When systemic signs of infection are present, appropriate anti-biotics should be prescribed for 7–14 days. Recurrent infection is not uncommon and may be due to inadequate treatment or tissue invasion (kidney, bladder, or prostate).

Of major concern is the prevention of bacteremia or septicemia since the organisms responsible for infection in the genitourinary tract are often resistant to the usual antibiotics and may produce the syndrome of septic shock. When this does occur, treatment must be aggressive with the use of intravenous fluids and antibiotics. Until the organism is identified, combinations of aminoglycosides, synthetic penicillins, and cephalosporins may be used, to be replaced by appropriate antibiotics depending on sensitivities. Baseline and sequential renal function tests and frequent serum antibiotic levels should be performed because of the nephrotoxicity of these drugs. At the moment, there is no clear evidence that high dose steroids are effective in changing the clinical outcome (6).

THROMBOEMBOLISM

The immobilized patient, particularly when neurologic deficit occurs in the lower extremities, is prone to develop thromboembolic complications because of a number of predisposing features. The paralysis, local vessel trauma, and hypercoagulability all set the stage for venous thrombosis. Such clots may become mobilized to produce emboli to the lungs, with the attendant morbidity including hypotension, hypoxemia, and cardiac arrhythmia. If the pulmonary emboli are large or when they occur in the elderly patient with pre-existing cardiopulmonary disease, death may occur. The diagnosis of pulmonary embolism is difficult because clinical features are often absent, particularly in this group of patients with sensory, perceptual, or communicative difficulties, so one must have a high index of suspicion, especially in those situations in which there is a sudden change in the clinical status of the patient. Unexplained worsening of spasticity, autonomic dysreflexia, tachycardia, dyspnea, or fever may be the only clues.

Laboratory aids may be of help in the diagnosis, such as arterial blood gases, especially if one has had values performed before the acute problem. A radionuclide ventilation perfusion scan is a better guide, but in questionable situations a pulmonary arteriogram is diagnostic (9). The electrocardiogram is usually nonspecific but occasionally may demonstrate the signs of acute right bundle branch block or diffuse myocardial ischemia. A chest x-ray more often is normal but may show a classic wedge-shaped pattern.

The treatment of choice is continuous intravenous infusion of 35,000–50,000 units of heparin in 24 hours, preceded by a bolus of 5,000–10,000 units. The flow rate should be adjusted to maintain the partial thromboplastin time (PTT) twice normal. After 5–7 days the heparin infusion may be replaced with oral warfarin, utilizing an initial loading dose between 5 and 20 mg of warfarin and thereafter appropriate dosages to keep the prothrombin time (PT) between 1.5 and 2 times the normal time (9).

Some clinicians feel that a lower extremity venogram should be done when the diagnosis of pulmonary embolism has been made, since additional clot may be present in a precarious proximal vein and potentially may cause recurrent pulmonary emboli. In such cases vena cava interruption by plication or umbrella instrumentation is suggested to prevent this possibility (8). The Greenfield filter is a device that is inserted into the inferior vena cava through a subclavian vein. This provides significant protection against recurrent emboli and is without significant complications.

Since the etiology of pulmonary embolism is usually a clot in the lower limb, it is important to make the diagnosis of thrombophlebitis. Unfortunately, since clinical signs are often absent in these patients, many rehabilitation centers use screening procedures in this high-risk group. The use of ^{125}I scanning, in addition to impedance plethysmography, has been a useful tool in identifying those patients who should have diagnostic venograms (4, 7).

The treatment of thrombophlebitis is intravenous heparin with the same technique used in pulmonary embolism, except that a bolus need not be utilized. Heparin should be continued for at least 5 days and replaced by oral warfarin for 2 to 3 months. The neurologically impaired patient has a higher incidence of complications of anticoagulants. A simple fall may produce mild intramuscular bleeding or, indeed, a more serious subdural hematoma. One must carefully evaluate the need for anticoagulation vs. the risk of serious complications when making a judgment about continued anticoagulation after discharge from the rehabilitation center. If the patient is at all unreliable or has significant ataxia so that there is reasonable risk of a fall, one should consider the safer but less effective procedure of subcutaneous heparin (5000 units every 12 hours) (1) or, indeed, the use of platelet inhibitors such as aspirin and Persantine® in combination.

GASTROINTESTINAL BLEEDING

The traumatized neurologic patient runs a higher risk for the development of stress ulceration in the gastrointestinal tract (5). The etiology is unknown but may involve altered mucosal physiology of the stomach and small intestine. These patients are often given corticosteroids, which add to the risk of ulceration. Bleeding may be massive and rapid with hematemesis or slower with the passage of black stools. Such patients may require heroic therapy with intravenous fluids, transfusions of blood, and close monitoring of the bleeding. It is best to have a gastroenterologist involved early for prompt diagnostic endoscopy, in addition to a surgeon, since bleeding may not be controllable medically.

The best preventative approach is the use of antacids and H2-histamine antagonists (e.g., cimetidine) in the high risk patient, especially in those who are expected to have multiple surgical procedures or require the use of steroids (10).

CARDIOVASCULAR PROBLEMS

Cardiovascular problems are common in patients who have had neurologic injury, since the degenerative vascular problems which predispose to stroke syndrome may also produce cardiac disease, particularly coronary atherosclerosis. Alternatively, the cardiovascular occlusion may be due to an embolus from the heart. Furthermore, the higher energy demands of activities for this population are further cause for cardiac difficulty. Congestive heart failure, the major problem, may present as pedal edema, subtle rales in the chest, dilated neck veins, and an S-3 gallop rhythm, or the syndrome of acute pulmonary edema with frothy bloody sputum and dyspnea. The diagnosis is not difficult clinically, when these signs appear. Laboratory documentation may be obtained through the chest x-ray, which will demonstrate cardiomegaly and pulmonary plethora.

In acute pulmonary edema, treatment will involve the use of parenteral diuretics, oxygen by nasal cannula, and cardiac glycosides. In mild congestive heart failure, the use of oral diuretics and gradual digitalization are indicated.

One can avoid unexpected congestive heart failure in these patients by taking a careful history. Dyspnea with activity, peripheral edema, and previous hospital admission for chest pain or congestive heart failure are indications of a possible precarious cardiovascular status. The physical examination and simple laboratory procedures such as the chest x-ray will be helpful in making a differential diagnosis.

Other problems which present themselves in these patients are angina pectoris and acute myocardial infarction. The patient who has coronary artery disease usually presents with a history prior to neurologic injury and may experience angina with the rehabilitation program. The use of nitrates, β-adrenergic blockers, and the newer calcium antagonists may be indicated. The extreme of this problem is the development of acute myocardial infarction, with its unrelenting chest discomfort and classic cardiac pain. These patients will require admission to an intensive care unit with close monitoring of rhythm and cardiac hemodynamics. In such circumstances a cardiologist certainly needs to be involved to optimize the care of such patients.

Cardiac arrhythmia may occur in this setting, representing a spectrum of problems from the more benign atrial premature contraction to ventricular tachycardia and ventricular fibrillation (2). The therapist may notice a change in pulse rate, or the patient may become symptomatic with lightheadedness. Baseline ECGs and ambulatory monitoring or, if available, telemetry during the most stressful daily activities will delineate the problem. Atrial arrhythmias may be treated with cardiac glycosides or quinidine. Ventricular premature beats may require Procaineamide® or Inderal®. A cardiologist should be consulted to assist in further management.

It cannot be overemphasized that a careful history will significantly reduce the emergent cardiac problem, since appropriate studies and treatment can be provided before the physical activity program proceeds. The cardiac patient, particularly when there is functional limitation due to angina or myocardial impairment, should be placed in a modified activity program with activities spread out through the day. There should be frequent rest periods during and after activity. Careful monitoring is necessary, with checking of symptoms and vital sign response. Those who were in failure should be weighed daily to assess possible fluid retention. Only if they tolerate such a program should they be allowed to progress to higher levels of activity with lesser concentration on monitoring.

AUTONOMIC DYSREFLEXIA

Autonomic dysreflexia (AD) or autonomic hyperreflexia (AH) is a "mass reflex" syndrome occurring in patients who have had complete spinal cord lesions at or above the T6 level. Actually, signs and symptoms of a mild degree can occur with lesions below T6 and in incomplete disease. Although the exact etiology of the syndrome is not clear, it appears that noxious visceral or cutaneous stimuli result in afferent impulses into the spinal cord giving rise to blood pressure elevation, pilomotor erection, and diaphoresis. In the intact spinal cord, these visceral responses are subdued or eliminated by regulatory discharges from the baroreceptors in the carotid artery, and the aorta is affected through the splanchnic outflow. In the spinal cord injured with lesions at T6 or above, the descending controlling stimuli have lost their efferent loop, which produces the "mass reflex" syndrome.

Clinically, headache and sweating are the most common symptoms, followed by nasal stuffiness, piloerection, and blurring of vision. Hypertension, bradycardia or tachycardia, ventricular premature beats, hyperhidrosis above the level of the lesion, and Horner's syndrome are frequent physical findings.

Aside from the physiologic interests of this syndrome, there are two clinically important features that will be considered. First, the precipitating event may, itself, cause additional problems that may be life threatening. Urinary bladder distention, for example, is the most frequent cause (76%) due to a blocked urinary catheter or calculus. Overwhelming sepsis may result if this distention is ignored while treatment is directed at the dysreflexia syndrome itself. Therefore, when presented with such a patient, one should make a rapid research for mechanical blockage of the urinary tract. Treatment of this alone will often result in complete interruption of the syndrome and avoidance of septic shock. Other treatable precipitants are severe constipation, pressure sores, fracture, and abdominal emergencies (e.g., appendicitis).

In some cases, there is no obvious precipitating event, and one needs to, therefore, consider the other issue of treatment. Pharmacotherapy has been helpful in the chronic recurrent varieties of the dysreflexia syndrome. One should comment that although the blood pressure response may be frightening, there have been only a few cases reported in literature where the patients have died from the hypertensive response. Phenoxybenzamine, pentolinium, mecamylamine, and guanethidine have been recommended in acute cases since they produce their response either through the sympathetic nervous system or at the ganglia. There are agents acting peripherally, such as diazoxide, hydralazine, or nitroprusside, which are direct arteriolar dilators and have been shown to be extremely helpful. Dosages are individualized, and it is recommended that vasopressors be available for those cases where uncontrolled hypotension results from overtreatment. In the prevention of autonomic dysreflexia, especially during surgical manipulative procedures such as cystoscopy and colonoscopy, preparing the patient with one of the agents listed above, using local anesthetics during cystoscopy or using generalized anesthesia, are usually effective measures in preventing uncontrolled hypertension.

ABDOMINAL EMERGENCIES

The problem of abdominal emergencies is compounded in the neurologically impaired patient because of the sensory or motor status or in the cortically damaged patient because of language impairment. Depending on the extent and level of the injury of the spinal cord patient, for example, abdominal pain and rigidity may be decreased or may be absent entirely. In the cortically brain-damaged individual, obtaining a careful history may be extremely difficult because of receptive and expressive impairment of language. In the presence of discomfort, anxiety will increase, further impairing language output.

The diagnosis, therefore, remains difficult, and one must utilize physical findings and sensitive laboratory procedures. In the spinal cord-injured patient, for example, although the most common causes of fever are urinary tract infection, followed by thrombophlebitis, if abdominal distension occurs, one should look carefully for a site of intra-abdominal inflammatory disease. In some instances, a sudden increase of spasticity in the lower extremities or autonomic dysreflexia along with the other findings would suggest major abdominal surgical disease. In the aphasic or brain-damaged patient, a sudden change in behavior with the appearance of abdominal discomfort and/or distention along with signs of inflammation, should alert the clinician to rule out intra-abdominal disease. In such patients, physical findings would be of the utmost importance since rigidity and tenderness will probably be present without, per-

haps, the localization of the able-bodied individual.

Where clinical presentation occurs, a careful laboratory survey is critical, including abdominal x-rays and intravenous pyelography. Free air under the diaphragm, calcification suggesting calculus in the gallbladder or kidney, and/or obstructive small bowel pattern may be diagnostic of a serious visceral problem. Another test which may be of help, especially in the spinal cord injured if there is no contraindication, is a peritoneal tap with analysis of the fluid. If the clinical suspicion is high and laboratory tests are suggestive, laparotomy may be the only means of ruling out surgical disease.

References

1. Blaisdell WF: Low-dose heparin prophylaxis of venous thrombosis: an editorial. Am Heart J 97:685–686, 1979.
2. Estanol BV, Marin OSM: Cardiac arrhythmias and sudden death in subarachnoid hemorrhage. Stroke 6:382–386, 1975.
3. Greenfield LJ, Zocco J, Wilk J Schroeder TM, Elkins RC: Clinical experience with the Kim-Ray Greenfield vena caval filter. Ann Surg 185:692–698, 1977.
4. Hull R et al: Combined use of leg scanning and impedance plethysmography in suspected venous thromboses. N Engl J Med 296:1497–1500, 1977
5. Kewalramani LS: Neurogenic gastroduodenal ulceration and bleeding with spinal cord injuries. J Trauma 19:259–265, 1979.
6. Kreger BE, Craven DE, McCabe WR: Gram negative bacteremia. IV. Reevaluation of clinical features and treatment in 612 patients. Am J Med 68:344–355, 1980.
7. Miyamoto AT, Miller LS: Pulmonary embolism in stroke: Prevention by early heparinization of venous thrombosis detected by iodine-125 fibrinogen leg scans. Arch Phys Med Rehabil 61:584–587, 1980.
8. Mobin-Uddin K, Utley JR, Bryant LR: The inferior vena cava umbrella filter. Prog Cardiovasc Dis 17:391–399, 1975.
9. Moser KM: State of the art: pulmonary embolism. Am Rev Resp Dis 115:829–852, 1977.
10. Priebe HJ et al: Antacid versus cimetidine in preventing acute gastrointestinal bleeding. N Engl J Med 302:426–430, 1980.

The Painful Sequelae of Injuries to Peripheral Nerves

B. T. SHAHANI and K. YIANNIKAS

Pain is essentially indefinable and cannot really be quantitated. Mountcastle has said that "Pain is that sensory experience evoked by stimuli that injure or threaten to destroy tissue, defined introspectively by every man as that which hurts." For physicians, pain control is often a difficult and frustrating venture. There has been a remarkable expansion of interest and knowledge in the scientific study of pain over the last 15 years, and clinical experience suggests that students, house officers, and practitioners have an inadequate understanding of this clinical problem and its management. A rational approach to the treatment of pain associated with nerve lesions requires an understanding of the neurophysiology of pain and the mechanisms involved in the pathophysiology of pain associated with various forms of peripheral nerve injury. The goals of this section of the chapter are to review the physiological substrate and mechanisms of pain in peripheral nerve injury and the current concepts in management.

THE MECHANISMS OF PAIN IN INJURIES TO PERIPHERAL NERVES

When one considers that all peripheral nerves contain large numbers of sensory nerve fibers it is surprising that traumatic nerve injuries are not painful more frequently. Occasionally, nerve damage is followed by spontaneous pain which is out of proportion to the extent of the injury. Thus, at one end of the spectrum is the painless nerve lesion, and at the other the spontaneous pain of incapacitating severity called *causalgia*. Both central and peripheral mechanisms are involved in the development of painful nerve pathology.

General Mechanisms

PERIPHERAL MECHANISMS

(a) Local structural changes in nerve fibers of the damaged segment render them more susceptible to physical deformation and ischemia.

(b) Involvement of the damaged segment of nerve in adhesions and scar tissue which may affect the blood supply.

(c) A sensitive neuroma at the site of a lesion in continuity or on the proximal stump of a severed nerve develops fiber sprouts within it that are spontaneously active, sensitive to pressure, and silenced by repetitive antidromic stimulation.

(d) The presence of hypersensitive degenerating or immature regenerating axons at the site of the lesion with unusual impulse generation and conduction properties. Abnormally myelinated degenerating or regenerating fibers have been shown to have increased excitability. Impulses are generated in these fibers in three ways: (i) spontaneous ectopic excitation; (ii) autoexcitation, i.e., firing from the site of ectopic excitation in an axon as a sequel to a previous impulse transversing the site of ectopic excitation; and (iii) the formation of artificial synapses (ephaptic).

Stable electrical fiber-fiber interaction may occur between pairs of injured axons, and this cross-talk may be long lasting. Furthermore, one cannot show that an observed small diameter fiber is not connected to a large diameter fiber; thus, neither the central connections of the observed fiber nor the physiological properties of its peripheral receptor can be determined.

These abnormally excitable fibers demonstrate abnormal sensibility to mechanical stimuli and to acetylcholine and noradrenaline. Korenman and Devor (5) found that sensory axons terminating in a neuroma produce a massive discharge when adrenaline or noradrenaline is injected into the peripheral circulation and suggested the presence of abnormal α-adrenergic receptors.

(e) Injury discharge. Ill-sustained injury discharge has been reported acutely following the section of peripheral axons and dorsal roots and may contribute to immediate pain associated with nerve lesions.

It thus appears that the peripheral component of pain is related to degeneration and/or partial regeneration of unmyelinated and small diameter myelinated fiber.

CENTRAL MECHANISMS

Recently, it has been shown that there are important alterations in the dorsal horn following peripheral nerve injury.

Ultrastructural Changes

Changes in afferent terminals in lamina 2 have been seen after sciatic nerve section in the rat. Peripheral section also leads to the appearance of nonneural "reactive cells" which accumulate in the dorsal horn by 3 days after sciatic nerve section or crush.

Biochemical Changes

Substance P, somatostatin, and acid phosphatase decrease after dorsal-root or peripheral nerve section. Capsaicin, which blocks conduction in A-delta and C fibers, also leads to depletion of substance P in the dorsal horn.

Electrophysiological Changes

The biochemical and histological changes correlate well with the reduction in the dorsal root potentials (DRPs) and failure of depolarization of the terminals of primary afferents (PAD) in the dorsal horn. The failure of PAD, which has been associated with presynaptic surround inhibition or block, may be associated with disinhibition and an amplification of otherwise weak afferent signals.

Receptive Field Changes

Devor and Wall (3) showed that dorsal horn cells in the cat, which had lost their normal afferent input as a result of peripheral denervation, adopted new receptive fields supplied by the nearest intact nerves. The majority of changes that occur are concentrated in the substantia gelatinosa. However, changes have also been reported in second order neurons suggesting that either other afferents sprout within the spinal cord or that previously existing but ineffective afferents become effective.

The relative contribution of peripheral and central mechanisms is difficult to assess, but there is no doubt that impulses from the periphery play a role, for discomfort is temporarily alleviated by peripheral local anesthesia. Furthermore, in grafted cases, recurrence of pain seems to take place synchronously with the reappearance of peripheral sensitivity. However, the peripheral mechanisms do not explain two crucial aspects of the problem: ongoing pain often recurs in the original area after complete transsection of the nerve, which denervates a larger area than the disordered one, and the pain and abnormal sensitivity are accurately duplicated after regeneration. It thus appears that patients transfer the source of abnormal processing of impulses from the periphery to more central structures.

A perplexing problem: certain humans repeatedly develop pains while others remain pain free after seemingly identical nerve injuries. The demonstration that subtle genetic factors can influence the development of anesthesia dolorosa in rats with ligation of a hind limb nerve may help to explain this; however, it needs further investigation.

Clinical Syndromes of Painful Nerve Lesions

PAIN RELATED TO DAMAGE OF NON-NEURAL TISSUE

Painful stimuli may activate a receptor of low threshold to some chemical or chemicals produced by tissue damage. Histamine has been shown to excite nociceptors (PMN) and C fibers in the cat, as has serotonin (5-HT), although moderate amounts of serotonin are not painful in human skin. Another group of proposed inflammatory mediators are the kinins, and bradykinin is found to be painful when injected into human skin. There is considerable evidence that prostaglandins are inflammatory mediators, and intravenous infusion of PGE_1 and PGE_2 produce sensitization to heat stimulation in nociceptive C-fibers from feline skin. Other agents implicated include angiotensin and substance P.

PAINFUL POLYNEUROPATHIES

Clinical patterns of neuropathy represent a continuum from the painless distal sensory loss to the severe burning pain, with dysesthesia and autonomic disturbances. Early work based on the *gate control theory* suggested that pain was due to the loss of inhibition normally provided by large diameter fibers. However, loss of large diameter fibers is not necessarily associated with pain. In Friedreich's ataxia, there is preferential loss of large diameter fibers without pain. On the other hand, Fabry's disease is associated with loss of small myelinated fibers and pain. Brown et al. (1) have shown that painful diabetic neuropathy is characterized by pathology of unmyelinated and small myelinated fibers. However, hereditary sensory neuropathy is associated with loss of small diameter fibers and analgesia. Dyck et al. (4) suggested that the painfulness in peripheral neuropathy

is associated with the rate and kind of nerve fiber degeneration. Pain was present in 19 of 25 patients with acute fiber degeneration and only in 5 of 34 patients with more chronic forms. Furthermore, abnormal pain sensation was found only when there was unequivocal pathology in small myelinated or unmyelinated fibers.

All combinations have been reported, and correlation of the remaining fiber diameter spectrum with symptomatology of neuropathies is not valid. The problem lies in the interpretation of biopsy specimens since anatomy does not always predict physiology. In experimental neuromas of the sciatic nerve of the rat, the fiber spectrum of the parent sciatic nerve is normal, but the small myelinated afferents conduct impulses from the neuroma. It is most likely that pain associated with peripheral neuropathy is related to degeneration (Wallerian or axonal) of unmyelinated and small myelinated fibers or to partial degeneration and regeneration.

PAIN ASSOCIATED WITH PLEXUS OR ROOT AVULSION

Avulsion lesions are invariably associated with distressing pain and most workers have found severe pain in a high percentage of patients with total paralysis. The pain, which takes some time to develop after the injury, is usually characterized by severe burning sensations accompanied by pins and needles in the distribution of the avulsed root (causalgia) and may be present in 25% of cases up to 4 years after the injury. The pain is most likely the result of central neuronal disturbances secondary to deafferentation and correlates well with reports of deafferentation syndromes following dorsal rhizotomies in animal studies. In cases with complete deafferentation, peripheral modulation techniques are unsuccessful.

PAINFUL NERVE LESIONS

Painful Neuroma

The site of injury to the nerve may be occupied by a tender neuroma, pressure or traction on which causes pain or other unpleasant sensations to radiate to the region originally innervated by the severed nerve. Large soft swellings usually contain highly sensitive regenerating axons which may have spontaneous impulse discharges.

Painful Entrapment Lesions

The incarcerated nerve fiber suffers from anoxia, compression, and accumulation of metabolites. Nerve fibers damaged in this way discharge spontaneously and are the source of pain in these lesions. Decompression releases the process, restores the circulation, and provides relief.

CAUSALGIA

On occasion trauma to a peripheral nerve, avulsion of the brachial plexus or roots, trauma to cauda equina, arachnoiditis, and certain types of peripheral neuropathy have associated pain in the upper or lower limbs which is so severe that it becomes incapacitating to the patient. Such pain is usually spontaneous and, although it waxes and wanes, it is continuous. It is most often described as a burning sensation and is often associated with an unbearable numbness, tingling, and coldness. Such pain is nearly always associated with neurological deficit, usually with an elevated somatosensory threshold, particularly to nociception. Hyperpathia is often present, and despite the fact that the lesions associated with causalgia are often incomplete, trophic changes contribute a striking feature of the condition. Characteristically, the onset of the discomfort does not coincide with the neurological insult but rather is delayed for days, even months. A variety of stimuli may intensify the pain or provoke severe attacks, and they commonly fit into two classes: (a) anything that increases the activity of the limb—mechanical, heat, cold, muscular activity; and (b) anything that increases the activity of the central nervous system—visual, auditory, or emotional stimuli. The pain often subsides within 6 months to a year

after the injury; however, it may be present for up to 4 years after the injury.

Neuronal interruption to relieve deafferentation pain is notable for its ineffectiveness at all levels of the nervous system. In a significant number of cases relief is observed from sympathetic block and subsequent sympathectomy. Campbell and Long (2) found that 40% of their patients with deafferentation pain enjoyed excellent results from transcutaneous nerve stimulation and, although the results are not clear, there is a definite tendency for stimulation in peripheral nerves, spinal cord, thalamus, and internal capsule that produces paraesthesia in the painful region to relieve deafferentation pain.

These features suggest that pain associated with deafferentation is a central phenomenon, and that biochemical, anatomical, and electrophysiological changes described earlier are a necessary substrate for this pain.

MANAGEMENT OF PAINFUL NERVE LESIONS

The treatment depends on the type of pain, its severity, and the degree to which it incapacitates the patients. In the case of pain associated with entrapment lesions, decompression of the compartment leads to symptomatic relief. The management of painful neuroma is dependent on whether the painful bulb is associated with a proximal stump or on nerves in continuity. Painful bulbs on nerves in continuity should be treated conservatively. Infiltration of the surrounding tissue with anesthetic will provide temporary relief and, usually, with the passage of time the bulb will become less sensitive. If the painful bulb remains, the nerve should be explored and the neuroma freed from adhesions or scar tissue predisposing to traction deformation during movement. In the chronically painful lesion, resection of the nerve and grafting usually end in a recurrence of the pain in a similar distribution to that before grafting. This is probably due to the development of secondary changes at a central level and the possible reformation of a new neuroma at the suture site. Excision of tender neuromas at the end of proximal stumps usually leads to new nerve bulb formation and is usually as painful as the first operation. Thus, although a single excision early in the course may be justified, repeat excisions are not.

The treatment of chronic pain associated with neuropathies, isolated nerve injuries, and nerve root avulsion is a difficult problem. Various programs report differing success rates; Maruta et al. (6), reviewing the 1-year follow-up of 200 patients, found that only 20% were successful. The recognition that chronic pain is a complex problem and is potentially modifiable at many levels of the nervous system has resulted in a number of important developments in pain research and treatment. Many new approaches have been developed to supplement the more traditional medical and surgical treatments for chronic pain. Rational treatment programs integrate therapy that is directed at multiple levels of the neuraxis, including supraspinal, spinal, and peripheral. The primary focus here is on some of the newer procedures being used, including transcutaneous electrical stimulation, acupuncture, and dorsal column stimulation.

Medications

ANALGESICS

Nonnarcotic

In general, aspirin is the most effective of the milder group of analgesics, which include paracetamol, dextropropoxyphene, etc., and which should be tried for the treatment of mild to moderate pain. These drugs probably cause relief by inhibiting prostaglandins and bradykinin at the receptor level.

Narcotics

The narcotic group of drugs (morphine, pethidine, and codeine) act at multiple levels of the nervous system, including diencephalon, frontal lobes, brain-stem, and spinal cord. These drugs act on opiate receptors and increase the threshold to noxious stimuli as well as modify the response to pain. Because of the possibility of dependence and addiction, they should be used sparingly in acute situations of intractable pain.

ANTIDEPRESSANTS AND SEDATIVES

Depression is a common feature in the symptom complex associated with chronic pain. In this situation tricyclic antidepressants may prove useful. Although not traditionally considered to be analgesic medication, tricyclic antidepressants, especially the methylated forms (imipramine, amitriptyline and doxopin), have been shown in animal studies to produce analgesia. The mechanisms of action are not well defined but may involve blockade of the pain-anxiety-depression-pain sequence by increasing cortical inhibition of sensory input, stimulation of central nervous system endorphins, and blockade of dopaminergic receptors or of reuptake of brain serotonin. There are good theoretical and experimental reasons for experiencing pain relief from tricyclics since zimelidine, a nontricyclic 5-hydroxytryptamine (5-HT) inhibitor, produces pain relief. Although phenothiazines generally do not have analgesic actions, methotrimeprazine, a phenothiazine derivative, may be a potent analgesic, but a mechanism for its pain relieving action has not yet been proposed. There has been some evidence to suggest that combinations of a tricyclic antidepressant with a phenothiazine is more effective than either drug alone, and their efficacy has been documented when used for treatment of painful neuropathies.

ANTICONVULSANTS

Anticonvulsants such as carbamazepine and phenytoin have been used for painful neuropathies, postherpetic neuralgia, and tic doloreux with notable success. The suggested rationale is the stabilization of neuronal hyperactivity.

PLACEBOS

Studies comparing placebo to various analgesics have found that the index of drug efficacy, the decrease in the amount of pain using an unknown drug vs. one of known analgesic effect, is a constant 0.55. Recent work supports the hypothesis that endorphin activity may account for placebo analgesia. The analgesia of narcotics and placebo seems to have a similar mechanism and with repeated use of placebos over longer periods of time, analgesia becomes less effective. Administration of naloxone, a narcotic antagonist, causes an increase in pain ratings in placebo responses.

INTRATHECAL MEDICATIONS

Recent work has suggested impressive pain relief in patients using 0.5 to 1.0 mg of morphine intrathecally or 1.0 to 3.0 mg epidurally. This technique promises great value in obstetric and operative analgesia, but its role in pain associated with nerve lesions is not determined. It appears to be highly specific for pain and is potentially rapidly reversible by naloxone. Yaksh and Rudy (10) has also suggested the effectiveness of intrathecal clonidine and baclofen, but these ideas are still in the experimental stage.

Physiotherapy (PT)

The role of PT is to:

(a) Institute a regime of massage, gentle manipulation, and passive movements
(b) Overcome venous and lymphatic stasis
(c) Encourage the use of the limb. Patients protect the painful limbs and immobilization of the hyperalgesic parts may lead to the development of trophic changes.

Naturally induced sensory inflow produced by different methods of treatment used in PT in some patients can be as effective in bringing relief as electrical stimulation.

Electrical Stimulation

Despite questionable features of the gate control hypothesis of Melzack and Wall (7), it has directed attention to the role of large afferent fiber stimulation in the control of pain and for suggesting possible avenues for clinical application of this method. This theory has led to the introduction of electroanalgesia procedures for the treatment of chronic pain—one at the periphery involving stimulation of the peripheral nerve trunk (transcutaneous electrical nerve stimulation or TENS) and the other based on stimulation of the dorsal columns of the spinal cord. Both procedures activate large fibers, thereby "closing the gate" to the small fiber traffic associated with the production of pain. Central mechanisms of action are supported by observations that TENS produces increases in CSF endorphins and that this analgesia is blocked by naloxone. Furthermore, TENS reduces cortical evoked responses to pain, and this effect is also reversed by naloxone. In addition to this central mechanism there is experimental evidence that some of the pain reduction following peripheral stimulation may be due to antidromic suppression of spontaneous discharge from the damaged nerve segment or neuroma.

In 1967 Wall and Sweet (9) first applied this concept to a clinical situation in the treatment of chronic pain and in the same year Shealy (8) used implanted electrodes to stimulate the dorsal columns of the spinal cord. Two major factors influence the effectiveness of TENS: (a) electrical characteristics of the stimulus and (b) optimal placement of electrodes.

The stimulus is adjusted to produce a tingling, vibratory, or numbing sensation. It should not be painful or cause muscle contraction. The pulse frequency varies from low frequency (2 Hz) to high frequency (60–120 Hz). Higher frequency is said to best stimulate the intraspinal gating mechanisms (no change in endorphin levels) whereas the lower frequency best stimulates endorphinergic mechanisms (increased CSF endorphins). Placement of electrodes is empirical, but stimulation is usually performed within the same segmental distribution as the source of the noxious stimulus. Within the region the operator may select the trigger points, muscle motor points, superficial peripheral nerves, or acupuncture points. Distal points such as median, ulnar, or radial nerve stimulation may be chosen for nonspecific stimulation.

TENS is well tolerated, the commonest side effect being skin irritation. The treatment is most effective in chronic pain associated with peripheral nerve lesions, root avulsion, and postherpetic neuralgia. It does not work well in central pain states and pain associated with sensory peripheral neuropathy. Although 60–70% of patients may respond to this form of treatment on a short-term basis, only 10–15% have long-term effects. There is a trend for patients with lower endorphin levels to have a better response to treatment.

Although *dorsal column stimulation* using implanted radiofrequency stimulating devices requires laminectomy for electrode implantation, a recent modification of this concept, *percutaneous epidermal stimulation*, can be placed without surgery. Both methods require highly skilled and experienced neurosurgical teams and sophisticated equipment to provide optimal electrode placement and are reserved for a selected group of patients for whom other modes of therapy have been unsuccessful.

Acupuncture

Melzack and colleagues (7) have shown there is a close correlation between trigger points and acupuncture points for pain. These similarities arise from observations that pressure at certain points is associated with particular pain patterns and that intense stimulation of these points may produce a prolonged relief of pain. Possible mechanisms include a gate control action and the release of endorphins, as acupuncture-induced analgesia can be reversed by naloxone and is associated with elevation of CSF endorphin levels. Acupuncture is performed by trained individuals using fine, hair-sized, stainless steel needles that are inserted subcutaneously and are either rotated manually or stimulated by an electric current. Localization of meridians may be determined from published atlases.

Surgical Procedures—Sympathectomies

If severe distressing pain persists in association with root and plexus avulsion (causalgia), the regional sympathetic ganglia should be blocked with local anesthetic to test the effect of pharmacologically interrupting sympathetic pathways. This may abate the pain temporarily and in a few cases may even give permanent relief. If relief is temporary then sympathectomy offers the best prospects of obtaining permanent relief. The preganglionic operation is preferred to the postganglionic one as it is more reliable and gives better results. The positive results support the hypothesis that damaged sensory axons develop ectopic α-adrenergic receptors that render them sensitive to sympathetic activity.

References

1. Brown MJ, Martin JR, Asbury AK: Painful diabetic neuropathy. Arch Neurol 33:164–171, 1976.
2. Campbell JN, Long DM: Peripheral nerve stimulation in treatment of intractable pain. J Neurosurg 45:692–699, 1976.
3. Devor M, Wall PD: The physiology of sensation after peripheral nerve injury, regeneration and neuroma formation. In Waxman SG: The Physiology and Pathobiology of Axons. New York, Raven Press, 1978.
4. Dyck PJ, Lambert EH, O'Brien PC: Pain in peripheral neuropathy related to rate and kind of fibre degeneration. Neurology 26:466–471, 1976.
5. Korenman EMD, Devor M: Ectopic adrenergic sensitivity in damaged peripheral nerve axons in the rat. Exp Neurol 72:63–81, 1981.
6. Maruta T, Swanson DW, Swenson WM: Chronic pain: which patients may a pain management program help? Pain 7:321–329, 1979.
7. Melzack R, Wall PD: Pain mechanisms: a new theory. Science 150:971–979, 1965.
8. Shealy CN, Morimer JT, Hagfors NR. Dorsal column electroanalgesia. J Neurosurg 32:560–564, 1972.
9. Wall PD, Sweet WH: Temporary abolition of pain in man. Science 155:108–109, 1967.
10. Yaksh TL, Rudy TA: Studies on the analgesic effects of intrathecal opiates, alpha-adrenergic agonists and baclofen: their pharmacology in primate. Anaesthesiology 54:451–467, 1981.

Aphasia

D. A. OLSON

Aphasia is a very individual problem. The term has different meanings for the patient with aphasia, the physician, nurse, or allied health professional, and the general public. The physician managing the aphasic patient must be aware of all of these implications.

The physician has many means of informally diagnosing aphasia. However, assistance can be obtained through the services of a qualified speech pathologist who is trained in the area of aphasia. The Academy of Aphasia and the American Speech-Language-Hearing Association are the two major professional organizations presently involved in assessment, remediation, and retraining of the aphasic patient.

Aphasia is not just a speech problem. The patient with aphasia has some difficulty (11) in understanding, speaking, reading, writing, and doing arithmetic and spelling. He finds it hard to organize speech for conversational purposes and to think clearly.

CAUSES OF APHASIA

Aphasia is caused by an insult to the brain (12, 13). A trauma, tumor, aneurysm, embolism, hemorrhage, or thrombosis within the brain is the most frequent cause of aphasia. Brain cells do not regenerate; the damage is permanent. Although the destroyed tissues are replaced by scar tissue, clinical experience has shown that the function of the injured brain is nevertheless partially restored. The specific means by which a damaged or a lost function is restored is not well understood or documented, but brain function is known to be highly adaptable, especially in younger patients. Early intervention with therapy programs—speech, physical, and occupational—can greatly support the pa-

tient's early spontaneous recovery and promote maximum possible restoration of functioning.

CARE OF THE PATIENT

Aphasia (a more correct term would be dysphasia, as few patients are totally aphasic) affects the total person. It affects the patient's abilities in all areas of functioning. It most dramatically strikes his language functioning, but behavioral, personality, emotional, social, and vocational changes should all be considered.

To begin to understand the aphasic person, the physician must first know or understand what that person was like before the brain damage occurred. Aphasia does not typically result in complete changes in the individual's manner of coping or behaving, but it does result in less ability to monitor, control, and manage himself efficiently. The patient needs structure and "controlled stimulation" to maximize recovery processes. A major impedance to recovery of the patient with aphasia is the tendency for the health professional to overstimulate the patient. Overstimulation can result from too frequent scheduling, too many people, or too many auditory and visual stimuli. However, *active controlled restimulation* of all areas of deficit must be planned and considered for the aphasic patient. Most aphasic patients have very limited endurance, and fatigue factors must be considered when therapy is planned and the results of that therapy are evaluated.

Each area of the patient's functioning abilities affected by aphasia must be considered in relation to other areas. The interrelationship of all areas of functioning necessitates a team approach to understanding and managing the aphasic patient. Being able to walk and talk again are frequently primary goals for the patient.

TERMINOLOGY

Terminology in the speech and language area is frequently confusing to the new professional. Terminology has been developed from several points of view. The area of neurology, the area of psychology, and the areas of speech and language have in some cases developed their own terminology, which is frequently confusing to other professionals assisting the aphasic patient. Therefore, a descriptive evaluation of the speech and language of the patient is frequently more helpful than many of the more formal terms applied to the patient.

A major subdivision among aphasic syndromes is by the type of speech output. That is, in the expressive aphasic, speech is impaired for imitation, word findings, sequencing, and production, and the resulting speech is nonfluent. In contrast, the more fluent forms of aphasia are characterized by good ability with articulation and frequent long combinations of words in a variety of grammatical forms. Formal and complete testing by the speech and language pathologist can assist the physician.

Few aphasic patients demonstrate only one aphasic type or a true aphasic category (3, 8). Most aphasic patients demonstrate a combination of expressive and receptive difficulties.

EXPRESSIVE APHASIA (BROCA'S APHASIA)

This type is typified by a lack of verbal output. Attempts to verbalize are minimal, frequently ungrammatical, and limited to simple nouns or concrete words. Frequently, the expressive aphasic cannot even initiate desired words. Memory problems, word-finding difficulties, organizational difficulties, and an inability to handle language in an organized fashion for communication purposes are frequent problems. The expressive aphasic lacks the ability to freely verbalize (dyspraxia), the ability to execute simple voluntary acts, and frequently the ability to write (agraphia). Dyscalculia, the functional loss of use of numbers or defects in the ability to calculate, is another expressive language area to be investigated. Another frequent problem is dysnomia or anomia, the difficulty in naming or using common names for articles, objects, or persons in the aphasic's environment.

RECEPTIVE APHASIA (WERNICKE'S APHASIA)

Patients with this disorder are typically very verbal individuals. An outpouring of words occurs, but the words have little meaning to the speaker or the listener. The patient frequently feels he is communicating, but he does not self-monitor his words, and the words have no meaning to him. Understanding and comprehension are basic to the development of all higher language areas. Therefore, the patient's ability to comprehend what he says himself and what others say in his environment is extremely important for the growth of other language areas. Receptive language problems, frequently called agnosias, may relate to inability to recognize and understand colors, size of objects, musical tones, numbers, or body parts.

CONDUCTION APHASIA

This condition is due to a possible disconnection of fiber tracks between the receptive and expressive areas of the brain (5). The patient has very fluent speech, but the fluency is somewhat meaningless, even though the patient shows some ability to understand and frequently has excellent reading abilities. An interesting aspect of this type of aphasia is that the patient is unable to repeat things correctly.

GLOBAL APHASIA

In the patient with global aphasia, all language forms, expressive and receptive, are so seriously affected that it is impossible to categorize him. Such a patient demonstrates the most severe type of problem and frequently has severe comprehension, expressive, and cognitive language difficulties. Global aphasia results from overall damage to the left hemisphere, the areas related to all aspects of language. Even in left-handed persons, all but 15% have a left hemisphere locus for language function.

CONSIDERATIONS IN EVALUATION

Physical Findings

The aphasic patient may also demonstrate hemiplegia or hemiparesis; pain in the shoulder and other physical problems may greatly affect the patient's ability to perform. Many patients are very disturbed by the associated sensory loss, such as that following a cerebrovascular incident. The patient's past history can be a major factor affecting his motivation and performance. The patient may be seizure-prone, or he may be affected by a heavy medication program. These and other physical problems can greatly affect his performance (1, 4).

Psychological Findings

Aphasic patients are people first, and therefore they can display the entire gamut of human behavior. However, certain psychological phenomena are exaggerated or emphasized by aphasia. Increased anxiety is perhaps one of the most observable signs. The aphasic is lost and confused and does not completely understand what has happened to him. Anxiety in a test situation or in any type of performance situation can greatly affect the patient's ability.

The examiner must support the patient as much as possible and attempt to rebuild confidence, which has frequently been shattered. Giving the patient sufficient time, responding to the patient as an adult, calling the patient by an appropriate title, whether it be Dr., Mr., Miss, or Mrs., and in general responding to the patient in a dignified fashion help to ensure a better response.

Limited attention span, poor concentration, hyperactivity, perseveration, regression, and depression are frequently major limiting factors. Psychological reactions are not the same in all aphasic patients. The patient's general personality typically does not change, but this lack of control, his lack of ability to cope, and his general confusion all contribute to an exaggeration of psychological symptoms which he was previously able to control.

Intellectual and Cognitive Functioning

Although in the majority of patients intellectual functioning is not destroyed, the patient's ability to use his intellectual abilities is affected. The brain-injured individual's motor and language problems affect his ability to respond to formal tests of intelligence. Therefore, informal methods of evaluation are frequently more revealing. Also, certain modes of behavior which would help the patient make maximum use of his intellectual abilities should be noted. For example, most aphasic patients have great difficulty in organizing material (2); they cannot pay attention for long periods of time, their judgment is disturbed, they easily shift from one activity to another, they are upset and concerned by new situations, and they cannot correct themselves, even though they may know the right answer. In a structured concrete one-to-one situation, with the patient given maximum time to respond, one can obtain a better impression of the patient's functional abilities.

The intellectual and cognitive functioning of the aphasic patient may well be inefficient, but if the examiner expects a delayed response, plans to give the patient extra time to respond, and allows the patient to speak with a much slower rate of speech, the patient's true ability may be revealed.

Speech

Although some patients show difficulty in producing certain consonants and vowels, the typical aphasic patient has more problems in the language areas. It is by defining his language abilities that we more clearly understand the aphasic patient. In the dysarthric patient, actual paralysis of some of the muscles of speech may occur. Swallowing and feeding difficulties may need to be managed by the nursing or speech-pathology staff. Dyspraxia, due to defective motor signals from the brain to the oral mechanism, may also be observed in many aphasic patients.

Language

Problems in language need to be considered in relation to the patient's ability to take in verbal stimuli and to understand it, as well as to give out verbal stimuli in an intelligible fashion. It is necessary to evaluate the aphasic patient's ability to read, to comprehend what is read, and to interpret the visual symbols he needs for functional reading. Also, evaluation covers his ability to handle numerical symbols as needed in arithmetic. Both the motor needs and the memory and cognitive needs for writing must be considered.

Social Impact

Aphasia has an impact not only on the patient but also on his family. Motivation and progress in aphasic patients are frequently very much related to the support system, whether it be spouse, family, or significant other. Role reversal between husband and wife is frequently necessary following aphasia. Difficulties in the patient's impression of his sexuality and the impression others in his environment have of him as an individual frequently cause serious problems for the aphasic patient. Limitations imposed by the aphasia contribute to a lack of stimulation and potential for retraining and growth. It is important that the aphasic patient have the opportunity for experiences similar to those he had before his stroke. That is, if he enjoyed playing cards or games or participating in sports, adjustments should be made so that he can participate in some form of these activities. Group counseling for family members, as well as for the aphasic patient himself, is frequently indicated.

PROGNOSTIC FACTORS IN APHASIA

There is little agreement on how recovery actually occurs in aphasia. Luria (9, 10) has no doubt presented a hypothesis of recovery in the clearest fashion. Although damaged brain cells do not regenerate, Luria suggests that recovery occurs as shock subsides in the brain following, say, a cerebrovascular incident. That is, damage is limited to one area, but shock is sustained by a much larger area of the brain. As the shock subsides, spontaneous recovery occurs. A second hypothesis states that secondary brain cells can take over the functions of primary brain cells, i.e., several areas can sustain the same functions; if the primary area is damaged, a secondary area can take over with time and retraining. A third hypothesis states that there is a complete reorganization of function in the brain. As this reorganization occurs, due to time and training and other factors, recovery is possible.

Clinically, several factors have been established that aid the physician or therapist in determining prognosis in recovery from aphasia. One of the more obvious indications is the time it takes a patient to recover. Rapid recovery immediately following a stroke or during the early months frequently is an indicator of a better prognosis. The earlier that changes are noted in speech, language, cognition and motor ability, the better the chances for functional improvement on the part of the patient. There also appears to be a tendency that the younger the patient, the better the prognosis. Furthermore, the less severely involved patient appears to progress better than the more severely involved patient.

Clinicians have noted that patients with trauma make better improvement than those with vascular deficiencies. In the recovery stages, the type of aphasia frequently changes. Global aphasics at times become more like receptive aphasics. Perceptive aphasics may change into expressive aphasics, and expressive aphasics into patients with anomia or word-finding problems. A prognosis can also be based on changes noted in the type of aphasia the patient presents.

Recovery (7) occurs over a long period of time following aphasia. The majority of recovery is perhaps noted most dramatically in the first three to six months or during the first year, but persons in contact with aphasic patients over long periods of time note significant changes in the aphasia years after the incident. Again, individual aspects of the patient and of his unique aphasia must always be considered by the physician and the therapist.

SUMMARY

The aphasic patient must be viewed from the perspective of the total problem. Aphasia affects the patient's speech and physical functioning most dramatically (6) but also affects other areas important to health, and intellectual, emotional, and economic needs. The goal of rehabilitation is to provide comprehensive care through obtaining appropriate medical and other health specialists to meet the needs of the patient. It is expected that as a result of this type of intervention, the aphasic patient will be asked to learn to perform up to the maximum of remaining capabilities. An increasing number of studies show that rehabilitation intervention has a significant positive effect on the improvement of aphasic patients. Not only have such patients shown improvement between the time of onset and the first examination, but studies also show that patients who begin therapy months or years after onset can show improvement. The aphasic represents a challenge to the physician, his family, and the rehabilitation team. However, appropriate intervention can result in significant improvements in the condition of a patient with aphasia and can assist in recoping with the world.

References

1. Abreu BC (ed): *Physical Disabilities Manual.* New York, Raven Press, 1981.
2. Basso A, Capitani E, Luzzatti C, Spinnler A: Intelligence and left hemisphere disease: the role of aphasia, apraxia and size of lesion. *Brain* 104:721–734, 1981.
3. Basso A, Capitani E, Vignolo LA: Influence of rehabilitation on language skills in aphasic patients: a controlled study. *Arch Neurol* 36(4):190–196, 1979.
4. Goldenson RM, Dunham JR, Dunham CS (eds): *Disability and Rehabilitation Handbook.* New York, McGraw-Hill, 1978.
5. Goodglass H, Kaplan E: *The assessment of aphasia.* Philadelphia, Lea & Febiger, 1972.
6. Hirschberg GG, Lewis L, Vaughan P: *Rehabilitation: a manual for the Care of the Disabled and Elderly,* ed 2, Philadelphia, Lippincott, 1976.
7. Jennett B, Teasdale G: *Management of Head Injuries.* Philadelphia, FA Davis, 1981.
8. Kottke FJ, Stillwell GK, Lehmann JF: *Krusen's Handbook of Physical Medicine and Rehabilitation,* ed 3. Philadelphia, WB Saunders, 1982.
9. Luria AR: *Restoration of Function after Brain Injury.* New York, Macmillan, 1963.
10. Luria AR: *Traumatic Aphasia: Its Syndromes, Psychology and Treatment.* The Hague, Mouton, 1970.
11. Mohr JP: The evaluation of aphasia. Curr Concepts Cerebrovasc Dis Stroke 16:29–32, 1981.
12. Rusk HA: *Rehabilitation Medicine.* St. Louis, CV Mosby, 1977.
13. Sarno MT: *Acquired Aphasia.* New York, Academic Press, 1981.

Special Resource

American Speech-Language-Hearing Association
10801 Rockville Pike
Rockville, Md.

CHAPTER ELEVEN

Musculoskeletal Problems

Mobility Problems of the Muscle-Joint Unit*

W. C. STOLOV

All physicians must deal with disturbances of the muscles, joints, and bones. Some of the commoner presenting problems will be described in this chapter.

Even an intact central and peripheral nervous system is severely compromised in the absence of sufficient integrity of the functional unit of the musculoskeletal system, namely, the joint and its associated structures. Ambulation is impossible if the hip, knee, and ankle joints have no motion, and no purposeful activity of the upper limb can exist if no motion exists at the shoulder, elbow, wrist, and hand joints, regardless of how intact the nervous system may be.

A joint is a union of two bones, and the nature of this union varies widely. The unions of most interest in disease and trauma are the synovial joints since almost all important joints of the appendicular skeleton are synovial. In this section the principles of joint range of motion,

joint stability, muscle tone, and joint contracture are reviewed, and the management of problems of joint instability and contractures are discussed. In addition, two special problems, burns and fracture aftercare, are highlighted.

PRINCIPLES

Joint Range of Motion and Stability

No two synovial joints (except for the obvious left-right symmetries) are exactly the same. True understanding, therefore, of each joint, requires complete knowledge of anatomical structure and associated periarticular tissues. All synovial joints, however, do have in common a number of components: (a) the articular cartilage at the bone ends; (b) the synovium which, with the cartilage, outlines the joint cavity; (c) the synovial fluid within the cavity; and (4) the capsule (Fig. 11.1). Joints also have ligaments crossing the union that are either reinforcements of the capsule or distinctly extra-articular. To complete the picture, the muscles

* Supported in part by Research Grant G008200020, NIHR, DOE, Washington, D.C.

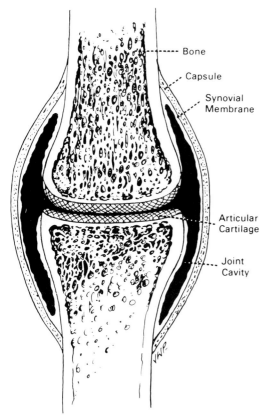

Figure 11.1. Schematic diagram of longitudinal section through a synovial joint. The size of the joint cavity (*black areas*) is exaggerated. Note that the synovial membrane reflects off the capsule along the bone to the edge of the cartilage. (Reproduced with permission from: C Rosse and DK Dawson. *The Musculoskeletal System in Health and Disease.* New York, Harper & Row, 1980).)

that cross the union and produce the movements must also be considered.

The assessment of joint *range of motion* (*ROM*) in the evaluation of joint integrity is a passive maneuver. With the patient relaxed, the examiner moves the distal bone of the union with relation to the proximal bone in the directions in which the examiner understands movement can be achieved in the normal. In addition to an actual measurement of the angles of the extremes of the movement and their comparison with standard expectations (see Appendix, Part II), the examiner also stresses the joint in planes or directions

not ordinarily possible. These maneuvers, together with inspection and palpation, allow the examiner to derive an understanding of the integrity of the joint.

Joints permit movements about a single axis (humeroradial, humeroulnar), about two axes (radiocarpal), or around multiple axes (the ball-and-socket joints of the glenohumeral and pelvifemoral articulations). The features that dictate the movements allowed and their extent include the shape of the articular surfaces of the two bones, the location and integrity of capsule and ligament attachments, the presence or absence of effusion or synovial hypertrophy and, in the extra-articular domain, the muscles crossing the joint. Passive joint ROM can also be compromised if the maneuver produces pain. Involuntary guarding (spasm) or volitional contraction by the patient of the muscle that elongates during the motion assessment must also be evaluated as a possible cause for reduced mobility. When a patient is asked to perform an active ROM, the range achieved may be further compromised by pain, weakness, and even functional inhibition.

Evaluation of the integrity of the shape of the joint surfaces usually requires radiological examination. Evaluation for the existence of a cavity occupying effusion or synovial hypertrophy usually requires palpation. Evaluation of the capsules and ligaments requires the passive ROM maneuver described. Evaluation of the muscles requires a somewhat similar maneuver.

Capsules, ligaments, and also tendons are specialized forms of connective tissue. They consist of cellular and extracellular components. The cellular component consists mostly of fibroblasts which are arranged in rows parallel to the collagen fibers that they elaborate. In addition to collagen fibers, the extracellular matrix consisting of water and proteoglycans that is sometimes referred to as the "ground substance." The gel provides polysaccharide complexes. The polysaccharides are called glycosaminoglycans, which are large molecules of various sugar polymers arrayed with hexosamines. The main glycosaminoglycans in capsules and ligaments include chondroitin 4 and 6 sulfate, hyaluronic acid, dermatin sulfate, and keratin sulfate.

The collagen fibers of ligaments and tendons are organized parallel to the axis of tension. Since collagen fibers are relatively inextensible, little to no force is required to draw them out from a folded or redundant position until they are at full length. At that point, they can sustain a great force without further extension bringing the bones of the joint union into strong compression. Ligaments are generally drawn out to full length only at one position within the range of motion of a joint.

In capsules, collagen fibers are oriented in a weave with many crossover points and form acute angles with the axis of tension. The development of tension within a capsule upon extension is somewhat different, therefore, than occurs within a tendon or ligament. When redundant, very little or no force is necessary to elongate the capsule until the collagen fibers become straight. At this point, further extension requires increasing force as the angular orientation of the collagen fibers with the line of stress becomes more acute. Since the collagen fibers in capsules are attached from bone to bone in a crisscross manner, at maximum extension they are still not fully parallel to the axis of stress. Capsules therefore exhibit a softer end point than do ligaments. Capsules are redundant in the midpositions of a joint's range and are only taut at the extremes. Thus, in a hinged joint, for example, the capsule on the flexor surface is taut on full extension, and the capsule on the extensor surface is taut on full flexion.

Synovial effusions, hemarthroses, and synovial hypertrophy by occupying the joint cavity reduce capsule redundancy in the midpositions. They will limit the extremes of motion simply because the capsule will draw to full length before the normally expected extreme motion is reached. Major effusions and synovial overgrowths might actually separate the opposing articular cartilage to further reduce redundancy in the midpositions.

Problems of the muscles crossing the joints are extra-articular causes of limited joint motion and must be distinguished from causes that are capsular, ligamentous, or intra-articular.

Joint stability is a concept that examines the questions, "How well do the opposing articular surfaces stay in contact at movement extremes?", "How well and with what forces do they stay in contact during active motion?", and "How well do they stay in contact when the joint union is stressed in directions a joint is *not* supposed to move?"

Perhaps the most important factor for joint stability is its basic architecture. Thus, for example, the deep acetabulum reinforced by the acetabular labrum provides a strong stable socket for the femoral head. On the other hand, the shallower surface of the glenoid, even with the labrum, does not effectively "hold" the humeral head. Synovial fluid surface tension and atmospheric pressure also add to the forces holding articular surfaces in approximation. In the lower extremities, particularly in the standing posture, gravitational forces contribute to joint stability. On the other hand, gravitational forces work to distract the upper extremity joints.

The concept of loose-pack and close-pack positions is useful in understanding when a joint may be less stable and more vulnerable. The *loose-pack* positions are those positions in a joint's ROM arc where the ligaments and capsules are slack. Stability or strong approximation of the articular surfaces in such positions depends upon the forces exerted by the muscles across the joint. Furthermore, in these loose-pack positions, the area in contact at the articular surfaces is generally low.

In loose-pack positions, if the muscles are also relaxed, the joints are more vulnerable and less able to resist an external force.

The *close-pack* position is that in which there are maximum contact between the articular surfaces and maximum tautness to the ligaments. Both features provide tight compression between the articular cartilages. In the close-pack positions the two bones, in essence, "become one." Thus, for example, the knee in full extension, the hip in full extension, and the elbow in full extension are in their most stable or close-pack position. On the other hand, the glenohumeral joint does not have very strong ligaments that draw taut in any of the motion extremes. Shoulder joint stability is, therefore, much more dependent upon active muscle contraction for maintenance of a close approximation of the articular surfaces.

The above review suggests methods by which joint stability can be assessed. This assessment requires, first, an understanding of the shape of the joint surface, the capsule locations, and the position in which the ligaments are usually taut. The assessment attempts first to distract the surfaces while in the loose pack position, with the muscles relaxed, to determine if the movement produced is greater than normal. This maneuver mostly assesses the capsule. In the next step, the examiner places the joint in its close-pack position when the ligaments should be taut, and then stresses the joint in the directions it is not supposed to move. This latter maneuver assesses mostly the integrity of the ligaments. Thus, the elbow in the extended posture is stretched medially and laterally to evaluate its collateral ligaments. Finally, the muscles across the joint are assessed for the integrity of their *origins* and *insertions* and for *strength*. Synovial joints are said to be subluxed or capable of subluxation if, on these relative movements, less than a normal surface area of contact of the articular cartilages results. Joints are said to be dislocated when there is no longer any contact of opposing articular surfaces. In the latter instance, frank capsular and ligamentous ruptures must occur.

Muscle Tone

The assessment of muscle tone is similar to that which is done to determine passive joint ROM. The tone of the muscle or muscles crossing the synovial joint is assessed by appreciation of the force necessary to move the distal bone relative to the proximal bone. The muscle or muscles assessed are those elongated by the movement. Since the movement is performed by the examiner, it is called a passive stretch or elongation. The magnitude of the force applied to produce the movement reflects the tension (tone) developed as elongation occurs. This tension may be assessed dynamically, that is, during the stretch, or statically, at some time after the stretch has ceased and the muscle has held at its new length.

Although the elongation is performed passively and the patient is asked to relax all of his musculature, there are situations where α-motor neuron discharge occurs. Examples include spasticity and the α-rigidity of Parkinsonism. Thus, one considers the state of the muscle as either being active or passive, the latter state existing when no α-motor neuron discharge is occurring either during or after stretch.

In *hypertonia* there is an increased resistance to the passive stretch. This can be appreciated dynamically as well as statically and may contain an active component. In spasticity, the hypertonia, has an active component and is dependent upon the rate of stretch. The faster the muscle is stretched, the greater the tension develops. In severe spastic states the active α-motor neuron discharge may persist at the new length. *Hypotonia* defines a decreased resistance to passive stretch and rarely has an active component, either dynamically or statically.

Contracture

If, on the performance of a passive ROM examination, full range is not achieved, then capsule or muscle contracture is suspected. A limitation of ROM can also be secondary to joint surface irregularities, synovial effusion, or synovial hypertrophy. While, sometimes, these situations are also referred to as joint contractures, the term should be limited to those situations where limitation of full range is secondary to capsule, ligament, or muscle problems. The term flexion contracture means limitation of extension and *vice versa*; the term that describes the contracture is opposite to the motion actually limited. Furthermore, the term deformity, sometimes used in place of contracture, is usually reserved for those situations in which the posture change is strictly due to a problem of bone. The following reviews only capsule and muscle contractures. The pathology and problems introduced by ligament contractures are similar to those of the capsules.

Capsule contractures are induced by prolonged posturing of a joint in the position that approximates the proximal and distal attachments of the capsule. Over time, changes within the capsule lead to the situation in which, when motion is finally allowed or attempted, the capsule draws tight before the end point of the range of motion expected in the normal can be reached. The capsule is said to be "shortened."

Akeson *et al.* (1) have demonstrated that total collagen does not change in capsule contractures produced by chronic flexion postures in animals, although turnover rates may increase. More specifically, water and glycosaminoglycan loss occurs. The effect is a reduced buffering action of the gel between collagen fibers and a greater likelihood of cross-linkaging of one collagen fiber to the next at the crossover points. Increasing crosslinks have been demonstrated and it has been postulated that they are facilitated by bridging by newly formed collagen fibrils. The net effect of binding at crossover sites

appears to be that the weave cannot be drawn out to normal length.

Muscle contracture also results from a chronic positioning of the joint or joints crossed that places the crossing muscle in a shortened posture. The mechanism, however, of this contracture is different than in capsule. Muscle contracture is said to be present when, on its elongation, insufficient length is achieved to produce a full range of joint motion, unless, of course, actual rupture of the muscle-tendon complex has occurred. This is akin to the appreciation of hypertonia, namely, a high resistance to passive elongation.

The entire muscle complex needs to be considered in the search for the reason for this inability. The complex includes the origin and insertion tendons, the origin and insertion aponeuroses, from and to which the muscle fibers and bone are attached, the muscle fibers themselves, and the architectural arrangement of these structures. Figure 11.2 schematically displays tension-length relationships that are illustrative. It shows the rest length, that length at which tension first is appreciated on elongation, and how

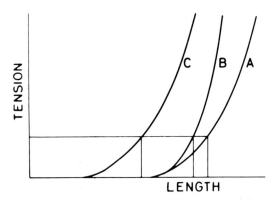

Figure 11.2   Schematic representation of the passive tension-length relationship of whole muscle-tendon complexes. *Curve A* represents the normal; *curve B* is a muscle exhibiting contracture manifest by a steep rise in tension with elongation; and *curve C* exhibits contracture by a shift in rest length to lower values. Muscles can also show combinations of *B* and *C* effects. Note at any tension the muscle lengths of *B* and *C* are less than those of *A* (i.e., contracture).

much additional length can be achieved with an increase in tension. If the tension rises too steeply, or the rest length has decreased to shorter values, the muscle length required for full joint range may not be achieved. Figure 11.3 illustrates an actual situation for normal muscle, and Figure 11.4 illustrates denervated muscle positioned in the shortened posture.

The muscle contracture produced by immobilization in a shortened posture appears to be a combination of origin and insertion aponeurosis changes in length as well as changes in muscle fiber length (4, 5) (Fig. 11.5). Of particular interest as the muscle remodels to its new length is an associated reduction of up to 25% in the adult rat and 60% in the baboon in the number of sarcomeres arrayed from end to end within the muscle fibers.

Since, in the clinical situation, the same maneuvers are used to determine the presence of capsule and muscle contracture, separation of the two is sometimes difficult. It is easiest for two joint muscles whereby appropriate positioning of the muscle of interest can be put on greater slack. Furthermore, capsule contracture end points are generally firmer and less pliant than muscle contracture end points. In many clinical problems, both capsule and muscle contracture occur.

The term *spastic contracture* refers to an inability to achieve a full passive range of motion because of active α-motor neuron discharge during stretch, and at the end of stretch contracture is of such a magnitude that the active tension cannot be overcome. If persistent for a long enough length of time, secondary true muscle contracture and capsule contracture may occur. Temporary nerve blocks that paralyze the muscle followed by the ROM test can usually be used to test for the presence of secondary contractures.

MANAGEMENT

Instability

When trauma creates acute joint instability via complete rupture of ligament or

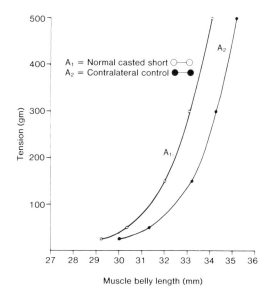

Figure 11.3 Effect of immobilization on contracture in normal rat gastrocnemius muscle after 5 weeks of positioning in knee flexion and ankle plantar flexion. Curve A1, tension-length relationship for immobilized muscle; Curve A2 normal control. At all tensions, length of A1 muscle is less than that of A2 due mostly to a shift in rest length.

capsule, modern approaches to treatment include early surgical repair, particularly in the relatively young. These repairs are often more than simple suture of frayed ends of torn ligaments and can also include the use of artificial materials or fascial transplants. The ligaments of the knee may well be treated with acute surgical repair. Since ligament and capsule connective tissue are relatively avascular, healing periods without surgery via approximation of torn structures and immobilization are 4 to 6 weeks or longer. Immobilization with or without surgery may induce secondary capsule and muscle contracture which then need to be corrected after mobilization is allowed.

More often than not, treatment of instability secondary to ligament and capsule laxity may be an appropriate progressive resistance exercise to strengthen the musculature about the joint to provide dynamic stability. Instability secondary to problems of the joint surface architecture

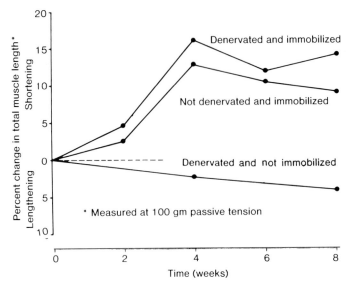

Figure 11.4.   Comparison of contracture produced in normal and denervated rat gastrocnemius muscle immobilized in shortened posture (see legend to Fig. 11.3). Denervated muscle shows greater shortening. Note that the denervated muscle that was not immobilized actually lengthened secondary to positioning in dorsiflexion during experimental period.

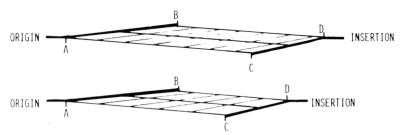

Figure 11.5.   Schematic longitudinal cross-section of rat soleus drawn to scale. (*Above*) Normal soleus; (*Below*) Soleus after immobilization in shortened posture for 5 weeks. Note that the contracture producing the shortening of AD was achieved by shortening of fibers (AC and BD) and shortening of insertion aponeurosis CD.

may lend itself to surgical correction and the use of artificial joints.

Capsule Contracture

Contractures are easier to prevent than to treat. Once present, their reversal requires restoration of lost water and proteoglycan and rupture of collagen cross-linkages. Inasmuch as chronic positioning in the shortened posture induced them, therapeutics are directed at promoting positioning in the extended posture. Thus, in capsule contracture in flexion, active motion of the extensor muscles and re-

sistance exercises to the extensor muscles promote contracture reduction. Prolonged passive stretch at low force also induces elongation. The latter is achievable by manual or sling traction. Furthermore, bivalved serial casts or splints progressively posturing the limb into extension with removal twice per day to allow the exercise activity can be useful. The direction of force application is specific; if incorrect, joint instability can be produced or pressure necrosis of articular cartilage can occur. Temperature elevation of the shortened structures during prolonged low force stretch also adds to permanency of the elongation (6).

Temperature elevation near and about joint surfaces (e.g., near capsules and ligaments) is best achieved through ultrasound diathermy (2). Recently, pharmaceutical attempts to inhibit proteoglycan loss during periods of immobilization of capsules in the shortened posture show promise to minimize capsule contracture formation (1).

Muscle Contracture

Muscle contractures are also managed by progressive positioning of the muscle into elongated postures. Chronic low force tension and elongation via serial casts or splints will induce remodeling to increasing lengths. This remodeling includes increasing elongation of origin and insertion aponeuroses and a relengthening of muscle fibers through restoration of lost sarcomeres and, hence, is a longer process. Relatively short-term stretching and heating are not therefore as useful, but it is possible that prolonged temperature elevation and increased blood flow might accelerate the metabolic process necessary, although this has not yet been definitely proven. In addition, since muscle atrophy occurs with immobilization, strengthening of the muscle that has undergone contracture should also occur to stimulate myofibril and sarcoplasm production. In progressive serial casting or splinting for the removal of capsule or muscle contracture, repositioning at least every 3–5 days is usually necessary.

Spastic contracture requires efforts to minimize the α-motor neuron discharge. In addition to oral pharmacological agents that reduce spasticity either at the spinal cord or muscle level, phenol blocks at motor points or at the muscle nerve can minimize the spastic component of the contracture. When capsule, ligament, and muscle contractures are extreme, surgical measures (e.g., soft tissue release, tendon lengthening, or osteotomy) may be necessary to restore range of motion.

SPECIAL PROBLEMS

Burns

Deep partial thickness burns, in which all of the epithelium and the dermis down to its deeper layer are involved, and the full-thickness burns, in which all dermis is destroyed heal by contracture of the wound with resultant major contractures and secondary joint immobility. Even with modern plastic surgical grafting techniques, much healing still occurs by wound contraction and scar formation. Burn scar has much cellular and capillary activity. The collagen, elaborated by the fibroblasts initially, is layed down in disordered bundles and whorls. Myofibroblast cells of unknown origin elaborate smooth muscle-like filaments which attach to the collagen bundles and contribute to wound contraction.

One of the goals of burn treatment during scar formation is minimization of this marked cellular activity and associated wound contraction and the avoidance of hypertrophic scar formation. The contracture tendency of hypertrophic scar may extend for up to 15 months; hence, even after wound closure, active treatment needs to be maintained to protect against disability development.

With regard to scar contraction, it has been demonstrated that application of continuous pressure minimizes scar hypertrophy and reduces the length of time it takes for scar maturation and for the contraction process to cease. Maintenance of continuous pressure daily for close to 24 hours until scar maturation is complete is necessary to protect against wound contraction. Pressures must be maintained about 25 mm Hg greater than capillary pressure. If pressure dressings are removed for cleaning or for exercise, no more than 1 hour should be allowed to elapse without resumption of compression. Pressure can be applied right after a graft and during the epithelialization process. Elastic garments, such as made by Jobst, and various face masks utilizing elastic garments, silastic molds or formed clear plastic masks are used and must continue to be used until full maturation has been achieved. Figure 11.6 illustrates the type of contracture and reduced mobility that can occur in neck burns treated without pressure garments. Figure 11.7 illustrates a total-contact clear plastic mask for providing continuous pressure in scar areas to soften and prevent scar hypertrophy and its attendant contraction. Joint contractures will develop secondary to hypertrophic scar of the skin tissue across a joint, even if the joint muscle unit is not involved in the burn itself. These secondary contractures are both muscular and capsular. If they do develop, then simply attending only to the skin will not restore full range of motion (3).

Joint contractures may also occur in burn management, secondary to convenience or neglect. Joints and attendant skin totally uninvolved in the burn process may end up being postured for too long a time in a single position, with the resultant secondary problems of muscle and capsule contracture as earlier described. An elbow that is always flexed, a shoulder that is always adducted, or a knee that is always flexed during the time the patient is in bed or is having his burns attended to are postures that are easily avoided.

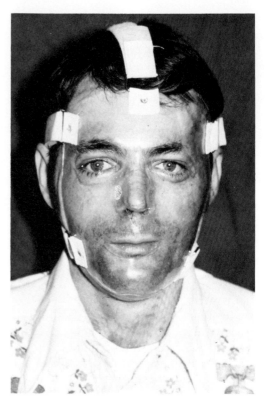

Figure 11.7 Clear plastic mask formed from silastic mold of the face provides continuous pressure to inhibit hypertrophic scar formation.

Joint contractures secondary to comfort are a more difficult problem to prevent. When movement or positioning is productive of pain, it is difficult to sustain the patient's cooperation. Much rapport among physician, therapist, nurse, and patient, as well as appropriate pain management, are all essential. (See also the section on *Burns* by Dr. Fisher in Chapter 14).

Fracture Aftercare

The guiding principle behind fracture treatment is maintenance or, rather, restoration of function, *not* necessarily the production of an anatomically correct union. The function goal, therefore, is a joint with full ROM, adequate stability, and sufficient muscular strength. Fractures are treated via closed reduction, or via open reduction with associated internal

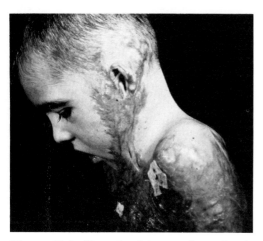

Figure 11.6 Hypertrophic scar formation in healed burned tissue managed without compression dressings produced this marked wound contracture into neck flexion.

fixation. Either approach requires immobilization for a length of time sufficient to secure a union that will hold if immobilization is removed and significant exercise is permitted. Immobilization after closed reduction is generally done with plaster casts, which invariably incorporate the joint proximal and distal to the fracture. In open reductions, internal fixation may be sufficient to avoid external immobilization. There is a trend toward earlier mobilization and more specificity in immobilization, as in the fracture bracing approach.

In addition to the often unavoidable problems of secondary capsule and muscle contracture, and disuse atrophy and weakness, care must be taken to avoid unnecessary soft tissue fibrosis. Extravasation of edema fluid occurs as a result of the original injury to the soft tissue secondary to the initial inflammatory response. Removal of this edema fluid, as well as extravasated blood, within 1 or 2 weeks through immediate resorption, usually preserves soft tissue integrity. If, however, removal requires organization and associated fibrous tissue replacement (brawny edema), adhesion problems affecting relative movement between muscles, bones, fascial layers, and bursae develop.

Limb elevation and active motion of muscles across proximal and distal joints not involved in the immobilization are two techniques that can be used early to achieve edema resolution. Where possible, massage to enhance the return flow circulation can help minimize early edema. Where permitted, isometric exercises within the case can further assist early edema resolution and prevent fibrous tissue formation. Ice packing in the first few hours after fracture helps control blood extravasation from ruptured vessels and soft tissue edema fom the initial inflammatory response.

As bony union begins to develop and the immobilization is discontinued, the problems that need to be dealt with include capsule and muscle contracture, residual edema (more likely now brawny), soft tissue adhesions, and muscle atrophy. A daily ritual of temperature elevation, massage, and active exercise often associated with elastic Ace wraps, assists the removal of the brawny edema and begins a reconversion of whatever fibrous adhesions may have occurred into a looser connective tissue. The active exercise is followed by progressive resistance exercises to restore normal muscle strength. In the appendages, whirlpool treatment is particularly useful because the heat and massaging action of the water can be coupled simultaneously with active exercise of the joints. In tissue with a relatively normal blood supply, whirlpool temperatures for the upper or lower extremity can be carried up to 110°F (43.3°C). For half-body immersion, temperatures should be kept to about 104°F (40°C) and at 100°F (38°C) for full-body immersion.

The principles of reversal of capsule and muscle contracture in postfracture management are the same as already discussed.

Physicians providing proper fracture aftercare management must be sensitive also to some of the complications of fractures that affect mobility, such as myositis ossificans, reflex sympathetic dystrophy, compartment syndromes, and associated nerve injuries.

References

1. Akeson WH, Amiel D, Woo SL: Immobility effects on synovial joints: the pathomechanics of joint contracture. *Biorheology.* 17:95–110, 1980.
2. Lehmann JF, deLateur BJ, Warren CG, Stonebridge JB: Heating of joint structures by ultrasound. *Arch Phys Med Rehabil.* 49:28–30, 1968.
3. Johnson CL, O'Shaughnessy EJ, Ostergren G: *Burn Management.* New York, Raven Press, 1981.
4. Stolov WC, Thompson SC: Soleus immobilization contracture in young and old rats. *Arch Phys Med Rehabil.* 60:556–557, 1979.
5. Stolov WC, Thompson SC: Soleus immobilization contracture in the baboon. *Arch Phys Med Rehabil.* 60:556, 1979.
6. Warren CG, Lehmann JF, Koblanske JN: Heat and stretch procedures: an evaluation using rat tail tendon. *Arch Phys Med Rehabil.* 57:122–126, 1976.

Muscle Pain and Myositis

E. A. AWAD

Muscle pain may be localized or generalized. Localized muscle pain may be due to: trauma (muscle strain, hematoma, tear), tendinitis, bursitis, anterior tibial compartment syndrome, muscle cramps, and psychogenic pain.

Generalized muscle pain may be due to myositis (polymyositis, dermatomyositis), myositis associated with malignancy, systemic lupus erythematosus, rheumatoid arthritis, scleroderma, or to infectious myositis (influenza virus, bacterial or parasitic), and polymyalgia rheumatica.

MUSCLE TRAUMA

Moderate traumatic injury due to direct blows or longitudinal stretching results in microscopic bleeding which leads to muscle spasm and restricted motion. More severe trauma may result in hemorrhage in the muscle. A hematoma may be palpable at the site of injury, or bleeding may track along tissue planes to a distant site. Excessive trauma may result in muscle tear leading to severe pain and muscle spasm. On palpation, there is acute tenderness and stiffness of the muscle. Myositis ossificans may result from muscle trauma and hematoma formation and usually occurs in the brachialis or quadriceps femoris muscles. The patient complains of localized swelling and pain, and there is limitation of motion. The hematoma is gradually ossified. Early x-ray examination is usually negative, although bone scan may be positive, and the serum alkaline phosphatase may be elevated. After 2–3 weeks, ill-defined radiodensities within the muscle may be demonstrated; these become more defined after several months.

In the early phase, treatment is by rest of the part involved, maintenance of the range of motion (ROM) and, later on, surgical excision of the ossified mass may be indicated after its complete maturation.

TENDINITIS

Inflammation of a muscle tendon is common; examples are supraspinatus and bicipital tendinitis. Cardinal symptoms are localized pain, tenderness, and limitation of motion, all of which usually follow overuse. The tendon is swollen at the muscle-tendon junction or its insertion into the skeleton. Treatment consists of rest, anti-inflammatory drugs, analgesics, passive ROM exercises within the limits of pain after application of ice massage in the acute stage or heat and massage in the subacute or chronic stages. Steroid injections at the point of maximal tenderness may be useful, although direct injection of a tendon may lead to rupture.

Acute or chronic inflammation of bursae in between muscles or tendons and the adjacent structures is common. Examples are the subdeltoid, trochanteric, and retrocalcaneal bursae.

COMPARTMENT SYNDROME

Acute compartment syndromes are usually complications of fractures or the reestablishment of circulation following occlusion. Chronic recurrent symptoms are usually exercise induced. Following excessive exertion, swelling of the muscles occurs, leading to increased pressure within the compartment. This leads to circulatory insufficiency which, in severe cases, may result in necrosis of the muscles. The patient complains of pain localized over the muscle belly, which may be tense and bulging. There is tenderness to palpation and weakness, and pain on passive stretch of the muscle.

Acute compartment syndrome is a surgical emergency requiring fasciotomy. If severe necrosis occurs, weakness and fibrotic contracture may result.

MUSCLE ACHES AND PAINS

Muscle Cramps

These are painful involuntary muscle contractions of brief duration which usually follow overexertion but may also be associated with hypocalcemia, sodium depletion, hypomagnesemia, or entrapment of the root or nerve innervating the muscle. Nocturnal cramps in the calf muscles are seen in the elderly and during pregnancy. The etiology is not understood but these patients may respond to quinine sulfate, supplementary calcium, ice massage, and stretching of the muscles affected.

Intermittent claudication usually occurs in the calf muscles during walking and is relieved by rest. Although the discomfort is often described as being like a cramp, true cramp does not occur. It is indicative of arterial insufficiency. Treatment is directed toward improvement of the peripheral circulation, which may be accomplished by a series of graded active exercises and elimination of aggravating factors such as smoking.

McArdle's Syndrome

This is a rare condition in which the patient complains of muscle aching in the calves during walking which becomes more severe with progressive ambulation. Cramps may develop, and stiffness follows activity. These symptoms disappear after a period of rest. Laboratory studies show a decrease in blood lactate and pyruvate levels after exercise, as opposed to the normal increase. This syndrome is due to phosphorylase deficiency, with the patient unable to convert glycogen into glucose-1-phosphate.

Psychogenic Muscle Pain

Pain may be an expression of functional disorders: depression, anxiety, neuroses, or conversion reactions. The patient complains of vague stiffness and pain, usually in the neck or back, which does not follow any anatomical pattern. Pain is poorly localized, not affected by rest, heat, or analgesics. The diagnosis is based on the absence of objective findings and the presence of manifestations of psychoneurosis.

POLYMYOSITIS AND DERMATOMYOSITIS

In polymyositis or dermatomyositis there is acute, subacute, or remitting nonsuppurative inflammation of the striated muscles, the connective tissue and, sometimes, the skin. At the onset, the patient complains of myalgia and muscle weakness which are symmetrical and diffuse; these symptoms gradually develop over a period of weeks or months and may follow a febrile illness. The weakness may begin in the upper or lower extremities. The patient complains of difficulty in climbing stairs or getting out of a chair, with a tendency to fall and difficulty getting up to the standing position. There is a generalized feeling of malaise. In the acute phase, the muscles are swollen and tender and later become atrophic.

In dermatomyositis, a rash over the face and knuckles as well as periorbital edema may be seen. In the childhood form, calcinosis of the skin may occur. The blood picture is usually normal; erythrocyte sedimentation rate is increased in 50% of the cases; there may be increased γ-globulins in the plasma proteins and increased urinary creatine. There is an increase in the creatine kinase in the serum, the level of which is a good indication of the severity of muscle damage. There may be an increase in the serum antibodies; anti-DNA is rarely present. Usually, there are high titers of antinuclear antibodies. Electromyographic (EMG) findings are usually helpful; however, they vary somewhat,

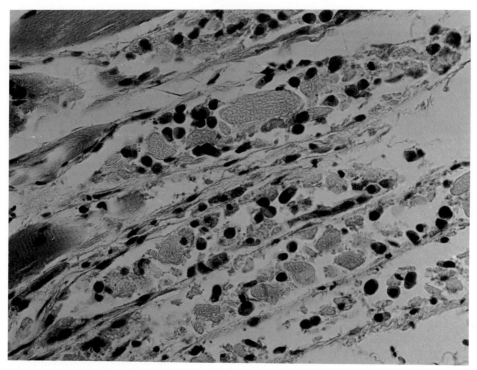

Figure 11.8   Acute dermatomyositis in a 20-year-old male showing coagulation necrosis and phagocytosis of muscle fibers.

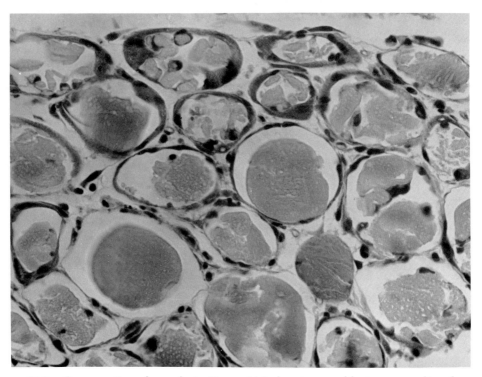

Figure 11.9.   Cross-section of muscle in Figure 11.8 showing myoblasts surrounding degenerating muscle fibers.

depending on the stage of the disease. As an EMG examination may raise the creatine kinase level in the serum, the blood work should be done first.

The diagnosis is usually established by muscle biopsy. The muscle to be biopsied should be moderately involved in the disease process, should show moderate weakness and tenderness, and should be accessible. Avoid muscles that have been tested by EMG previously since the needle probing may lead to localized inflammatory changes and muscle fiber degeneration. Avoid also muscles routinely used for injections such as the deltoid and gluteus maximus. The biopsy in polymyositis or dermatomyositis shows extensive inflammatory infiltrates, primarily of lymphocytes (Figs. 11.8 and 11.9).

Cellular infiltrates may surround small blood vessels or may be diffuse in between the muscle fibers. In the acute stage, there are necrosis and severe degeneration of the muscle fibers with phagocytosis and regeneration. Myoblasts are seen surrounding the necrotic fibers and have grown to form small rounded muscle fibers with central vesicular nuclei and basophilic cytoplasm.

Treatment during the acute stage is by rest in bed and passive range of motion exercises. During the subacute stage, active exercises are initiated carefully. The goal is to maintain the muscular strength and to prevent joint contractures. During the chronic stage, the patient should resume activity but should avoid fatigue. Prednisone (60–100 mg daily) should be administered, with gradual reduction of the dosage, according to the patient's clinical status, muscle strength, and serum enzyme changes.

POLYMYALGIA RHEUMATICA

The characteristic features are generalized muscular pain and stiffness, especially in the shoulder girdle, neck, and back muscles; these symptoms are usually seen in middle aged or elderly women and are associated with a very elevated erythrocyte sedimentation rate. The serum enzymes, EMG, and muscle biopsy are normal. In some patients it may be associated with temporal arteritis. These patients respond dramatically to corticosteroid treatment.

Myofascial Pain Syndromes

D. G. SIMONS

Myofascial trigger points (TPs) are sharply circumscribed, tender, irritable spots in muscle that are among the most common, yet poorly managed, causes of musculoskeletal pain and dysfunction seen in clinical practice (13). They account for many headaches, shoulder pains, and backaches. Where the patient complains of pain is often not the site of the abnormality. Pain can be referred

from muscle, just as diseased viscera refer pain to distant somatic areas (1). Few patients with myofascial pain discover the source of the pain themselves, nor do their physicians, unless they are familiar with the referred pain patterns.

Acute or chronic muscular strain can activate an irritable TP focus in the muscle or its connective tissue. A myofascial syndrome is characterized by referred pain, local and referred tenderness, and a tense shortened muscle with resultant stiffness and limitation of motion, weakness and, sometimes, autjonomic dysfunction (15). The TP is located in a tense band of muscle fibers that shorten the muscle, increase its tension, and is detected by cross-fiber palpation of the muscle (15). Passive stretch increases the tension on this band and is painful (4), as is a strong voluntary contraction of the muscle, especially in the shortened position (14).

The TP has also been called muscular rheumatism, fibrositis, fibrositis syndrome, myalgia, myalgic spots, myogelosis, nonarticular rheumatism, and interstitial myofibrositis, to name a few (9, 10). Myofascial syndromes are often misdiagnosed and mistreated as, for instance, bursitis, tendinitis, arthritis, radiculopathy (8), and psychogenic illness.

ETIOLOGY

The etiology is unknown, and no theory fully accounts for all the characteristics. The hard nodules or bands palpable in the tender muscle are not simply due to deposition or inflammation of connective tissue (fibrositis), as once thought; they are not due to gelling of muscle colloids (myogelosis); are not due to nerve-propagated contraction of a group of muscle fibers; nor primarily to exudates of mucopolysaccharides. Muscles with strongly active TPs showed nonspecific dystrophic changes (11). Nonpropagated contracture of affected muscle fibers (11) with associated sensitization of muscle pain afferents (5) is a promising possibility.

Kellgren (2) demonstrated that skeletal muscles throughout the body can refer pain to other locations when stimulated by the injection of 0.1 or 0.2 ml of 6% saline solution. His results have been amply confirmed (15). Recent experiments have shown that cat muscles are well supplied with A-delta and C-fiber pain afferents (5) and that in man some of these muscle pain fibers also refer pain to areas remote from the muscle (7).

DIAGNOSIS OF MYOFASCIAL TRIGGER POINTS

The following diagnostic characteristics help to distinguish myofascial syndromes from the myopathies considered earlier in this chapter. When asked what started the pain, some patients can remember in detail the specific movement associated with the acute onset. This movement helps to identify the muscle involved.

Myofascial TPs *refer pain* in a consistently predictable pattern characteristic of each muscle. The patterns of referred pain from skin and scar tissue are not so predictable (15). Myofascial referred pain is not constrained to a segmental distribution. There may be pain only on movement, but when severe, there also may be spontaneous rest pain. Several muscles may refer pain to the same reference zone. Recognition of single-muscle and multiple-muscle pain patterns is the key to identifying which muscles are most likely to be causing the pain. Occasionally, the chief complaint of the patient with TPs is restricted movement, weakness, or referred autonomic phenomena, rather than pain.

Myofascial pain is generally dull and aching. Nonpain phenomena may appear in the pain reference zone as vasomotor activity, sweating, or increased motor unit activity.

Exquisite spot tenderness to digital pressure (often with a jump sign by the patient) (3) is nonspecific but is *always* found at a myofascial TP. Two phenomena frequently can be elicited from TPs: (a) a local twitch response of the muscle, elicited by snapping palpation, or by needling the TP, and (b) reproduction of at least part of the patient's pain by pressure on, or needling of, the TP. Findings *indicative* of myofascial TPs but less diagnostic include nonreproducible pain reported in characteristic patterns; a history of sudden onset closely associated with acute muscular strain, or of gradual onset associated with repeated or sustained contractions; restriction of the stretch range of motion of the affected muscle; a palpable taut band in the muscle; and elimination of the signs and symptoms of TP activity by therapy directed specifically at the responsible TPs. In general, the more active the TP, the more complete and clear-cut are the above findings. The more of these indicative findings one observes, the surer is the diagnosis.

When perpetuating factors are present, therapy provides only temporary relief. TPs that develop in the pain reference zone of the primary TP are called *satellites. Secondary* TPs develop in other muscles of the myotatic unit shared with the primary TP (15).

TREATMENT

This irritability of the TP may be inactivated by stretching the muscle to its *full* normal range of motion. However, pain and reflex spasm must be blocked to obtain full stretch (13). An active TP also can be inactivated by probing it with a dry needle or, less painfully, by injecting it with 0.5% procaine (14). Deep pressure or deep massage produce more prolonged discomfort during treatment but are effective in muscles that are within reach (8, 15). Identification and resolution of any perpetuating factors are essential for prolonged relief.

Treatment of an acute single-muscle syndrome in a patient free of perpetuating factors can be simple, the response dramatic. Management of a chronic, multilayered syndrome with several perpetuating factors is a worthy and rewarding challenge to the talented physician. Specific myofascial treatment techniques include stretch and spray, ischemic compression, and injection, which are combined with teaching patients how to prevent and manage recurrences themselves (15).

Beware! Symptomatic relief of chest or abdominal pain by the specific myofascial therapies of stretch and spray, ischemic compression, and TP injection does *not* exclude serious visceral disease (15).

Stretch and Spray

This technique is valuable for complex cases, when many muscles in one region of the body are involved and their TPs are interacting strongly with one another. On the other hand, it is a simple, quick, and relatively painless way to clear up a single-muscle syndrome and is frequently used immediately after injection to ensure inactivation of all TPs in that muscle.

To inactivate TPs by stretch, the muscle must be extended to its full normal length. However, during simple stretching, pain and reflex spasm of the muscle stops further movement. Patient relaxation and vapocoolant spray help to block the spasm, permitting gradual stretch with spray, e.g., the trapezius (Fig. 11.10). To obtain complete relaxation of the muscle being stretched, the patient must be positioned *comfortably, totally* relaxed and well supported. A stream of vapocoolant spray (Fluori-Methane®) is applied in one direction only and in parallel sweeps to avoid excessive cooling, such as frosting of the skin. Fluori-Methane® (Gebauer Chemical Co., Cleveland, Ohio) is much preferred to ethyl chloride, which is a potentially lethal general anesthetic, flammable, explosive, and colder than desirable. The path of spray should cover the entire length of muscle, extending toward and over the referred pain pattern. The cold shock and impact stimulus of the skin inhibits pain from, and reflex spasm of, the muscle being stretched (13). Hot moist packs may be used to *rewarm* the skin, followed immediately by a full range of active motion. For details, turn to *Appendix I* (pp. 313–320) where Plates I–VII cover the most significant areas.

In Plates I–VII of *Appendix I*, each box juxtaposes the pain pattern most com-

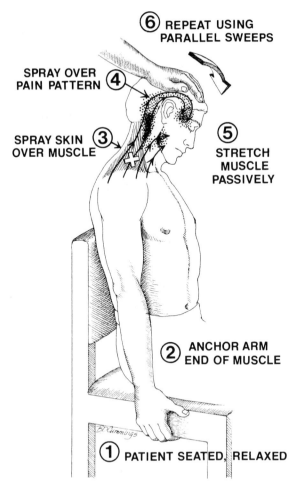

Figure 11.10.   Stretch and spray technique. The supine or, in this case, seated patient is well supported and made comfortable. For the trapezius and scalene muscles, the patient grasps the chair to anchor the shoulder end of the muscle. The operator holds the patient's head reassuringly and moves it gently while the patient is encouraged to relax the neck and body muscles, including the other arm. The stream of vapocoolant is directed in unidirectional parallel sweeps, first covering the muscle fibers, then over the referred pain pattern of the muscle. A hot pack rewarms the skin, and immediately the patient moves the muscle through its full (short and long) range of movement to restore normal use.

monly referred by a muscle next to a drawing of how to stretch that muscle. Matching the patient's pain with the pain patterns in *Appendix I* shows which muscles to examine.

Ischemic Compression

Ischemic compression (Shiatsu, finger pressure, acupressure, or myotherapy (8)) is a simple and effective but somewhat painful technique for inactivating TPs. It can be used by patients to inactivate accessible TPs overlying bony structures.

To perform ischemic compression, the operator or patient presses precisely on the TP (point of greatest sensitivity) with a steady, *moderately* painful force. After many seconds, when the pain starts to ease, increasing pressure is gradually added. When the TP stops hurting (after one or two minutes), the pressure is released. With release, first blanching, then reactive hyperemia of the skin are evident; the local TP tenderness, as well as any pain referred from that TP, may be relieved. Treatment may be repeated daily.

Injection

Injection is most useful when a limited number of TPs remain that are unresponsive, or inaccessible, to other modes of therapy. The effectiveness of dry needling and injection of TPs with pure isotonic saline (13, 15) attests to the importance of mechanically disrupting and flushing the TP zone, but these methods are often more painful to the patient than injection of 0.5% procaine without epinephrine (13).

After injection, prompt application of a hot pack often augments the range of motion and markedly reduces postinjection soreness that may last a day or two. Finally, having the patient use the newly treated muscles through their *fully* shortened and *fully* stretched range of motion is essential to *establish* in the patient's mind the normalized function of those muscles. This full range of motion is maintained by a home program of stretching exercises.

PERPETUATING FACTORS

When it becomes clear from the history, laboratory results, or a temporary response to therapy that perpetuating factors are important, those factors must be identified and resolved. Otherwise, the TPs can reactivate within hours or days after treatment. Simply correcting the perpetuating factor or factors may provide relief of pain and the recovery of full function *without any* specific myofascial therapy. When patients have multiple contributory factors, the completeness of relief depends on how well *all* factors are resolved. Perpetuating factors fall into several major categories.

Structural Inadequacies (e.g., short leg, small hemipelvis leading to scoliosis).

Poor Posture. This often results from poorly designed furniture (lack of lumbar support in most chairs).

Immobility. Prolonged immobilization of muscles left in a markedly shortened position aggravates myofacial TPs, as when sleeping huddled at night or sitting slumped forward.

Constriction of Muscles. Constriction of a muscle's circulation by tight bands, such as a tight collar or necktie, bra shoulder strap, or garters, increases its irritability.

Nutritional Inadequacies (Vitamins and Minerals). "Low normal" vitamin levels are usually ignored because their potential contribution to myofascial pain syndromes is not well known, because few of these patients have other signs, symptoms, or serum levels that qualify as a vitamin deficiency, and because many physicians erroneously believe that a "good" American diet ensures completely adequate vitamin levels. The myofascial pain of patients with vitamin B_1, B_6, folic acid, or B_{12} levels in the low–normal range often responds dramatically to vitamin therapy *without patients receiving any specific therapy for their muscles.* Vitamin C and the above B-complex vitamins are critical to normal muscle function. Deficiencies interact. Folic acid is essential for the utilization of vitamin B_{12}, and replacement of low levels of folic acid alone will drop the serum B_{12} level to seriously deficient levels if it is already inadequate, and *vice versa.* It is wise to maintain the desired level with a supplement of vitamin C, B-complex vitamins, and minerals that provide at least one recommended daily allowance (RDA). Within the pharmacological dose range of 10 times the RDA, toxicity of *water-soluble* vitamins is not a concern.

Low serum calcium (ionized calcium is the most significant form) and low serum potassium aggravate TP activity. Iron and the trace elements Mg and Zn are essential for normal muscle function. Inadequacies of these elements should be corrected.

Endocrine-Metabolic Impairments. Patients with mild to moderate clinical symptoms of hypothyroid function and low normal (lower quartile) levels of serum T_3 and T_4 frequently have hyperirritable muscles. This is a relatively common finding among myofascial pain patients who are refractory to myofascial treatments and who have adequate vitamin levels (14). Thyroid medication may need to be continued for life and must be checked regularly for adequacy of dosage. The increase in metabolism by the hormone will increase blood pressure, vitamin B_1, and estrogen requirements. Therefore, adequate stores of vitamin B_1 *must* be ensured before starting thyroid therapy, and may eliminate the need for it. Overmedication with thyroid can cause cardiac irregularities. When *impaired energy metabolism* is present, muscles are more vulnerable to developing active TPs and are refractory to treatment during periods of *hypoglycemia* and when the patient is *anemic.*

Sleep Disturbance. Myofascial pain patients commonly report disturbed sleep. A study of patients with myofascial TPs demonstrated electroencephalographic evidence of abnormal sleep in most of them (B. Baker, personal communication). Disturbed sleep decreases pain tolerance and encourages depression. Our first approach to improve sleep is the inactivation of TPs causing sleep-disturbing pain, e.g., in the subscapularis or posterior deltoid muscles. Then, if necessary, we prescribe a sleep-inducing drug such as 50 mg of Dramamine or Phenergan orally, ½ hour before bedtime. L-tryptophan (1 mg) or chlorpromazine (5 mg) may be effective and have been studied in relation to this problem.

L-tryptophan is a precursor of serotonin in the brain. Increased brain serotonin (5-hydroxytryptamine) results in sleep or sleep-like behavior in animals and reduces the amount of decreased slow wave and rapid eye movement (REM) sleep.

Moldofsky and Lue (6) monitored the sleep of patients with the "fibrositis syndrome." Although they defined this condition differently, probably most of their patients had myofascial TPs. They found that these patients had increased α-activity during their nonrapid eye movement sleep and an overnight increase in measurable muscle tenderness and subjective pain symptoms.

Other Factors. Other factors that must be identified and resolved include any other factor that impairs energy metabolism, foci of chronic infection (the teeth, sinuses, or urinary tract), an active allergic state, and psychological distress. Depression should be treated promptly and *adequately* to achieve prompt full pain relief. Anxiety-tension, secondary gain, and sick behavior interactions between patients and the others important in their lives usually must be altered if present (15).

ACKNOWLEDGMENTS

The author is deeply grateful to Barbara D. Cummings for the drawings, to Janet Travell, M.D., for her help in reviewing the text and drawings, to June Rothberg, R.N., Ph.D., and to Bruce Baker, M.D., for their critical review of the manuscript.

References

1. Berges PU: Myofascial pain syndromes. *Postgrad Med* 53:161–168, 1973.
2. Kellgren JH: Observations on referred pain arising from muscle. *Clin Sci* 3:175–190, 1938.
3. Kraft GH, Johnson EW, LaBan MM: The fibrositis syndrome. *Arch Phys Med* 49:155–162, 1968.
4. Macdonald AJR: Abnormally tender muscle regions and associated painful movements. *Pain* 8:197–205, 1980.
5. Mense S, Schmidt RF: Muscle pain: which receptors are responsible for the transmission of noxious stimuli? In Rose FC: *Physiological Aspects of Clinical Neurology*, Oxford, Blackwell, 1977.
6. Modofsky H, Lue FA: The relationship of alpha and delta EEG-frequencies to pain and mood in "fibrositis" patients treated with chlorpromazine and L-tryptophan. *Electroencephalogr Clin Neurophysiol* 50:71–80, 1980.
7. Ochoa JL, Torebjörk HE: Pain from skin and muscle. *Pain (Suppl)* 1:88, 1981.
8. Prudden B: *Pain Erasure: the Bonnie Prudden Way.* New York, M. Evans, 1980.

9. Reynolds MD: Myofascial trigger point syndromes in the practice of rheumatology. *Arch Phys Med Rehabil* 62:111–114, 1981.
10. Reynolds MD: The development of the concept of fibrositis. *J Hist Med Allied Sci* 38:5–35, 1983.
11. Simons DG: Muscle pain syndromes. Parts I and II. *Am J Phys Med* 54:289–311, 1975; 55:15–42, 1976.
12. Simons DG, Travell JT: Myofascial trigger points: a possible explanation. *Pain* 10:106–109, 1981.
13. Travell J: Myofascial trigger points: clinical view. In Bonica JJ, Albe-Fessard D: *Advances in Pain Research and Therapy*. New York, Raven Press, 1976, pp 919–926.
14. Travell J: Identification of myofascial trigger point syndromes: a case of atypical facial neuralgia. *Arch Phys Med Rehabil* 62:100–106, 1981.
15. Travell J, Simons DG: *Myofascial Pain and Dysfunction: The Trigger Point Manual*. Baltimore, Williams & Wilkins, 1983.

Arthrosis

R. L. SWEZEY

The arthroses include diseases and disorders that either exclusively or characteristically cause joint pain or dysfunction. They may involve a single joint—monarticular (sepsis, gout, secondary osteoarthritis); a few—pauci-articular (juvenile rheumatoid arthritis, pseudogout, Reiter's syndrome, rheumatic fever); or many, often symmetrically involved joints—polyarticular (rheumatoid arthritis, primary osteoarthritis, or degenerative joint disease). In some disorders systemic or local extraarticular manifestations are predominant; for instance: systemic lupus erythematosus, sarcoidosis, ulcerative colitis, polymyalgia, viral hepatitis, scleroderma, dermatomyositis, psoriatic arthropathy, and acromegaly. It is therefore essential that a thorough history and physical examination be performed if joint disease is evident or suspected.

Clinically, one can identify articular involvement by observing any of the cardinal signs of inflammation occurring in the precise anatomical location of a joint. Swellings may be caused by synovial effusions and capsular edema or by bony-cartilaginous proliferation (osteophytes). There is associated tenderness on palpation of the entire circumference of the joint margin and/or pain elicited by passive range of motion in all planes of motion of the joint. Laboratory, radiographic, radioactive isotope, and other studies are often helpful but not always. X-rays and laboratory tests, for instance, may be normal in the presence of joint disease (pseudogout, scleroderma), and laboratory or isotope studies may be falsely positive in the absence of articular involvement (cirrhosis, old age).

Definite rheumatoid arthritis, in the *A.R.A. 1958 Revision of the Diagnostic Criteria* (3) requires at least five of the following:

1. Morning stiffness.
2. Pain on motion or tenderness in at least one joint (observed by a physician).
3. Swelling (soft tissue thickening or fluid, not bony overgrowth alone) in at least one joint (observed by a physician).
4. Swelling (observed by a physician) of at least one other joint (any interval free of joint symptoms between the two joint involvements may not be more than 3 months).
5. Symmetrical joint swelling (observed by a physician) with simultaneous involvement of the same joint on both sides of the body (bilateral involvement of midphalangeal, metacarpophalangeal, or metatarsophalangeal joints is acceptable without absolute symmetry). Terminal phalangeal joint involvement will not satisfy this criterion.
6. Subcutaneous nodules (observed by a physi-

cian) over bony prominences, on extensor surfaces, or in juxta-articular regions.

7. X-ray changes typical of rheumatoid arthritis (which must include at least bony decalcification localized to or greatest around the involved joints, not just degenerative changes). Degenerative changes do not exclude patients from any group classified as rheumatoid arthritis.

8. Positive agglutination test—demonstration of the "rheumatoid factor" by any method which, in two laboratories, has been positive in not over 5% of normal controls—or positive streptococcal agglutination test.

9. Poor mucin precipitate from synovial fluid (with shreds and cloudy solution).

10. Characteristic histologic changes in synovial membrane with three or more of the following: marked villous hypertrophy; proliferation of superficial synovial cells, often with palisading; marked infiltration of chronic inflammatory cells (with lymphocytes or plasma cells predominating) with tendency to form "lymphoid nodules"; deposition of compact fibrin, either on surface or interstitially; foci of cell necrosis.

11. Characteristic histologic changes in nodules showing granulomatous foci with central zones of cell necrosis, surrounded by proliferated fixed cells, and peripheral fibrosis and chronic inflammatory cell infiltration, predominantly perivascular.

Criteria 1–5 must be continuous for at least 6 weeks for a *definite* diagnosis. *Probable RA* may be diagnosed if at least one of categories 1–5 is continuous for 6 weeks. *Possible RA* and the formidable list of exclusion criteria are best considered by rheumatology specialists.

TREATMENT

Once it is determined that an arthrosis exists, its nature can be established, and therapy can be planned. A diagnosis of rheumatoid arthrosis (RA) suggests a number of pharmacological therapies. However, if the elbows and a fourth proximal interphalangeal joint (PIP) are the only joint sites involved, the elbows show no evidence of active inflammatory disease, and there is but minimal contracture of the PIP joint, the treatment will differ enormously from that of a generalized chronic progressive deforming erosive polyarthritis further complicated by a peripheral neuritis and pulmonary effusion and anemia.

An acute monarticular attack of gout (podagra) readily responsive to NSAIDS or colchicine requires no rehabilitative therapies, but a chronic osteoarthritic knee or first carpometacarpal joint may require very specific rehabilitative therapeutic interventions. In the treatment of many arthritic disorders, pharmacological therapy, including anti-inflammatory drugs (salicylates, NSAIDS, local, and occasionally systemic steroids) or remittitive agents (gold, hydroxychloroquine, penicillamine) in rheumatoid arthritis are required. Surgical management ranges from early synovectomy to late reconstruction of severely damaged joints and periarticular structure. Noninvasive rehabilitative therapies provide another mainstay of the management of arthritic disorders (11).

A mnemonic, MEMORIES (Modalities, Exercise, Movement considerations, Occupational therapy, Rest, Immobilization, Education, and Social) may be helpful (13).

MEMORIES should not be a "seed catalog" of treatment options memorized and applied by rote rather than with reason. Selective indications for therapy exist for specific articular problems. Some of them are covered in greater detail elsewhere in this book.

Modalities

The first to be considered are the modalities employed for the control of pain and to facilitate exercise therapy, e.g., heat, cold, electrical stimulation, diathermy traction, hydrotherapy.

Exercise, Motion, and Stretching

After pain control is established, exercise can be instituted. The first priority of exercise is usually gentle stretching to prevent any loss of range of motion (ROM). In an acute severe inflammatory arthropathy, even the slightest joint motion may not be tolerated. If the acute arthropathy is self-limiting and noncrippling by nature, e.g., acute gout, no exercise is required. In more indolent or destructive and deforming arthropathies such as rheumatoid arthritis or variants of RA, early introduction of ROM exercises is necessary to preserve as much ROM as possible. This may be accomplished by 1–3 assisted joint motions to the extent of motion tolerated in one or two sessions daily. Once there is the possibility of increasing ROM, active and assisted stretching consisting typically of 3–5 repetitions of joint motion per session in 2–3 sessions daily is prescribed. It is important to remember that repeated passive or active motion increases joint inflammation (2), so the exercise prescribed should be sufficient to accomplish its purpose and should not be more, lest it be counterproductive.

Rules of thumb for exercise are: that an exercise should not cause significant pain and any pain brought on during an exercise should subside within 2 hours and no increase of pain attributable to exercise should be present on the day following the exercise sessions. All exercise must be precisely prescribed, taught, and performed. All exercise programs must be reviewed to ensure proper compliance and must be revised as needed by changes in the course of the joint problems—either improvement, regression, or failure to improve.

In an indolent or quiescent articular disorder in which contractures require stretching to regain lost motion, stretching exercise sessions can be prescribed hourly for 5–10 stretch repetitions of 6 to 10 seconds each in duration. Some patients better tolerate 1–2 repetitions of a more prolonged—20 to 60 seconds—stretch at each session. In general, a prolonged or "static" stretch is preferred. The patient should be taught what part of the joint is being stretched and where to feel the stretching sensation. He should be given concrete exercise performance guidelines, e.g.,

"reach up to the top of the door" or "repeat this exercise three to five times until you get your best stretch and then do one more 'to be sure.'"

There is a practical limit to each patient's tolerance for exercise and one may have to make a triage-type judgment in order to determine where to best focus the exercise effort in order to obtain an optimal level of function (13). Remember too that, although mobility of joints can often be improved or maintained by exercise, joints that are subluxated as a consequence of a destructive arthrosis cannot be restored to normal joint alignment by exercise.

Inhibition of joint motion as a consequence of painful joint disease invariably leads to some degree of muscle deconditioning and, when prolonged, to frank disuse atrophy (see Chapter 12). *Muscle strengthening exercises* are instituted as soon as it is established that joint mobility can be maintained on the stretching regimen and that the impact of additional strengthening exercise will not increase pain or lead to further loss of joint mobility—this is particularly true when the shoulder joint is involved.

In order to strengthen muscles undergoing disuse (type II) atrophy the exercise must be designed to cause minimal pain. This can be accomplished efficiently with an isometric contraction of the muscles acting on an arthritic joint by placing the inflamed joint capsule under the least amount of tension (loose-pack position) (10, 11). Not only does this minimize painful inhibition of the force of static contraction required to create a strengthening stimulus, but it also avoids the joint irritation that occurs with movement. The isometric exercise has the advantage of brevity and minimal discomfort to the patient, although the contraction should be held at the maximum strength possible for approximately 6 seconds/muscle group. It need be repeated but twice daily.

The functional implications of isometric exercises are those associated with anaerobic "weight lifting" activity such as arising from a chair, walking short distances, putting on clothes, or pouring from a tea kettle. Once joint mobility and strength have been restored to their potential, general *conditioning* exercises should be considered. In almost all cases, swimming and exercises in warm water provide the most ideal environment. Repeated motion or forceful stresses to an impaired joint will usually precipitate or aggravate symptoms and may lead to further joint damage, but if the joint disorder is self-limiting, nondestructive, and resolved, no special precautions for exercise are required.

Movement

Mobility issues for arthroses present a few unique problems. Canes and crutches are often extremely helpful in reducing weight-bearing stresses, but patients may need convincing before they will use them. Platform handle adaptations for crutches or walkers and enlarged crutch and cane grips modified to reduce strain on arthritic hands and arms can further enhance the use of these mobility assistive devices. For the severely involved patients, special wheelchair (7) and automobile adaptations may prove necessary (1, 8).

Occupational Therapy

Occupational therapy considerations are discussed in Chapter 8. Careful assessment of the arthritis patient is made in terms of total functioning, which should include not only what the patient can or cannot do, but also what to do or not to do in order to minimize pain and promote healing of this diseased joint. To the extent that training and joint protection and protective body mechanics are successful and necessary assistive devices have been employed, the need for potentially more toxic medication or aggressive surgery may be minimized.

Rest

Rest is therapeutic in many systemic disorders. For the systemically ill patient with arthritis or for the patient who is in chronic pain, sufficient rest to prevent exhaustion is mandatory. For the severely ill this may require most of the day in bed. For some patients a nap or two during the day will suffice, and many patients can function on a normal workday schedule without specific rest periods. Attention to rest position and posture, both sitting and lying, is important to prevent the formation of joint contractures. A firm supportive mattress, no pillows under inflamed knees, periodic prone positioning to minimize hip contractures, and supportive firm but padded seating should be provided.

Immobilization

Immobilization is a form of rest as well as support to a specific joint area. Severe or moderate joint inflammation can be kept in check by thermoplastic positioning splints or plastic casts. When splinting is used, the joint should be positioned for optimal function and away from the usual deformity (e.g., knee in extension, wrist in mild dorsiflexion) in the event that ultimately a full range of motion cannot be restored. Splints should be removed so that ROM exercises can be used once or twice daily to preserve motion. Functional or working splints support joints to minimize strain while permitting as much movement of involved adjacent joints as possible. The static wrist splint, the first carpometacarpal thumb-stabilizing splint, and the weight-bearing ankle-foot orthosis for ankle and proximal tarsal joint disease are useful (13).

Static splints or braces have not been shown to be of value in preventing or correcting deformities due to articular destruction in arthritis joints. The temptation to apply a splint that "might help" should be tempered by the burden of its cost and inconvenience to the patient. A splint or brace should demonstrably relieve pain or improve function to justify its prescription. There may be a role for dynamic (spring, or elastic, or turnbuckle assisted) bracing in the management of soft tissue contractures.

Education

Education of the patient as to the nature of his disorder, its prognosis, and what he is to do about it is essential for compliance to a therapy regimen (6, 14). The patient must know how many pills to take, how to position himself in bed, how many repetitions of each specific exercise he should do, when he needs to do more, or when to quit any or all of the above (9). Handouts and audiovisual presentations with patient information are helpful, but the patient usually needs individualized instruction, and the physician or therapist needs demonstrable confirmation from the patient that he truly understands how to take care of himself. Resources, including pamphlets and other supplemental educational materials, can be obtained through the Arthritis Foundation (3) and the Canadian Arthritis Society (4).

Social Factors

Psychosocial factors must be addressed in all patients with persistent joint pain or dysfunction. Deformities of the hands are often more difficult for the patient to accept than the pain or dysfunction. Prescribed splints or braces can be rejected unless they are presented to the patient in a sensitive manner. Hand splints worn at night and sexual activity are often incompatible. Sexual positions and the timing of sexual relations to minimize pain must be explicitly discussed (5, 6). Self rejection, divorce, drug abuse, isolation, family alienation, economic loss threatened or real, depression and self-destructive non-compliance with therapy regimens are all issues that may need skilled psychological and social counselling (15).

A comprehensive or holistic approach to the patient with an arthritic disorder is clearly necessary for proper management in many instances. But all of the management components must be rationally planned and carefully tailored to the patient's needs for a carefully designed and integrated, comprehensive program.

Surgical Intervention

Joint replacement surgery does not end in the operating room. Careful rehabilitation ensures the best results and requires close cooperation between the surgeon and the rehabilitation team.

References

1. American Automobile Association. *Vehicle Controls for Disabled Persons.* Washington, D.C., 1973.
2. Agudelo CA, Schumacher HR, Phelps P: Effect of exercise on urate crystal induced inflammation in canine joints. *Arthritis Rheum* 15:609, 1972.
3. Arthritis Foundation, Atlanta, Ga., USA.
4. Canadian Arthritis Society, Toronto, Canada.
5. Ehrlich GE: Sexual problems of the arthritic patient. In Ehrlich GE: *Total Management of the Arthritic Patient,* chap 9. Philadelphia, JB Lippincott, 1973.
6. Fries JF: Arthritis—*A Comprehensive Guide.* Reading, Mass., Addison Wesley, 1979.
7. Kamenetz HL: Wheelchairs. In Licht S, Kamenetz HL: *Orthotics Etcetera,* chap 21. New Haven, E. Licht, 1966.
8. Kent H, Sheridan J, Wasko E, June C: A driver training program for the disabled. *Arch Phys Med* 60:273–276, 1979.
9. Lorig K, Fries JF: *The Arthritis Help Book.* Reading, Mass. Addison Wesley, 1980.
10. Machover S, Sapecky AJ: Effector isometric exercise on the quadriceps muscle in rheumatoid arthritis. *Arch Phys Med* 47:737, 1966.
11. McCarty DJ: *Arthritis and Allied Conditions.* Philadelphia, Lea & Febiger, 1979.
12. Muller EA: Influence of training and or inactivity on muscle strength. *Arch Phys Med* 51:449, 1970.
13. Swezey RL: *Arthritis: Rational Therapy and Rehabilitation.* Philadelphia, WB Saunders, 1978.
14. Swezey RL, Swezey AM: Educational theory as a basis for patient education. *J Chronic Dis* 29:417, 1976.
15. Wolff BB: Current psychological concepts in rheumatoid arthritis. *Bull Rheum Dis* 22:656, 1971 and 1972.

Regional Pain Problems

R. CAILLIET

Notwithstanding the phenomenon of referred pain and tenderness described earlier in the chapter, musculoskeletal pain of a region may imply irritation or inflammation of the particular tissues of that region. The irritation may be direct trauma or indirect injury from faulty use. Direct trauma is evidenced from the history, but indirect trauma may be due more to a subtle action such as posture, faulty or excessive activities, or minor anatomical structural changes.

Regional pain problems implicate stress upon a *pain-sensitive tissue* within a joint structure. The structure of that joint must be understood from a functional standpoint, and each tissue component that is capable of causing pain must be evaluated as to its contribution to the pain and dysfunction.

Evaluation of the patient with regional pain, as has been made clear in Chapter 3, must include: (a) By history, the site of pain as pointed out by the patient. The history must elicit the mechanism of the incident by which the joint sustained an injury or by which pain has been subsequently elicited. The position or movement of that joint causing pain should be clearly determined. (b) By examination, the appearance of the joint being investigated and the passive movement of that joint may reveal the deviation from normal. Also, active movement, that is, the movement actively performed by the patient or improperly performed by the patient, will be helpful. By reproducing the specific pain with specific motions, the mechanism of joint pain and the tissue site of pain can usually be established. (c) Specific tests, as indicated in earlier chapters, may verify what the history and physical examination have implicated.

These tests include X-rays, computerized scans, electrodiagnostic tests, nuclear medicine techniques, blood chemical tests, and responses to various forms of treatment such as interruption of nervje pathways by nerve blocks, sympathetic nerve interruption, spinal-paraspinous nerve injections, or various other modalities. Specific problems of specific regions require specific diagnostic tests.

All regional pain problems transmit pain through a common pathway. Modifications or elimination of pain may be accomplished by direct or related approaches upon various sites of this pathway. A detailed discussion of the pain problems affecting individual bodily regions is beyond the scope of this section. Emphasis will be placed on a few common clinical examples and the functional anatomy that helps to understand them.

HEAD AND NECK

Head pain may be attributed to either intracranial or extracranial sources. The intracranial sources of pain may be neurological or vascular. Surprisingly, intracranial sources of pathology are frequently not painful. Symptoms such as vision, hearing, or neurological impairment are more frequent. For instance, subdural hematoma resulting from trauma may cause visual disturbances, mental aberration, vertiginous episodes of lightheadedness or dizziness but usually not pain.

The *extracranial sources of pain* are numerous and may be vascular, musculoskeletal, or neurological. The vascular sources include migraine and temporal arteritis. The former are due to vasospasm or vasodilation, frequently described by the patient as unilateral and "throbbing," and are associated with gastrointestinal symptoms (nausea, vomiting) and vertigo. In temporal arteritis, the temporal arteries are frequently tender and palpable, and show evidence of inflammation and are often associated with polymyalgia rheumatica.

Far more frequent sources of pain, however, are pains in the head and neck originating from the cervical nerve roots that emerge between the cervical vertebrae. Head pains can result from irritation of the C1, C2, and C3 branches, emerging from intervertebral foramina to run through musculofascial tissue of the neck. The upper cervical nerve roots form the greater occipital nerves from which pain may be hemicranial in the distribution of the dermatomes. The pain is frequently accompanied by sensitivity and tenderness of the involved scalp, and underlying subcuticular tissues.

Neck pain, felt in the neck and upper extremities, can result from irritation of the cervical nerve roots. These nerves emerge through foramina between vertebral bodies and have a specific dermatome and myotome distribution. The foramina are narrowed on neck extension, lateral bending, and rotation to that side and are opened in flexion and movement away from the involved side; these movements being performed should reproduce and relieve the patient's symptoms (particularly pain and paresthesiae) respectively, if mechanical nerve root irritation or radiculopathy is the source.

The commonest cause of these neck-head pains are direct trauma, such as a rear end accident, causing the so-called "whiplash" type of injury (Fig. 11.11). Here the history is one of trauma with the head bouncing forward and backward in an abrupt manner with resultant neck pain, head pain, and frequently referred hyperesthesia and paresthesia in the upper extremity in the distribution of the affected nerve root. Examination will frequently reveal painful limitation of the

neck ROM caused by muscle spasm protecting the underlying neck joints and ligaments, and neurologic deficit (sensory, motor, or reflex) in the nerve root's distribution. Subsequently, the neurological diagnosis may be confirmed by electromyography, if symptoms persist or become aggravated.

SHOULDER

The complex of upper arm movement involves a composite movement of numerous joints of the shoulder girdle: (a) *glenohumeral joint*, where movement of the humerus is within the glenoid fossa; (b) *suprahumeral joint*, with movement of the humerus within the compartments formed by the acromion and the overlying coracohumeral ligament; (c) *acromioclavicular joint*, the movement of the clavicle as it supports and positions the scapula; (d) *scapulocostal articulation*, which allows movement of the scapula upon the rib cage to ensure the scapular movement phase of the scapulohumeral rhythm; (e) *sternoclavicular joint*; (f) the movement of the sternum articulating upon its *sternocostal joints*; and (g) movement of the ribs as they articulate proximally with the vertebral bodies. Examination of the shoulder must evaluate all of these joints as the potential causative site of pain.

The commonest site of pain is the glenohumeral joint. This is a complex joint controlled by the rotator cuff muscles (supraspinatus, infraspinatus, teres minor, and subscapularis) which proceed under the acromion to attach to the humerus and act in conjunction with the deltoid to abduct, elevate, and externally rotate the arm. During this movement the space between the overhanging acromion and coracohumeral ligament and the rotating greater tuberosity of the humerus is very small and filled with sensitive tissues— the cuff, its nerves, and the blood supply. Faulty use of the arm, such as overhead elevation without the appropriate external rotation, may frequently cause an

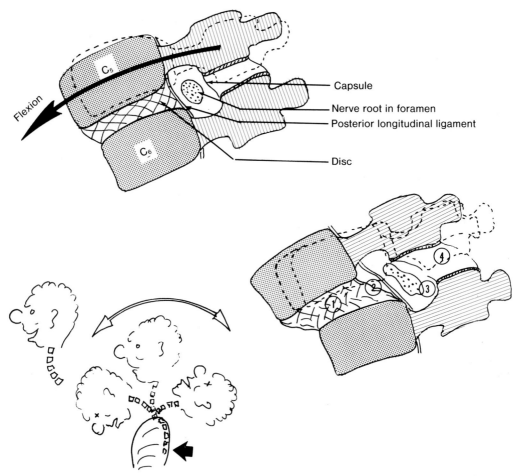

Figure 11.11. "Whiplash" injury mechanism. Normal flexion is indicated in the upper *drawing*; the lower *drawings* illustrate the extreme forceful flexion caused by a rear collision. In the latter, the following structures may be injured: (*1*) Intervertebral disc. (*2*) Posterior longitudinal ligament. (*3*) Nerve root. (*4*) Apophyseal joint.

acute inflammation of the cuff tendons. The tendons undergo inflammation and become swollen. At this particular point of abduction, pain is felt at the site of the greater tuberosity immediately under the overhanging acromion, and movement is limited by virtue of the fact that during abduction, external rotation and overhead elevation of the inflamed tendons, which are swollen, cannot pass adequately under the overhanging acromion; limitation as well as pain results (Fig. 11.12). As the cuff is also an external rotator, pain is noted as is weakness in external rotation of the arm, as when the

arm is held to the side with the elbow bent and external rotation attempted.

The subdeltoid bursa, which lies immediately adjacent to and above the supraspinatus tendon, frequently becomes secondarily inflamed; subsequent subdeltoid bursitis, as well as supraspinatus tendinitis, occurs (Fig. 11.12). The symptoms are the same.

In the event of a fall or a direct blow upon the abducted arm, the cuff may be torn. Here, there is immediate acute pain with subsequent and immediate inability actively to abduct, elevate, and externally rotate the arm. The patient has the ability

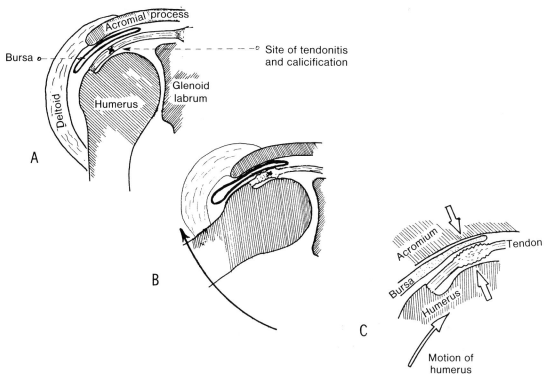

Figure 11.12.   Pain in shoulder during abduction due to inflamed supraspinatus tendon.

to hold the arm abducted when the examiner is able to replace the cuff function by passively abducting the patient's arm. Confirmation of tear is made by arthrography in which joint injection of dye will depict the communication via the tear from the glenohumeral capsule into the subdeltoid bursa.

Pain at the acromioclavicular joint may be due to direct trauma or severe traction upon the arm. In this condition, elevation of the scapula (shoulder shrugging) with simultaneous palpation of the acromioclavicular joint will produce pain, frequent limitation, and often crepitation. Local tenderness is present. With severe injury and loss of the coracoclavicular ligaments, a downward displacement of the acromion on the clavicle may be visible. X-rays may depict dislocation of the acromioclavicular joint with a weight on the wrist and the arm held dependent.

Pain between the scapula and the chest wall is frequently noted and is essentially muscular, insofar as the scapula is held to the chest wall exclusively by muscle, except at the acromioclavicular joint. The most common sites of pain are the levator scapulae and the rhomboid muscles which are stressed by faulty rounded shoulder posture or occupations that hold the arm in a forward elevated position. This causes sustained muscular contraction of not only the trapezius but also the levator scapulae, rhomboid, and supraspinatus muscles. Tenderness can be found in these muscles, but (as discussed earlier in this chapter) local tenderness does not always indicate a local disorder.

ELBOW

The elbow consists of the humeroulnar joint, the humeroradial joint, and the proximal radioulnar joint. Any of these three joints may be involved in the causation of pain. The humeroulnar joint permits flexion and extension of the elbow.

The most common cause of pain and limitation is direct trauma, such as a fall on the extended or semiflexed arm. Pain will result from the fact that the tissues of the capsule become stressed.

The forearm movements of *pronation and supination* occur at the proximal and distal radioulnar and humeroradial articulations. Direct trauma can cause fracture or tearing of the ligaments that hold the joints together. Pain is felt on passive or active pronation, and supination and tenderness can be elicited over the involved tissues.

At the lateral epicondyle, the extensor muscles of the forearm that extend the wrist and fingers attach, and it is at this point that any forceful movement, be it continued stress or acute trauma, may cause pain and tenderness, causing a "tennis elbow" or, more properly termed, *lateral epicondylitis* (Fig. 11.13). In this condition there is tenderness and pain on active contraction of the wrist and finger extensors. Pain can also be elicited by passively stretching these muscles—flexing the wrist and fingers and pronating the forearm with the elbow extended.

WRIST AND HAND

The wrist, the articulation between the radius and the proximal carpal bones, is a gliding-joining complex that moves in a combination of flexion-extension with simultaneous radial and ulnar deviation. This movement requires laxity and flexibility of the capsular structures. The wrist may be severely sprained when movement exceeds the physiological range of motion. The history here is of trauma, usually a fall. Pain can be elicited on passive and active movement of the joint with some swelling being noticed as well.

In a Colles' or Smith's fracture of the distal radius and ulna, the wrist joint distal to the fracture is indirectly involved only in that the ligaments, the capsule, and even the alignment of the bones are temporarily disrupted, and treatment re-

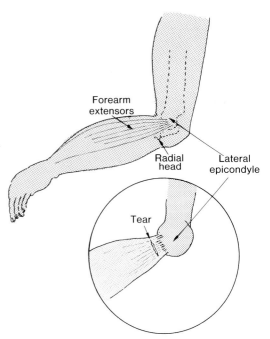

Figure 11.13.   Lateral epicondylitis.

quires immobilizing this joint. Consequently, after fracture healing, the joint between the carpal bones and the radius is frequently stiff and painfully limited.

The hand's clinical problems relate to its prehensile function, which requires good normal muscular mechanisms and intact sensory input from the fingers to create good integrated neuromuscular action. Any direct or indirect trauma to the hand must be carefully evaluated as to the full passive and active range of motion of all the digits and normal sensation of all the fingers—not only light touch but proprioception and perception of heat and cold as well.

Thumb

The proximal joint of the thumb, the carpometacarpal joint, permits circumduction, flexion, extension, adduction, and abduction. All may be impaired from any direct injury to the thumb. Primary or secondary arthritis may result in pain, limitation, and crepitation. Examination requires that the thumb be fully moved in all its movement and that the patient be asked to oppose the thumb to the little fingertip, or to the first fingertip, forming a large "0." This implies that the thumb has been able to "palmar abduct" and at the same time has the muscular coordination and strength to oppose the index or little fingers.

Fingers

Digits 2–5, i.e., the four fingers, move in a flexion-extension plane primarily, but they simultaneously must have some degree of abduction, adduction, and rotation to allow the hand to rotate in a fingertip-to-fingertip movement. In ligamentous injury, the joint shows swelling, painful movement, as well as tenderness, and lost range of motion.

The tendons that extend or flex the fingers also require smooth gliding movement with normal synovial lubrication. Any inflammation of these tendons resulting in tendinitis may cause pain and crepitus on active or passive motion, tenderness, swelling, and limitation of motion. Sensory impairment is frequently elicited by entrapment of the median nerve at the palmar level (carpal tunnel syndrome). This can occur in the carpal tunnel region, from trauma, or from inflammation of the tissues within the tunnel, such as rheumatoid arthritis or tendinitis. The median nerve sensory distribution is from the thumb to the middle of the ring finger; paresthesias result in this area. Weakness of the muscles of the thenar eminence and first and second lumbricals may become apparent. The symptoms may be reproduced by maintaining the flexed wrist position for a period of 30–90 seconds—the Phalen test. Confirmation is frequently necessary by nerve conduction studies and electromyography.

LOW BACK

Low back dysfunction and impairment may be due to trauma, degeneration, or abuse of the intervertebral articulations of the L4-L5-S1 region. The erect posture is that of a mild lordosis supported on an oscillating sacrum. The commonest cause of static low back pain is an increase in lumbar lordosis, and the history is that of low back pain after prolonged standing. Examination reveals a lordotic posture, and the symptoms can be accentuated by passively hyperextending the patient's low back. Relief of the pain by lumbar flexion is supportive evidence. X-rays may reveal an increased sacral angle or frank abnormalities, such as a congenital malformation, spondylolisthesis, spondylolysis, or a disc space narrowing.

Kinetic back pain may be seen in the person who bends, stoops, and lifts improperly. Normal forward flexing includes a reversal of the lumbar lordosis with a simultaneous rotation of the pelvis about the hip joints. This movement is restricted by soft tissue limitation, such as tight muscles, ligaments, and fascia. The back can become painful due to this inflexibility. The history is of low back pain after prolonged repeated flexion. The examination reveals the failure of the back to properly reverse its lordosis and simultaneously rotate the pelvis around the hip joint.

The most common cause of kinetic low back pain, however, is faulty bending in the act of lifting. In this particular instance the patient has lifted either with the legs unflexed or has returned to the erect position by prematurely reassuming the lordosis before the pelvis is totally derotated around the hip joint. This faulty mechanism may result in low back pain, ligamentous stress associated with the forceful apposition of the posterior zygoapophyseal or facet joints. If there is a rotatory component, tearing of the annular fibers of the disc can result.

Low back pain can result from stress upon the ligaments and muscles of the posterior articulations, stress by pressure upon the posterior longitudinal ligament, or from irritation of the nerves in their intervertebral foramina. The intervertebral foramina, bounded superiorly and inferiorly by the pedicles and posteriorly by the facet articulations, narrow down and encroach upon the emerging nerve roots on a lumbar extension and especially upon hyperextension.

Combined lateral bending and hyperextension of the low back will compress the nerve roots as they emerge through the foramina. Consequently, during the examination one may attempt to reproduce not only back pain but nerve root pain into the lower extremities. The examination requires observing the spine in its erect posture and in its attempted flexion and re-extension, performing tests of straight leg raising and related root tension signs to determine the freedom of the nerve roots as they emerge through the lower intervertebral foramina. One must do a neurological examination for all the myotomes, dermatomes, and reflexes involved.

Investigations may be lumbosacral spine films, bone scans, computerized tomography, or invasive procedures such as myelography, discography, and epidural venography. Electromyography and reflex studies may be used to test the adequacy of the nerves that emerge through the lumbosacral intervertebral foramina.

HIP JOINT

The hip joint is one of the most congruous joints of the body in that the convex surface of the femoral head almost matches the concave surface of the acetabulum. This joint moves in a spherical manner and is deeply seated and well-supported by a confining capsule. The hip permits stance, ambulation, and stooping and thereby requires flexion, extension, abduction, adduction, and internal rotation. All of these become limited if the articular cartilages of the opposing surface become roughened by disease or trauma.

The examination here is to confirm the history of the patient who has pain in the region of the hip joint, mostly groin and anterior thigh, after prolonged standing or repetitive motion. A limp may occur from pain or limited range of motion. Examination requires checking of motion and testing the musculature about the hip joint to determine the presence of spasm or weakness. Confirmation of the hip pathology is possible with routine x-rays in most cases.

KNEE JOINT

There are two articulations in the knee: the femorotibial and the patellofemoral. The femorotibial articulation allows primarily a flexion-extension movement but with a very important rotatory component of internal rotation of the tibia early in flexion. This movement is facilitated by the contour of the condyles, the ligaments, and the menisci. Pathology in the knee may result from direct trauma external to the knee such as a blow against the extended leg in standing or from internal damage in which flexion-extension is done improperly with inadequate or improper rotational torque.

The history should explore the trauma that the patient has sustained. The examination of the knee evaluates the medial and lateral collateral ligaments performed with the knee fully extended and at 20–30° flexion by varus and valgus movement of the lower leg upon the fixed thigh.

The normal cruciate ligaments prevent anterior and posterior shear. Tears are usually associated with sudden stops or from excessive twisting and turning as on the athletic field. The history is that of pain and effusion or hemarthrosis, and differentiation from tears of the medial and lateral collateral ligaments by the performance of the "drawer sign," which reveals an excessive amount of mobility in anterior-posterior shearing movements. Rotational instability may also be present and may be confirmed by the "pivot shift" series of physical maneuvers.

The menisci within the knee joint present pathology that can be both painful and disabling. As the menisci must move smoothly with the articulating tibia and femur, crepitation, limitation or "locking" may occur if the menisci are damaged.

The *patellofemoral articulation* is a frequent source of pain. During flexion-extension there is simultaneous compression of the patella against the femoral condyles due to quadriceps contraction. The symptoms are those of pain and crepitation in the region of the patella, elicited mostly on deep knee bends, stair climbing, and descent, with the examination revealing a crepitation and pain on forceful passive and active movement of the patella against the femur. Compression of the patella against the femur with simultaneous contraction of the quadriceps elicits the pain, and reflex quadriceps inhibition will be noted in conditions such as chondromalacia patellae: early degenerative changes of the patellofemoral articular cartilage, often predisposed by abnormalities of patellar alignment or tracking (e.g., in genu valgum).

ANKLE

The ankle joint is the weight bearing articulation of the foot in which the talus articulates within the mortise formed by the tibial and fibular malleoli. Movement of the tibial mortise joint is plantar- and dorsiflexion, but the structure of the talus locks the talus into the mortise on dorsiflexion and unlocks it in plantar flexion. Any lateral or medial movement of the foot in the ankle mortise is limited strictly by the lateral and medial ligaments. Injuries to the ligaments of the ankle occur usually on marked inversion or eversion of the foot in a plantarflexed position. This position permits the talus to be flexible within its mortise, and the ligaments themselves that normally restrict the movement become strained and damaged.

The history is that of a twisting of the ankle, usually twisting in (inversion), with ligamentous sprain occurring and causing pain on the lateral aspect of the ankle. Effusion is usually noted. There is tenderness and pain on passive stretch of the involved ligaments, and there may be excessive inversion due to talar tilting which may only be detected by stress radiography.

FOOT

The foot is comprised of many joints and ligaments, e.g., the talocalcaneal joint and the talonaviculocuboid joints. The tarsal bones and metatarsals form the longitudinal arches which are reinforced by the plantar fascia (Fig. 11.14). A foot that pronates and everts excessively shows depression of the medial longitudinal arch, commonly called a "flat" foot. In the hyperpronated foot all of the articulations of the foot become loose; ligamentous strain occurs, causing discomfort and pain. The posterior tibial tendon, which normally is not a supporting structure, becomes supporting and may become tender. The plantar fascia becomes excessively stretched, with consequent pain in the plantar aspect of the foot. Examination of the standing person shows a depression of the longitudinal arch. Tenderness may be present at the posterior tibial and medial ligamentous structures of the ankle and foot.

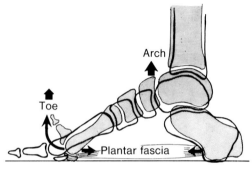

Figure 11.14.   The plantar fascia is an important tie-beam for the longitudinal arch of the foot.

Forepart of the Foot

Pain in the forepart of the foot under the metatarsal heads (commonly called metatarsalgia) may result from a pronated foot which is permitting the transverse metatarsal arch to depress and more weight bearing to be imposed on the second and third metatarsal heads than normally. On examination, observe the pronated foot, the spreading of the toes, and the tenderness being elicited under the heads of the second and third (and occasionally fourth) metatarsals.

A condition of interdigital neuritis, known as Morton's neuroma, may occur in which the nerves between the metatarsal bones as they proceed into the digital nerves become compressed between the metatarsal heads (Fig. 11.15). Tenderness is elicited in the cramped shoe position that brings the metatarsal bones together or may be present after prolonged walking. The examination consists of palpating for tenderness *between* the metatarsal heads, the site where the nerves are located and also having subjective as well as objective evidence of neuropathy with numbness of the toes of that region. If

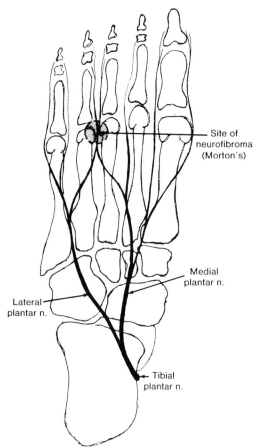

Figure 11.15. Morton's neuroma.

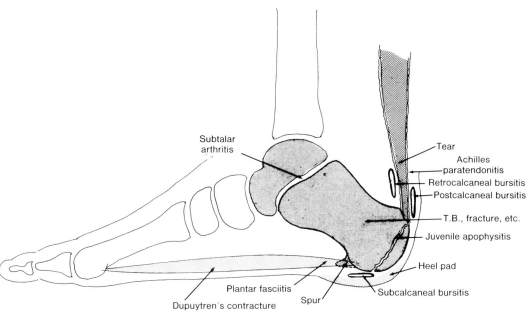

Figure 11.16. Sources of pain at the back of the foot include several types of bursitis, tears, and calcaneal spur.

pressure upon the nerve suggests the diagnosis, injection of the nerve with a lidocaine anesthetic frequently relieves the symptoms and supports the diagnosis.

A common source of pain is in the big toe at the first metatarsophalangeal joint. This is a condition that occurs if there is marked varus of the first metatarsal and valgus of the proximal phalanx, ending in a condition known as hallux valgus, or bunion toe. The examination reveals the marked angulation of the proximal joint of the big toe. There is frequently crepitation on movement, and pain and tenderness.

Heel and Posterior Half of Foot

A number of conditions that are painful occur in the back of the foot and heel (Fig. 11.16).

CONCLUSION

In regional pain problems of the musculoskeletal system, an extensive knowledge of functional anatomy is mandatory. The history suggests the anatomical site and depicts the possible mechanism of injury. Observation with manual examination determining the joint integrity, ligamentous stability, and muscular function is necessary to determine the exact source of pain and, therefore, the diagnosis of the regional pain problem. Laboratory confirmation may be necessary.

Amputations

S. N. BANERJEE

Amputation of an extremity is often a life-saving measure or relieves the misery of intolerable pain, but it creates severe physical and emotional disability which requires the attention of rehabilitation personnel for the functional and psychosocial well-being of the patient.

The practice of amputation has a long history (1). It made its greatest progress in response to the demands imposed by the two world wars. Before World War II, the residual limb was considered to be a passive structure, but afterwards myoplasty became the more standard procedure for amputations at various levels. Now, the surgeon reconstructs the residual limb for providing power and proprioception in order for the amputee to use a prosthesis successfully. Immediate application of a prosthetic device to the lower extremity amputees has become widely used in the past two decades (2). This method of applying a rigid plaster dressing to the residual limb immediately following surgery has revolutionized postoperative care and prosthetic fitting following amputation. Modern amputation surgery makes it possible to achieve satisfactory healing of an amputation stump at the lowest possible level (especially in patients suffering from peripheral vascular disease) which has a significant effect on the final outcome of rehabilitation management.

INCIDENCE OF AMPUTATION

There were 311,000 persons in the United States in 1971 with major extremity amputation (3), and the annual incidence of major extremity amputation was 43,000. In 1970, the amputation rate in Canada was 30.5/100,000 population (4), and there has been no significant change in recent years (6). Western Europe has similar rates.

Influence of Age

Different age groups show a characteristic pattern. The incidence in the first year of life is around 20/100,000 population, and this drops to about 10/100,000 population at the end of 1 year and remains fairly stable until about 15 years of age. This high incidence during the first year of life is possibly related to congenital amputation. From age 15 onwards, there is a gradual rise in the rate of amputation, possibly related to injury resulting from exposure to work situations and highway traffic. At 55 and upwards, there is a sharp increase primarily related to peripheral vascular disease (4, 5). There is a distinct male preponderance of amputees in all age groups.

LEVELS OF AMPUTATION

The relative distribution of amputees according to level of amputation (Table 11.1) varies widely because it is dependent on cause of amputation, surgical technique, postoperative care, etc. Although in amputee clinics one sees more lower extremity amputees than upper extremity amputees, hospital medical records do not support this observation, primarily because patients with minor toe or finger amputation rarely attend amputee clinics. The ratio of lower to upper extremity amputation in Canada in 1975 was 2.4:1. If one excludes the minor amputations, the ratio climbs to 16:1 (6). Glattly (7) reported that 85% of all amputees surveyed in the U.S. had major lower extremity amputation.

The specific level of amputation, especially in lower extremities, is influenced, among other factors, by the philosophy with regard to amputee care in that particular institution. Sarmiento et al. (8), while reviewing lower extremity amputation at the University of Miami between

Table 11.1
Distribution of Levels of Amputation

Levels	Glattly (7) (1964)	Statistics Canada (1975) (6)
	%	%
Shoulder disarticulation	1.1	0.07
Elbow disarticulation and above elbow	4	2.3
Wrist disarticulation and below elbow	9.4	2.4
Hip disarticulation	1.8	1.2
Knee disarticulation and above knee	45.2	45
Below knee	36.8	38
Syme amputation	1.87	10 (includes foot)

1960 and 1968, found reversal of ratios between amputation performed at above-knee and below-knee levels (8). Significant change in achieving healing in a lower level of amputation may be attributed to meticulous care during amputation surgery, application of rigid dressing on the operating table, and close monitoring of wound healing during the postoperative period. Similar trends have been reported by Burgess et al. (9) and others.

CAUSES OF AMPUTATION

In the industrialized nations of the West, peripheral vascular disease secondary to atherosclerosis is the leading cause of amputation (5, 10). However, in many developing countries, infection and Buerger's disease appear to be the predominant causes of amputation.

PREOPERATIVE ASSESSMENT

As most amputations are elective procedures, a detailed preoperative assessment is essential. This permits a determination of the level of amputation and a prediction of the ultimate functional outcome, which can be extremely helpful to the patient and his family in coping with the amputation, as well as for future planning of accommodation, vocation, etc. The preoperative assessment should take into account the patient's overall medical status because atherosclerosis can affect other body systems which may affect the patient's ability to use a prosthesis. A detailed examination of the musculoskeletal system may reveal the presence of joint contracture, muscle weakness, sensory impairment, etc.; these should be treated during the preoperative phase. Sometimes, the presence of a fixed contracture of a joint proximal to the level of amputation may make prosthetic fitting impossible, and a higher level of amputation may be required. However, joint contracture usually can be at least partially reduced to a point where prosthetic fitting can be carried out adequately.

All patients facing amputation surgery are overwhelmed with the prospect of losing a part of their body, and they feel helpless in terms of their future ability to function adequately in their social and vocational environment. During this phase both patient and family require considerable support from all health care workers involved. Sometimes a visit by another amputee who has gone through similar procedures may be of extreme help to the patient. However, the other amputee should be chosen carefully to match the patient's age and expected level of functioning after prosthetic fitting. Otherwise, the visit may raise unrealistic hope. In addition to the assessment by the surgeon planning to perform the surgery, the patient should be assessed by a physiatrist and other members of the rehabilitation team, particularly a physical therapist, occupational therapist, and social worker. This early contact with the rehabilitation team ensures easy transition from the acute to the rehabilitation phase of treatment.

AMPUTATION SURGERY

Amputation of an extremity is no longer considered a failure of treatment but rather the beginning of a new phase in which most patients can be restored to a fairly high level of functioning through proper rehabilitation management. Following amputation surgery, the residual limb will be responsible for activating the prosthesis and should be pain-free and have adequate neuromuscular integrity and a full range of joint movement. For it to be a dynamic end organ, the surgeon must have a thorough knowledge of prosthetic fitting, biomechanics of current prosthetics, and the possible functional outcome in each level of amputation (see Chapter 7.)

Ideally, amputations are done by a limited number of specialists who do most, if not all, of the amputations in larger communities and regional centers. As most amputations are done today for peripheral vascular disease (Figs. 11.17 and 11.18), the utmost care must be taken in handling tissue, avoiding excessive dissection, and achieving adequate hemostasis. The surgeon tries to achieve the lowest possible level of amputation at which adequate healing is guaranteed, especially in the case of the lower extremity of an elderly patient with peripheral vascular disease. In these patients every effort must be made to preserve the knee because very few elderly patients with above-knee amputation become functional ambulators.

SELECTION OF AMPUTATION LEVEL

The surgeon is guided by various types of information in order to make a decision on the selected level of amputation. In cases of trauma or tumor, primary considerations are the extent of the tissue injury and viability, location, and pathological nature of the tumor. However, in the case of an elderly person with peripheral vascular disease, the adequacy of blood supply at the selected level becomes the major guiding factor. The adequacy of blood supply can be determined from the history and physical examination, assisted by arteriography, but arteriography in the

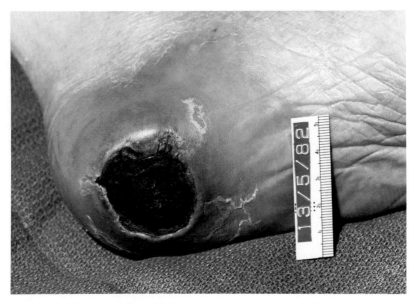

Figure 11.17. Necrotic nonhealing heel ulcer in an 82-year-old diabetic requiring B/K amputation.

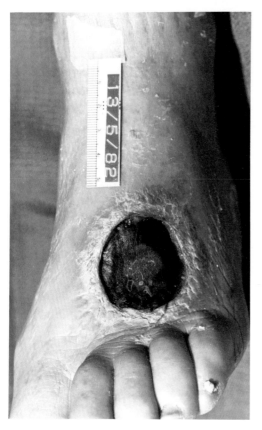

Figure 11.18. Nonhealing ulcer on the dorsum of the foot of an 80-year-old diabetic requiring amputation.

presence or absence of peripheral pulses is not always an accurate predictor of the healing potential of an extremity, usually underestimating the vascularity (9, 11). Burgess *et al.* (9) also noted that the presence or absence of the popliteal pulse did not influence the healing of a below-knee stump. Because of the limitations of arteriography and clinical signs, various other investigative methods had been used to predict healing, especially in cases of peripheral vascular disease.

Measurement of distal arterial pressure by Doppler ultrasound or strain-gauge plethysmography has been found to be reliable in predicting healing following surgery (12). Besides arterial pressure, wound healing is also dependent on skin blood flow, which can be measured by xenon-133 radioisotope clearance, but there is no unanimous agreement regarding the critical value of skin flow which will guarantee healing (13, 14).

Other factors must be taken into account. For example, if an elderly patient is in extremely poor health and has multiple contractures in the affected extremity with no potential to be ambulatory following amputation, a higher level of amputation may be wise and humane to avoid multiple procedures.

POSTOPERATIVE CARE

Following surgery, wound healing is a prime concern of the surgeon because, in a patient with peripheral vascular disease, wound necrosis is not an uncommon problem and requires a higher level of reoperation.

Rigid Plaster Dressing

Now widely accepted is the method of wound care carried out by applying a rigid plaster dressing over the residual limb in the operating room (15–17). After drying of the plaster, a pylon may be attached (Fig. 11.19), making it possible for some amputees to ambulate within 48 hours of surgery. In patients with peripheral vascular disease with a lower limb amputation, early weight bearing is delayed, depending on the general medical health of the patient and on wound healing (17); this results in healing at the below-knee level in 75% of unselected patients (Fig. 11.20).

Although wound healing is not a significant problem in upper extremity amputations (since they are seldom needed), similar postoperative care by applying a rigid plaster dressing can lead to early fitting of a prosthesis. It is possible to attach a hook as a terminal device which can be activated by a shoulder harness and Bowden cable in the early postoperative period. This allows an upper extremity amputee to carry out bimanual tasks immediately following amputation and tends to increase the chance of acceptance of the final prosthesis by the amputee.

Edema Control and Promotion of Healing

Besides application of plaster casts in the operating room, other methods of edema control and facilitation of wound healing have been tried with a fair degree of success.

Air Splint. A pneumatic prosthesis may

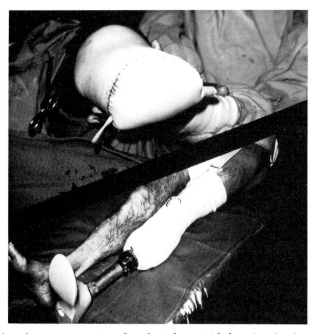

Figure 11.19.   Below-knee amputation fitted with a rigid dressing (*top*) and temporary prosthesis (*bottom*) at time of surgery. (From Banerjee, S. N. (ed.), *Rehabilitation Management of Amputees.* Baltimore, Williams & Wilkins, 1982.)

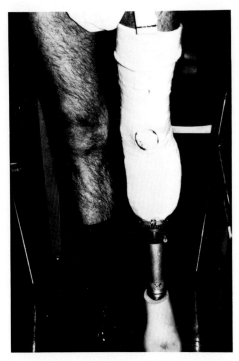

Figure 11.20. Limited weight bearing in an immediate postsurgical prosthetic fitting. Reproduced with permission from SN Banerjee (2) (ed): *Rehabilitation Management of Amputees.* Baltimore, Williams & Wilkins, 1982.

be applied in the operating room for control of edema, as well as for early weight bearing. It consists of an inflatable plastic bag mounted on an aluminum frame connected to a prosthetic foot. The air pressure is maintained around 25 mm Hg; after 48 hours, dressings are changed, and patients are allowed to carry out partial weight bearing. All patients in Little's (18) series achieved primary healing of the wound.

Unna's Paste. Ghiulamila (19) advocates application of Unna's paste to the residual limb on the operating table as a compressive bandage to promote healing and prevent edema. No untoward complications have been noted, and most patients have achieved primary healing of the surgical wound (19).

Controlled Environment Treatment. In this method the residual limb after surgery is placed in a transparent plastic bag that is connected through a flexible hose to a console containing an air compressor which controls temperature, humidity, timing, and sterility of the air circulating through the plastic bag (Fig. 11.21). The residual limb is kept in this environment 24 hours/day until complete healing of the wound is achieved. The method requires some further improvement before it can be applied on a routine basis (20).

REHABILITATION PHASE

With proper preoperative care and achievement of healing at the lowest possible level through meticulous care during surgery and the postoperative period, the patient is well on the way to the next phase of treatment—rehabilitation. Rehabilitation care for amputees is usually provided through a multidisciplinary amputee clinic team on either an inpatient or an outpatient basis. Many elderly patients are too disabled with other medical problems to be able to attend outpatient treatment, so they may require hospital admission. However, many younger patients can be adequately treated through the outpatient amputee clinic.

During the rehabilitation phase, patients are assessed by all members of the amputee clinic team, which includes a physician, physical therapist, occupational therapist, prosthetist, nurse, psychologist, and vocational counselor. Following complete assessment, specific problems are identified, and an integrated treatment program is outlined and reviewed on a weekly basis at team meetings. The overall care of the patient is usually directed by a physician specialist with knowledge and competence in all aspects of amputee care.

The patient must become an integral part of this team and should be encouraged to make suggestions for treatment, depending on specific needs. The patient's family also should be involved in the treatment, as many patients will require support from their family after discharge

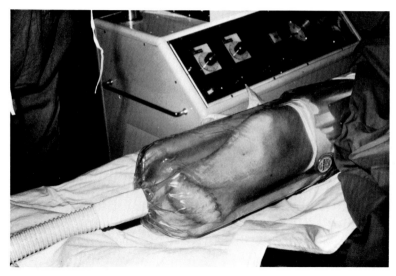

Figure 11.21.   Controlled environment treatment dressing envelope for a below-knee amputation immediately after surgery. (Reproduced with permission from: SN Banerjee (ed): *Rehabilitation Management of Amputees*. Baltimore, Williams & Wilkins, 1982.)

from the hospital. Without patient and family involvement, treatment will be less than satisfactory. The ultimate aim of rehabilitation is to allow the patient to function both physically and emotionally at the highest possible level and to reintegrate with family and community. However, both the patient and the rehabilitation team must be realistic, regarding what is achievable through the present state of our knowledge in order to avoid the "bionic man" syndrome.

FUNCTIONAL OUTCOME FOR VARIOUS LEVELS

Lower Extremity

Most patients with a unilateral below-knee (or below-elbow) amputation can expect to achieve a level of physical functioning very close to that before amputation. However, amputations above knee or above elbow create varying degrees of difficulties in carrying out certain activities. The young unilateral above-knee amputee can expect to function independently in all areas of activities of daily living and can participate in many sports activities which do not require much running. True running is not possible for an above-knee amputee because true running requires an amputee to bear weight on a flexed knee. An elderly unilateral above-knee amputee will have significant restrictions regarding his ability to walk on rough ground or climb stairs, although some vigorous elderly patients master these activities. For lower extremity amputees there is a need for development of better knee units for elderly amputees which would allow more elderly amputees to be independent ambulators with an above-knee prosthesis.

Bilateral below-knee amputation would appear to create significant difficulty, but many patients, young or old, are able to function independently with two prostheses. Of course, their walking speed is somewhat slower than that of unilateral amputees, and their endurance is more limited.

Most bilateral above-knee amputees do not become functional ambulators with two articulated above-knee prostheses because of a significant increase in energy expenditure, even for level walking. Most elderly patients with bilateral above-knee amputation are better off with an appropriate wheelchair rather than trying to walk with two articulated prostheses. There are situations where elderly bilateral above-knee amputees need to walk a short distance, e.g., in order to be able to live in their own homes; they can be fitted with "stubbies," which are really weight-bearing sockets without knee joints. The energy expenditure of walking with "stubbies" is much less than with articulated prostheses.

Upper Extremity

Patients with proximal upper extremity amputation, including above-elbow and shoulder disarticulations, will certainly benefit from a powered-prosthesis but, at present, the available powered elbow units do not provide optimal function because of frequent breakage and significant delay in operation. It appears that many amputees benefit from appropriate prosthetic fitting and training, but functional replacement for upper extremity function is still quite limited. Considerable work needs to be done in design and development of upper extremity components and terminal devices which provide optimal function.

References

1. Vitali M, Robinson KP, Andrews BG, Harris EE: Amputations and Prostheses. London, Bailliere Tindall, 1978.
2. Banerjee SN (ed): Rehabitation Management of Amputees. Baltimore, Williams & Wilkins, 1982.
3. McCollough NC, III, Shea JD, Warren WD, Sarmiento A: The dysvascular amputee: surgery and rehabilitation. Current Probl Surg, October, 1971.
4. Surgical Procedures and Treatments. Ottawa, Statistics Canada, 1970.
5. Hansson J: The Leg Amputee: A Clinical Follow-up Study. Acta Orthop Scand Suppl: 69, 1964.
6. Surgical Procedures and Treatments. Ottawa, Statistics Canada, 1975.
7. Glattly HW: A Preliminary Report on the Amputee Census: Selected Articles from Artificial Limbs. R. E. Kreiger, 1970.
8. Sarmiento A, May BJ, Sinclair WF, McCollough III, NC, Williams EM: Lower extremity amputation. Clin Orthop. Related Res. 68:22–31, 1970.
9. Burgess EM, Romano RL, Zettl JH, Schrock RD: Amputations of the leg for peripheral vascular insufficiency. J. Bone Joint Surg., 53:874–890, 1971.
10. Glattly HW: Aging and amputation. Artificial Limbs 10:1–4, 1966.
11. Murdoch G: Research and development within surgical amputee management. Acta Orthop Scand 46:526–547, 1975.
12. Wagner FW Jr: Orthopedic rehabilitation of the dysvascular lower limb. Orthop Clin North Am. 9:325–350, 1978.
13. Kostiuk JP, Wood D, Hornby R: The measurement of skin blood flow in peripheral vascular disease by epicutaneous application of 133 Xenon. J. Bone Joint Surg. 58A:833, 1976.
14. Moore WS, Henry RE, Malone JM, Daley MJ, Patton D, Childers SJ: Prospective use of xenon-133 clearance for amputation level selection. Arch Surg 116:86–88, 1981.
15. Berlemont M, Weber R, Willot JP: Ten years of experience with the immediate application of prosthetic devices to amputees of the lower extremities on the operating table. Prosthet Int 3:8–18, 1969.
16. Weiss M et al: Physiologic amputation, immediate prosthesis and early ambulation. Prosthet Int, 3:38–44, 1969.
17. Burgess EM, Romano RL, Zettl JH, Schrock RD: Amputations of the leg for peripheral vascular insufficiency. J Bone Joint Surg 53A:874–890, 1971.
18. Little JM: A pneumatic weight bearing temporary prosthesis for below-knee amputees. Lancet 1:271–273, 1971.
19. Ghiulamila RI: Semirigid dressing for postoperative fitting of below-knee prosthesis. Arch Phys Med Rehabil 53:186–192, 1972.
20. Burgess EM, Pedegana LR: Controlled environment treatment for limb surgery and trauma. (A preliminary report). Bull Prosthet Res 10(28):16–57, 1977.

CHAPTER TWELVE

General Deconditioning

T. Kavanagh

For centuries before the advent of antibiotics the cornerstone of medical treatment was bedrest. The physician, lacking a specific agent to destroy the invading pathogen, relied largely on the patient's natural defenses. If these were to be successful, the body needed to direct all its energy into the fight. Only activities vital to bodily function were permitted. Strict bedrest seemed the logical answer. Little, if any, movement was permitted—except the mandatory daily bowel movement. Even this was performed between the sheets, with the patient perching precariously on the ubiquitous bedpan (an endeavor, ironically, later found to be more energy-consuming than using the toilet). At the time, the arguments in favor of this approach seemed irrefutable: it complied perfectly with a cardinal requisite of all medical treatment, "*primum non nocere*"—do no harm.

By the late 1940s isolated reports began to appear in the medical literature suggesting that prolonged bedrest might give rise to physical changes which were counterproductive. Further evidence accumulated in succeeding decades made it increasingly apparent that a combination of recumbency and limitation of movement robs the body of its ability to cope with its normal environment and every-

day pattern of activity (1–3). Paradoxically, many of the signs and symptoms of this deconditioned state often had been confused with the manifestations of the very disease for which bedrest was prescribed. Healthy subjects confined to bed for weeks and months become just as quickly deconditioned as sick patients.

While bedrest plays only a small part in the treatment of illness today, in recent years the problem of deconditioning has been highlighted by the finding that it also results from the weightlessness of spaceflight (4). Since this can pose difficulties for the astronaut, not only during the flight itself but also on return to earth's gravitational field, research is continuing to discover ways of dealing with the situation. Apart from actual exposure to simulated space conditions, the commonest methods of inducing an exaggerated deconditioning effect in healthy volunteers are prolonged bedrest and prolonged water submersion. Major data on the subject have also accumulated from the American Gemini, Apollo, and Skylab missions, as well as the Soviet Union's Vostok and Soyuz flights.

Severe muscle or nerve diseases, such as paralytic poliomyelitis, by their very nature enforce a high degree of physical limitation and, so, are irrevocably linked with all or part of the deconditioned state. This must be taken into account when caring for or treating such conditions. Deconditioning changes may also be localized to a limb or limbs as a result of immobilization from casting, nerve section, or tenotomy.

Finally, we might consider the effects of our modern life-style, with all of its technological substitutes for muscular effort, as an insidious but equally relentless deconditioner of the human body. Indeed, it has been suggested that our current sedentary way of life might be linked to what have been referred to as "hypokinetic" diseases, i.e., diseases occurring as a result of a paucity of physical effort and bodily movement. They include coronary artery disease, obesity (and its attendant predilection for diabetes, accidents, and hypertension), various forms of osteoarthritis, autonomic disorders (insomnia, constipation), increased susceptibility to infections, a general feeling of malaise, and psychoneurotic reactions (5).

CLINICAL MANIFESTATIONS OF DECONDITIONING

Cardiovascular System

Studies on the effect of extended bedrest in healthy volunteers show considerable disturbance in cardiovascular performance. A standard submaximal level of physical effort is now accomplished at a higher heart rate and a lower stroke volume and cardiac output. While maximal heart rate is not affected, maximal stroke volume and cardiac output are reduced. This results in a drop in maximal O_2 consumption. Concomitant with these changes there is a reduction in plasma volume, red cell mass, and heart size (6).

The practical result of these cardiovascular changes is a deterioration in capacity for physical work. The deconditioned subject develops a higher heart rate and becomes breathless and distressed at effort levels which, in the conditioned state, could be accomplished with ease. The highest workload previously attained is now considerably reduced.

An even more disabling result of the cardiovascular deconditioning is the development of orthostatic intolerance, or postural hypotension, i.e., an inadequate blood pressure adjustment to sudden assumption of the upright position. Normally this maneuver requires considerable reflex alterations in the circulation of the splanchnic and peripheral venous capacitance vessels. When the conditioned individual suddenly stands up, the blood pressure remains steady, the heart rate increases by a few beats only, and the cerebral circulation is maintained. During prolonged bedrest or spaceflight, the cardiovascular system no longer has to work against gravity, and so loses some of the reflex efficiency associated with an adequate cardiodynamic response to the upright position. Sudden standing or upright tilting on the tilt table is met with a marked fall in blood pressure and an increase in heart rate together with other signs of autonomic imbalance, e.g., sweating, pallor, restlessness, and even fainting (7).

Musculoskeletal Manifestations

Long-term bedrest, water submersion, or spaceflight result in deossification of the weight-bearing bones of the skeleton (8, 9). This loss of both the organic and inorganic fractions of bone leads to a true osteoporosis which can be severe enough to be seen on simple x-ray. More sophisticated radiological techniques such as photon scanning or wedge densitometry will detect early demineralization changes in the os calcis within days of the subject being confined to bed or immobilized in a cast.

A further feature of prolonged immobilization of the whole body, or an individual limb, is pronounced loss of muscle strength and bulk (2, 10). Bedrest subjects show this particularly in the muscles of the back and also the legs, where the anterior tibial and the gastrocnemius-soleus groups are affected the most. Confinement to bed can cause a 10–15% loss of muscle strength each succeeding week. An arm encased in a plaster cast will lose 36% of its strength within 10 days.

Thermoregulation

A frequent clinical observation is that bedridden patients require higher than normal room temperatures in order to feel comfortable. Put simply, they "feel the cold" more than those who are up and about. After 8 weeks of a 16-week bedrest period, healthy subjects were found to experience a feeling of coldness, despite comfortable room temperatures and humidities, and their resting rectal temperatures fell below normal. During exercise, however, core temperatures rose more rapidly and to higher levels than usual, and took a correspondingly longer period to return to normal. Finally, sweating occurred more readily and at lower skin temperatures than prior to the bedrest (11, 12).

PHYSIOLOGICAL CHANGES ASSOCIATED WITH DECONDITIONING

Cardiovascular System

Table 12.1 summarizes some of the above and other effects. The reduction in blood volume which occurs with prolonged bedrest is also a feature of spaceflight. The mechanism is largely the same in both situations. On lying down, or encountering a zero gravity environment, some 600–700 ml of blood (11% of the average total blood volume) shifts from the legs and splanchnic circulation to the upper body, namely, the thorax. The initial effect of this sudden increase in central blood volume is an augmentation in cardiac output through the Frank-Starling mechanism. The cardiopulmonary mechanoreceptors, particularly those in the atria, are thus activated, with resultant inhibition of the vasomotor center and a decrease in peripheral vessel sympathetic tone. It is this peripheral vasodilation

Table 12.1.
Effects of Deconditioning

Measure	Effect	Prevention
Plasma volume	↓	Negative pressure to lower body, upright exercise
Tilt-table (orthostatic) tolerance	↓	Negative pressure to lower body, upright exercise
Cardiac volume	↓	Supine or upright exercise
Heart rate		
resting	↑	Supine or upright exercise
at submaximal work	↑	Supine or upright exercise
at maximal work	Nil	Supine or upright exercise
Stroke volume		
resting	↓	Supine or upright exercise
at submaximal work	↓	Supine or upright exercise
at maximal work	↓	Supine or upright exercise
Cardiac output		
resting	Nil	Supine or upright exercise
at submaximal work	↓	Supine or upright exercise
at maximal work	↓	Supine or upright exercise
A-V O_2 difference		
resting	Nil	Supine or upright exercise
at submaximal work	↑	Supine or upright exercise
at maximal work	Nil	Supine or upright exercise
$\dot{V}O_2$ maximum	↓	Supine or upright exercise
Nitrogen excretion	↑	Supine or upright exercise
Calcium excretion	↑	Weight bearing, longitudinal pressure

which inhibits secretion of antidiuretic hormone from the posterior pituitary, increases renal blood flow, and inhibits release of renin and aldosterone. A significant water diuresis occurs as well as a consequent drop in plasma volume (13).

These adjustments are evident within a few days and continue to occur throughout the first month. Ultimately, the cardiovascular system appears to stabilize to the new hydrostatic pressures, and a reduction in heart size, stroke volume, and cardiac output is seen.

The orthostatic intolerance associated with deconditioning can be largely accounted for by the reduction in plasma volume. Sudden standing causes a reversal of the above events. Of the already depleted total blood volume, 500 ml (or more) are displaced from the upper body to the legs. The ensuing drop in cardiac output and blood pressure is largely unopposed because of inadequate compensatory sympathetic constriction of the capacitance vessels. Credence to this explanation is given by a series of experiments in which, after 4 weeks of recumbency, the lower body was encased in a waist-high airtight container, and the interior pressure was reduced by a vacuum pump so as to expose the legs to a negative pressure of −30 mm Hg. This resulted in sodium and water retention, expansion of plasma volume, and almost complete maintenance of orthostatic tolerance (14). A similar tube-like device was used in the NASA Skylab missions, with lower negative body pressure being applied regularly as part of the pre- and inflight routine. Orthostatic tolerance was largely maintained, and was regained more quickly in the days following return to earth's 1-g conditions (15).

Whether or not hypovolemia is responsible for all of the adverse cardiovascular changes still presents some uncertainty. For example, while application of lower body negative pressure can be shown to reverse postural hypotension, it failed to prevent the reduction in maximum O_2 consumption (16). Conversely, prolonged periods of chair rest, wherein gravity and shifts in central blood volume are not major factors, have nevertheless been shown to result in a decreased plasma volume (17). This suggests that absence of physical effort and subsequent reduction in muscle volume may also play a part. Exercise has also been shown to ameliorate some of the unpleasant side effects suffered by the astronauts as a result of the initial sudden increase in central volume, e.g., distention of head and neck veins, and facial edema. Here, however, the benefit is probably due to an increased blood flow to the working muscles, with a consequent reduction in central blood volume.

Some researchers believe that the adverse hemodynamic characteristics of deconditioning are due, at least in part, to a direct deleterious effect of inactivity on the myocardium itself. This is supported by the finding that imposed bedrest after a period of hard physical training is accompanied by rapid regression of the training-induced increase in left ventricular end-diastolic volume and posterior wall thickness (6).

Metabolic Changes in Bone

The changes in the bone structure are accompanied by a negative calcium balance. This occurs independently of calcium intake. Urinary calcium levels begin to rise within a day or two of the commencement of bedrest, and then increase rapidly in the next 5 to 10 days until, by the 24th they are approximately twice as high as the initial values. Thereafter, they level off, and only begin to return to normal when the body regains the upright posture.

A number of well designed and carefully executed experiments have shown repeatedly that this defect in bone metabolism is due to a lack of weight bearing (2, 8, 9). No amount of muscular activity, either in the supine position or in the weightless environment of space, will compensate for the stimulus of pressure applied through the longitudinal axis of the skeleton.

In the early days of training for weightless flight, recumbent volunteers were subjected to longitudinal pressure through the skeleton by means of a spring device which, acting through the shoulders and the soles of the feet, exerted a load equivalent to body weight (Fig. 12.1). This was found to be effective in reducing the excessive urinary calcium loss. Recently, it has been discovered that rate of change of loading is more important than peak load (18); in later space flights the astronaut has carried out a maneuver involving pushing off with both legs, in a series of jumps, against the dynamic axial resistance of the springs. However, while there is now no doubt that the negative calcium balance of recumbency is due to the absence of longitudinal pressure on the bones and not due to physical inactivity, there are still some unexplained areas. For instance, why is it that some studies on poliomyelitis paraplegic patients fail to reveal any reversal of negative calcium balance by the use of techniques to apply longitudinal pressure (19, 20)? It may be that some muscle contraction is still required for the full benefit of axial pressure to be obtained.

Nitrogen Balance and Tissue Protein

Increased nitrogen excretion in the urine as well as a lowering of creatine tolerance, is also seen during immobilization and is accompanied by a significant loss of muscle mass and strength (10). Here the stimulus is lack of movement, a situation seen clinically as well as experimentally when immobility is attained by means of plaster casting. The situation is not affected by protein intake, since protein loss continues even when caloric intake has been balanced to meet energy expenditure needs. The loss of nitrogen commences by the 5th day of immobilization and reaches its maximum by the 10th day. It appears to be due to reduced synthesis of tissue protein rather than increased breakdown (21).

Thermoregulation

Little is known, as yet, regarding alterations in thermoregulatory mechanisms. However, it seems most likely to be associated with changes in the peripheral circulation, heat conductance of the skin, and sensitivity of sweat reflex. All of these are probably a measure of the decreased plasma volume (11, 12).

Pathologic End Results

Finally, certain well-recognized patho-

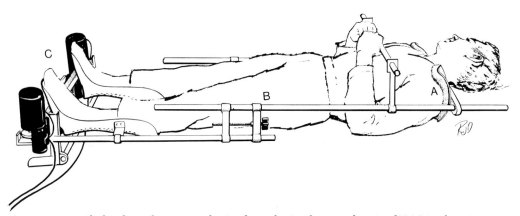

Figure 12.1.   Skeletal axial pressure device for reducing hypercalcuria of NASA pilots. Pressure points are: (A) shoulder stirrups; (B) bilateral screw device to simulate axial loading of body weight; (C) the spring loader which is screwed down to apply the compressive load to soles of the feet. (Courtesy of Dr. C. A. L. Bassett, College of Physicians and Surgeons, Columbia University, New York, N.Y.)

logical conditions arise from the deconditioned state. These include renal stones and soft tissue ossification (consequent upon the negative calcium balance and increased urinary calcium), as well as venous thrombosis and pulmonary embolus (due to the hypovolemia, combined with lower limb "blood-pooling" from immobility).

PREVENTION OF DECONDITIONING

From the above we can conclude that different mechanisms are at work in the various manifestations of the deconditioned state. Preventive measures must take this into account.

Regular exercise is of paramount importance in maintaining optimum physical work capacity, either during prolonged recumbency or space flights. All recent Skylab and Soyuz spaceflight crews have carried out regular in flight training regimens, using bicycle ergometers, treadmills, and hand devices. They all reported an improved sense of well-being from exercise, and testing confirmed that cardiovascular fitness had been well maintained. One hour daily of treadmill walking or working the pedals of the bicycle ergometer, either in the upright or supine position, is sufficient to prevent any appreciable loss in physical work capacity, maximal oxygen consumption, and muscle strength (22, 23).

Upright exercise will also partially prevent the development of postural hypotension although, as we have seen, this is more readily dealt with in space flight by regular applications of lower body negative pressure. The acute effects of falling blood pressure experienced by astronauts when they land and exit from the spacecraft under 1-g conditions are prevented by wearing an inflatable waist-high suit which exerts a pressure of 90 mm Hg at the ankles and 10 mm Hg at the waist.

Muscle strength and mass can be maintained by the dynamic type of exercise carried out with the arms and/or legs on the bicycle ergometer or treadmill. Resistance exercise, using weight and pulley circuits or a system of springs, may be more appropriate for other muscle groups. Maximum isometric contractions can also be used to achieve the same effect, probably at less frequent intervals than isotonic work (24).

The increase in urinary calcium excretion and consequent development of osteoporosis is avoided by quiet standing for 2 to 3 hours daily. Sitting in a chair will not suffice. Where standing is not possible, an oscillating bed can be employed. As we have seen, the astronauts used spring-loaded pressure on the skeleton to achieve the same effect. In the clinical setting, an interesting application of this principle has been used in the rehabilitation of patients who have been confined to bed for some time or who have developed osteoporosis of the lower limbs as a result of prolonged immobilization in a plaster cast. The method involves the use by the patient of a spring-loaded sling which provides a stirrup for the feet and a set of handles which allows the patient, by using both arms, to exert the prescribed amount of compression through the appropriate axis of the skeleton (25). There also has been increasing interest in the effects of electrical currents on bone formation and development, as well as reduction of osteoporosis of disuse; the potential for future development is intriguing.

GENERAL RECONDITIONING

Early mobilization, the more frequent use of physical and occupational therapy in the recovery phase, and the virtual demise of prolonged bedrest as a major therapeutic tool has well-nigh led to the disappearance of severe cases of deconditioning. Nevertheless, from time to time we do come across such cases, particularly in those suffering from chronic disabling disease, e.g., poliomyelitis, muscular dystrophy, or prolonged immobilization after bone fractures. A reconditioning program then becomes mandatory and, while the detailed approach will vary depending on the degree of disability, the following provides a general guide.

Cardiorespiratory System

General overall endurance, or stamina, is a pre-requisite for any exercise lasting for more than a minute. In order to obtain improvement in cardiovascular fitness, we require an endurance-type training program. Not only the type of activity, but also the intensity, duration, and frequency of workouts must be fully defined. The simplest and cheapest of all endurance activities is walking, and so it is usually our first choice as a mode of training. An alternative is stationary bicycling. Where leg power is absent or minimal, a bicycle ergometer, operated by a combination of leg and arm power or arms alone, can be used (Fig. 12.2).

Other endurance-type activities, such as swimming or cross-country skiing, can be considered but present a problem because they require special skills and are difficult to quantify.

The intensity of effort required for a particular training program is calculated as a percentage of maximum effort. The latter is expressed in terms of heart rate or oxygen consumption. To attain endurance fitness the training intensity should be between 50 and 70% of maximal oxygen consumption, or 65–75% of maximal heart rate. The latter is largely dependent on age, decreasing with advancing years; maximum oxygen consumption, or aerobic power, is not only a measure of age but also of the individual's level of endurance fitness. Both values can be established accurately by carrying out a maximum, or submaximal, exercise test on the bicycle ergometer, or treadmill. While this is always desirable in the interests of scientific precision, it may sometimes constitute a problem in the day-to-day limitations of clinical medicine. In such

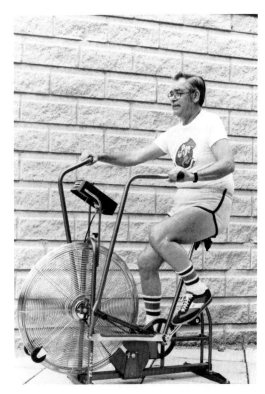

Figure 12.2.   Combined arm and leg exercise on a bicycle ergometer.

situations, we can concentrate on heart rate only, and obtain an approximate value for this by using a formula (26) based on the subject's age:

Maximum heart rate (beats/min)

$$= 210 - (\text{age in years} \times 0.65)$$

This formula is probably justified when, apart from deconditioning, the subject has no evidence of heart disease. Having calculated the maximum heart rate, we now take 70% of this figure and then ascertain the level of exertion required to achieve it, using either a trial walk, bicycle ergometer, or the treadmill, depending on our chosen mode of training.

To prescribe a suitable endurance training intensity for a 45-year-old male:

Training heart rate

$$= [210 - (45 \times 0.65)] \times 70/100 = 126 \text{ beats/min}$$

A trial demonstrates that 126 bts/min is

achieved by a workload of 50 watts on the bicycle ergometer or, say, 3 miles/hour of walking on the level.

As fitness improves, a higher intensity of training will be necessary in order to achieve the same heart rate. As for the duration of the workout, most authorities are now agreed that for development of endurance fitness, it should be between 30 and 60 minutes daily. Initially, a 30-minute session may be beyond the patient's capability, in which case one can then prescribe shorter workouts, building up to the desired duration as tolerance improves. Where there is pronounced weakness, we can employ the interval training method. This consists of 1 minute of exercise at the desired intensity, followed by 1½ minutes of rest until the requisite total exercise time is achieved, or until the heart rate fails to return to 60% of maximum by the end of any 90-second recovery period.

Beware that in the early stages of an endurance training program, the severely deconditioned patient may show evidence of cardiovascular stress. Anginal-type symptoms, facial pallor, excessive sweating, lightheadedness, nausea, or irregular heart rhythms are all indications that the intensity and/or duration of workout is excessive.

As for the frequency of these workouts, the consensus is that it should be in excess of three times weekly. Although competitive athletes will train twice daily for 7 days/week, such a draconian regime is unnecessary for the average person. Five times per week seems ideal for most of us. Three times per week will maintain the status quo, and less than that will result in deterioration.

Musculoskeletal System

Assumption of the upright position and increased weight-bearing will allow gravity to exert its pressure on the axial skeleton, thus strengthening bone tissue. Actually, 45 minutes of quiet standing, four times daily, effectively reverses calcium loss and thus reduces disuse osteoporosis.

Isometric and isotonic strengthening routines can be prescribed for individual muscle groups. Again, the intensity, duration, and frequency of training sessions have to be defined. There is some dispute as to the relative value of static, as opposed to dynamic muscle loading, and as to whether or not submaximal or maximal isometric effort is the more effective. However, a common approach is that of DeLorme and Watkins, which is based on relatively low resistance and high repetition weightlifts [27]. In this regime, the maximum weight which can be lifted 10 times through a prescribed range and without rest between lifts is termed the Ten Repetition Maximum (10 RM). Either one-half or three-quarters of this value is used as the basic training unit for 10 lifts, e.g.,

10 lifts with ½ 10 RM
10 lifts with ¾ 10 RM
10 lifts with 10 RM
30 lifts, 4 × weekly
Reassess and progress 10 RM weekly

CONCLUSION

It should be obvious from all of the above that the conditioned state can only be attained by a suitable program of regular physical activity. Most of the changes resulting therefrom are not permanent. If physical demand is reduced or removed, then functional capacity rapidly deteriorates:

"All is flux, nothing stays still."

References

1. Cuthbertson DP: The influence of prolonged muscular rest on metabolism. *Biochem J* 23: 1328–1345, 1929.
2. Deitrick JE, Whedon GD, Shorr E: Effects of immobilization upon various metabolic and physiologic functions of normal men. *Am J Med* 4:3, 1948.
3. Taylor HL, Henschel A, Brozek J, Keys A: Effects of bed rest on cardiovascular function and work performance. *J Appl Physiol* 2:223, 1949.
4. Berry CA et al: *Man's Response to Long-Duration*

Flight in the Gemini Spacecraft. Gemini Midprogram Conference. Washington, D.C., NASA SP-121, 1966.

5. Kraus H, Raab W: *Hypokinetic Disease: Diseases Produced by Lack of Exercise.* Springfield, Ill., Charles C Thomas, 1961.

6. Saltin B, Blomqvist B, Mitchell JH, Johnson RL, Jr, Wildenthal K, Chapman CB: Response to submaximal and maximal exercise after bed rest and training. *Circulation* 38 (Suppl 7): 1968.

7. Birkhead NC, Blizzard JJ, Daly JW, Haupt GH, Issekutz B, Jr, Myers RN, Rodahl K: *Cardiodynamic and Metabolic Effects of Prolonged Bed Rest with Daily Recumbent or Sitting Exercise and Sitting Inactivity.* Technical Documentary Report AMRL-TDR-64-61, Aerospace Medical Research Laboratories, Wright-Patterson Air Force Base, Ohio, August 1964.

8. Issekutz B, Jr, Blizzard JJ, Birkhead NC, Rodahl K: Effect of prolonged bed rest on urinary calcium output. *J Appl Physiol* 21:1013–1020, 1966.

9. Hattner RS, McMillan DE: Influence of weightlessness upon the skeleton: a review. *Aerospace Med* 38:849–855, 1968.

10. Whedon GD, Deitrick JE, Shorr E: Modification of the effects of immobilization upon metabolic and physiologic functions of normal men by the use of an oscillating bed. *Am J Med* 6:684–711, 1949.

11. Greenleaf JE, Reese RD: Exercise thermoregulation after 14 days of bed rest. *J Appl Physiol* 48:72–78, 1980.

12. Shvartz E, Bhattacharya A, Sperinde SJ, Brock PJ, Sciaraffa D, Haines RF, Greenleaf JE: Deconditioning-induced exercise responses as influenced by heat acclimation. *Aviat Space Environ Med* 50:893–897, 1979.

13. Gauer OH, Henry JP, Behn C: The regulation of extracellular fluid volume. *Annu Rev Physiol* 32:547, 1970.

14. Stevens PM, Lamb LE: Effects of lower body negative pressure on the cardiovascular system. *Am J Cardiol* 16:506–515, 1965.

15. Johnson RL et al: Lower-body negative pressure: third manned skylab mission. In: *Proceedings of the Skylab Life.* Sciences Symposium, vol II. Washington, D.C., NASA TMX-58154, JSC-09275, 1974.

16. Stevens PM, Miller PB, Lynch TN, Gilbert CA, Johnson RL, Lamb LE: Effects of lower body negative pressure on physiologic changes due to four weeks of hypoxic bed rest. *Aerosp Med* 37:466, 1966.

17. Lamb LE, Johnson RL, Stevens PM: Cardiovascular deconditioning during chair rest. *Aerosp Med* 35:646, 1964.

18. O'Connor JA, Lanyon LE: The effect of strain rate on mechanically adaptive bone remodelling. *Orthop Trans* 6:240–241, 1982.

19. Plum F, Dunning MF: Effect of therapeutic mobilization on hypercalciuria following acute poliomyelitis. *Arch Intern Med* 101:528–536, 1958.

20. Whedon GD, Shorr E: Metabolic studies in paralytic acute anterior poliomyelitis. II. Alterations in calcium and phosphorus metabolism. *J Clin Invest* 36:966–981, 1957.

21. Schonheyder F, Heilskov NSC, Olesen K: Isotopic studies on the mechanism of negative nitrogen balance produced by immobilization. *Scand J Clin Lab Invest* 6:178–188, 1954.

22. Johnston RS, Dietlein LF: *Proceedings of the Skylab Life.* Sciences Symposium, vols. 1 and 2. Washington, NASA TMX-58154, JSC-09275, 1974.

23. Academy of Sciences, USSR: *Basic Medical Results of the Flights of the Soyuz-13, Soyuz-14 (Salyut-3) and Soyuz-15 Spacecraft.* Washington, NASA Technical Translation, NASA TT F-16,054, 1974.

24. Hettinger T: *Isometrisches Muskeltraining.* Stuttgart, Georg Thieme, 1968.

25. Bassett CAL: Effect of force on skeletal tissues. In Downey JA, Darling RC: *Physiological Basis of Rehabilitation Medicine.* Philadelphia, WB Saunders, 1971, pp 312–315.

26. Spiro SG, Juniper E, Bowman P, Edwards RHT: An increasing work rate test for assessing the physiological strain of submaximal exercise. *Clin Sci Mol Med* 46:191–206, 1974.

27. DeLorme TL, Watkins AL: Technics of progressive resistance exercise. *Arch Phys Med Rehabil* 29:263, 1948.

CHAPTER THIRTEEN

Disability

Activities of Daily Living

M. E. BRANDSTATER

This chapter on *disability* is devoted to the complex of considerations that together make up the whole person in the total environment of home, social surroundings, and work-places.

Everyone, whether disabled or not, must regularly carry out certain tasks and activities to live, and to participate in society. These essential personal activities of self-care are called activities or daily living (ADL). They comprise activities such as getting out of bed, bathing, dressing, eating, drinking, evacuation of the bladder and bowels, and locomotion (whether it be achieved through walking or by pushing a wheelchair). If a physically disabled patient fails to achieve functional independence in any one of his self-care activities, he cannot be completely self sufficient but remains dependent on someone else to assist him. Such dependency may be the critical factor determining whether the disabled person is able to work, live at home, or travel, and it can have a major bearing on the individual's quality of life.

EVALUATION OF ADL

The evaluation of a patient's ability to perform self-care activities independently should be made systematically using a comprehensive list of all essential ADL. For clinical purposes, the list can be a simple checkoff to identify those activities with which the patient has difficulty. Staff in special rehabilitation units often evaluate their patients according to a standard protocol (7), observing performance in detail and assigning a score on a defined rating scale (Table 4.1).

Evaluation of the patient's performance in attempting ADL should be made by direct observation, not simply from a verbal report from the patient. Direct observation ensures accuracy and reveals the factors contributing to functional difficulty, such as muscle weakness, poor coordination, limited joint mobility, and perceptual impairment.

THERAPY TO IMPROVE INDEPENDENCE IN ADL

The details of the patient's performance in ADL are interpreted in the context of the patient's known locomotor status, *i.e.*, joint range of motion (ROM), muscle strength, and coordination. The information from both the ADL evaluation and the locomotor assessment forms the basis for decisions on which specific treatment would be best to help the patient achieve functional independence in ADL.

Therapy consists of two separate but interrelated phases, namely, interventions to correct locomotor deficits (e.g., loss of joint ROM) and instruction in and practice of the various self-care activities themselves. Adequate muscle strength is required for tasks such as rolling over in bed, pulling oneself up into the sitting position, sitting pushups to transfer position, and standing up. Weakness of the specific muscle groups involved in those tasks, namely, the trunk, abdominals, shoulder girdle, and hip and knee extensors, makes the respective task difficult or impossible. Strength is increased in these and other specific muscles through repetitive exercises carried out against resistance.

Significant joint contractures (discussed elsewhere) can interfere with many physical tasks and prevent completion of ADL. Once they have developed, persistent and sometimes aggressive treatment is required for their correction, e.g., serial casting or surgery. They are best treated by their prevention through proper limb positioning and performance of regular systematic ROM exercises.

Impaired motor coordination may interfere with completion of many tasks, e.g., feeding or sitting and standing due to poor balance. The most effective therapy for improving coordination is repeated practice, beginning with simple exercises and as skill improves, progressing to more complex tasks.

Brain-damaged patients may have difficulty in ADL because of perceptual deficits, confusion, or poor memory. The ability to attend, learn, and remember is obviously an important prerequisite for acquisition of new skills and techniques, for safe use of devices, and for operation of equipment such as a wheelchair.

Once a patient achieves independence in a certain self-care activity, he is expected to incorporate that activity into the personal daily routine while continuing the rest of his rehabilitation program.

Some patients, although quite independent in ADL, are passive and tend to wait for nursing or other staff to assist them in self-care activities. However, assistance should only be given when patients need it. An understanding but firm and consistent approach by all staff is necessary. When patients actively cooperate by regularly using their newly learned skills in ADL, they receive the following therapeutic benefits: regular practice improves strength, coordination, and skill, making task performance progressively easier; motivation increases as the patient observes progress; more precise discharge plans can be made because the patient and family know the level of functional independence; and it is more likely that patients will continue to function independently following discharge.

TRANSFERS

A transfer is the act of changing one's position in space within a small area, such as bed mobility and getting in and out or up and down from chairs, floor, tub, toilet, car, or wheelchair. The transfer situation presents many sources of potential hazard to the patient. He may fall because he misjudges distances. A patient in a wheelchair may forget to apply its brakes, or may stumble over the footrests. He may inadvertently injure his leg by scraping it over sharp edges, especially if the leg is anesthetic. Safety is therefore an important issue to be stressed during training. The patient should know the various transfer maneuvers well and should know of and avoid hazards.

Transfers are physically demanding of patients. A patient should be able to maintain the sitting position without postural hypotension. He must be able to roll over in bed and pull himself up into the sitting position, which requires strong abdominal or elbow flexors. Strong shoulder depressors and adductors (especially latissimus dorsi and pectoralis major) and triceps for elbow extension are required for sitting pushups by which the patient moves about in the sitting position. Sitting pushups on soft surfaces are best carried out by pushing with closed fists. For patients with hemiplegia, good function in one arm is necessary for independence.

Proper equipment is essential. The wheelchair should have good brakes on both sides and should have swinging detachable footrests. For sitting sliding transfers, the armrests must be detachable. The surfaces should be firm and at the same height. Grab bars are very useful in the bathroom to provide stability and leverage for transfers on and off the toilet, and into and out of the tub. They should be firmly fixed on the wall at the proper angle and height for the patient. The problem of getting up out of the bathtub can be avoided if the patient transfers onto a wooden stool in the bath or onto a board that is level with the bath top.

An elevated chair or toilet seat attachment saves the ambulant patient from getting down and then being unable to return to standing. Brain-damaged patients may be inattentive or may have perceptual deficits or poor balance. Quadriplegic patients with the neurological level above C7 do not have a functional triceps muscle to fix the elbow, although they may learn to lock the elbow in hyperextension. Specific techniques for different forms of transfer are used in all rehabilitation units, such as the standing pivot transfer or the one-man quadriplegic lift (2, 4, 8).

FEEDING

To feed himself, a patient must be able to grasp the food or utensil, must have adequate range of joint motion in the upper limb, and must have adequate muscle strength and coordination. Utensils with a large variety of adaptations are available to facilitate feeding, and some are shown in Figure 13.1. Built-up handles are often

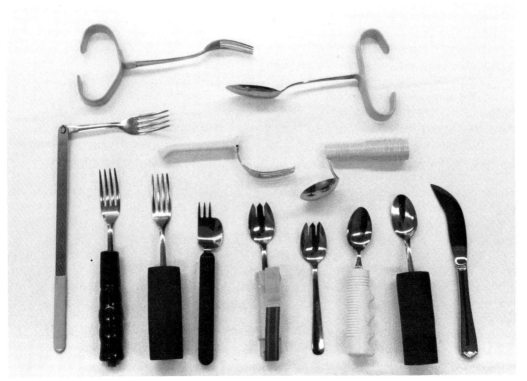

Figure 13.1. Some examples of utensils that have been adapted for patients with impaired grip.

helpful when grip range is impaired due to arthritis, and a utensil-holding device such as a universal cuff shown in Figure 13.2 helps to neutralize the grip weakness in quadriplegia. Special feeding aids (e.g., the mobile arm support in Figure 6.15) have been developed for patients with severe weakness of shoulder abduction and elbow flexion. Careful selection of the device to properly match the disability of each patient is essential. A feeding device is of value only if it permits the patient to feed himself independently, and if it is incorporated into the patient's daily routine.

Patients may have difficulty swallowing food or fluids, the possible effects being drooling, leakage from the mouth while chewing, retention of food in the mouth, nasal reflux, or aspiration. Whatever the problem, its cause and mechanisms should be analyzed to determine the best approaches to treatment. When aspiration is occurring due to dysphagia (recognized by coughing spells and lung changes) great care should be taken over the details of therapy. It is useful to have a nutritionist work with nursing and speech pathology to monitor the intake,

to maintain nutrition and hydration, and to provide optimal consistency taste and temperature of the food for swallowing. It is useful to consider also the patient's ability to take or administer their own medications.

DRESSING

Dressing and undressing require considerable joint mobility, coordination, and manual dexterity for activities which include putting the arm through a sleeve, balancing while bending over, buttoning garments, and tying laces. The patient's reach must extend to every part of his body and to the floor to retrieve items of clothing which may be inadvertently dropped. The patient must be able to don and doff splints or artificial limbs as well as clothing.

Patients with severe physical disability, e.g., hemiplegia, benefit from detailed instruction in new techniques for dressing. Adaptations to clothing are frequently necessary to help a patient achieve independence. It is easier to fasten clothing in the front than in the back and to use Velcro® or elastic instead of buttons or zippers. Some standard features are being incorporated into certain lines of clothing made commercially, but custom modification to individual items are still sometimes necessary. Long-handled reachers (Fig. 13.3) are useful for retrieving items of clothing, and many other devices are available. Resource books are available with description of devices and clothing adaptations to assist in planning an appropriate dressing strategy for a given patient (4).

PERSONAL HYGIENE

Maintenance of personal hygiene involves cleanliness and grooming, and includes the specific activities of washing, brushing teeth, using a handkerchief, shaving, applying make-up, combing hair, and attending to bladder, bowel, and menstrual care. A disabled individual

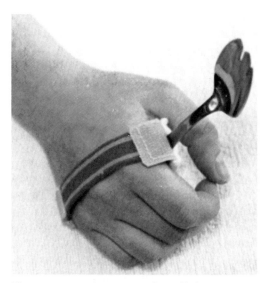

Figure 13.2. A universal cuff for patients with weak grip, e.g., quadriplegia. A pocket holds the handle of the utensil.

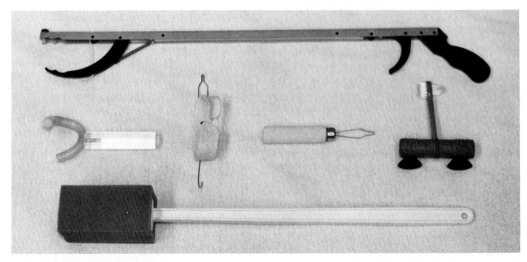

Figure 13.3.   Special devices to assist patients to reach, to wash, to do and undo buttons, and to open doors.

must have an adequate grasp and reach to carry out these activities. When the grasp is weak, a tooth brush or razor can be held by a holding device attached to the hand, such as a universal cuff or splint.

Each patient must acquire a satisfactory method for attending to bladder and bowel evacuation. Failure to keep the perineum clean and dry often leads to rashes, infections, or ulceration of the skin. Bladder incontinence in the male is best controlled by external drainage using a condom catheter and a plastic bag strapped to the leg as a reservoir. Because external drainage is not possible in the female, the options for control of incontinence are use of absorbent pads and waterproof overpants, intermittent self-catheterization or indwelling catheter. The management of neurogenic dysfunction of the bowel and bladder are described in Chapter 10.

Bowel management is best established through restoration of normal bowel function and regular evacuation. Normal function is promoted by a high residue diet and judicious use of medications when necessary. It is important to avoid constipation, impaction, and diarrhea. Disabled individuals usually schedule a certain period at the same time each day for bowel care. If a stimulus is needed to promote evacuation, a glycerine suppository may be used, or the anal sphincter may be dilated with the gloved finger. Suppository inserters and anal dilators are available for patients with inadequate range or strength. Reaching aids capable of holding toilet tissue are also sometimes necessary.

The rehabilitation goal for each patient is achievement of independence in all aspects of personal hygiene. Not only must the patient be able to carry out specific self-care techniques and manage the related activities such as transfers, but also he needs to learn to plan his schedule to allow completion of what are often very time-consuming tasks.

DISORDERS OF COMMUNICATION

Language may be defined as the comprehension and transmission of ideas and feelings through symbols, using sounds and gestures. The term speech refers to the motor aspects of verbal expression, i.e., articulation. Aphasia is a disorder of language (described in Chapter 10), and dysarthria is a disorder of speech due to weakness, spasticity, or incoordination of one or more of the muscles used in speaking; language function is usually intact.

Individuals who have loss of voice production due to a disorder of the larynx or its innervation have dysphonia, or difficulty in phonation.

Some persons are profoundly disabled in the communication domain; they are dependent on others and are often viewed as being mentally defective, existing as fringe members of their society. Adults who lose the ability to communicate often regress. Because of the physical and psychosocial impact of impaired communication, patients need detailed evaluation and treatment by a speech pathologist, along with appropriate interaction and support from the whole rehabilitation team.

If speech is so dysarthric that it cannot be understood, communication can often be helped with instruction to the patient to speak more slowly, to repeat, to say one word at a time, or to spell the word. The patient can point to a list of words or letters on a chart, or write the word. Communication may be aided by the use of various devices with switch controls and word coding, depending on the needs and capacity of the patient. Automatic dial telephones and answering devices may be useful for some disabled patients.

Blissymbolics is an exciting new communication system, especially useful for verbally handicapped children (5). It uses symbols as a communication mode. The symbols are pictorial and have a rational basis, which makes learning their meaning easy. They have no sound reference, and therefore they represent the same meaning in any language. Symbols may be arranged in groups to provide an extended repertoire of representations for things, actions, feelings, relationships, and ideas. Each symbol is drawn within a square, as shown in Figure 13.4. The selection of symbols and their layout on the communication board is determined by the needs and pointing skill of the individual. Many nonverbal children who had previously been judged as having no potential for communication have

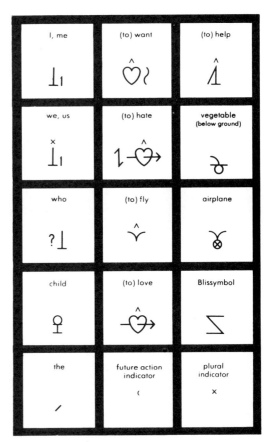

Figure 13.4. Some examples of the pictorial symbols used in the Bliss communication system.

learned to use blissymbolics and become effective communicators.

A crucial factor for the communicatively impaired patient is the role of spouse and family. Difficulties can be minimized when those close to the patient understand the nature of the problem and are prepared to invest the time, effort, and psychological support necessary to encourage and develop communication.

TRANSPORTATION AND DRIVING

An individual must be mobile if he expects to participate in the usual activities of everyday living in the community. He needs to leave his home to travel to work or school, shop, visit friends, or enjoy entertainment. Most people require some form of public or private transportation.

For the disabled, lack of suitable transportation can represent a major barrier to full independence. Some communities have developed special public transportation systems for the disabled, and these have been of immense benefit, although rarely have they met all needs. The private automobile continues to be the most important form of transportation. Whether a disabled patient is able to drive a car safely and legally therefore becomes a very important question in the context of overall independence.

The complex activity of driving a car may be analyzed according to the physical and mental demands on the individual. The tasks of opening the door, getting inside, starting the engine, releasing the brake, operating the controls, and steering require a certain degree of muscle strength, coordination, dexterity, balance, mobility, and sensation. Mentally, an individual must be attentive and be able to process information, must be able to learn to drive and know the highway laws, must have good perception of depth, spatial relationships, and figure-ground, and must have adequate visual acuity, field of vision and night vision, auditory discrimination, and judgment.

The medical evaluation should be directed at identifying those features which could be relevant to driving ability such as seizures, unstable diabetes, medications, physical endurance, attention span, judgment, visual field loss, and musculoskeletal function in the upper and lower limbs. An occupational therapist usually provides therapy to improve transfers and skill in operating controls and recommends adaptive equipment.

Some patients require no special equipment other than power steering and brakes, and automatic transmission. Hemiplegic patients may require moving the accelerator control and gear shift to the opposite side. Paraplegic patients and some double lower limb amputees require

hand controls for braking and acceleration. Quadriplegic patients also need hand controls plus adaptations for operation of the horn, lights, and ignition. They may need a special transfer board and cushion and must wear a chest harness. The only way high spinal cord-injured patients can become fully independent is through use of a van with motorized lift. Such specially adapted equipment is now commercially available.

The problems of brain-damaged patients are more complex and are less easy to define and resolve. Patients with reasonable skills should be given every opportunity to establish their capacity to drive. Because safety is so important, patients should be assessed very carefully and monitored closely during training sessions. A driving simulator is a useful aid to evaluation and training but cannot replace the on-the-road work. In patients who are borderline candidates (e.g., those having had a stroke) it is wise to postpone a final decision, allowing the patient both to improve further and to adjust emotionally to the disability. Such a patient will often do much better when re-evaluated 3–6 months later.

LOCOMOTION

Locomotion is the ability to move from one position in space to another, whether it be by walking, running, hopping, crawling, or moving by means of a wheelchair. Only walking is considered in this section. During normal human walking, smooth forward progression of the body is achieved through a series of angular motions of the lower limbs. While one leg bears weight, the other swings forward, producing an alternating, symmetrical, cyclic pattern of coordinated movements. An individual gait cycle is completed when one lower limb passes through successive swing and stance phases. It is convenient to describe and analyze gait according to these two phases, swing and stance.

Gait can only be evaluated in the clinic

when the observer is familiar with the patterns of movement seen during normal locomotion. The important angular motions occurring during the swing and stance phases in normal gait are summarized in Tables 13.1 and 13.2. For a satisfactory swing, the toe and foot must clear the ground, and there must be full reach to obtain a good step length. During stance, the individual must have suffi-

cient stability to maintain a secure upright posture on the single limb (1, 3).

Pathological gait is evaluated in two stages. First, the patient is carefully observed while walking, with and without shoes and walking aids as the case may dictate. The patient should preferably be dressed in shorts. Each body segment is systematically reviewed as the patient walks, and a written record is made of

Table 13.1.
Normal Locomotion Swing Phase (6)

	INITIAL SWING	MID-SWING	TERMINAL SWING
PELVIC ROTATION	BACKWARD 5°	NEUTRAL	FORWARD 5°
HIP	FLEXION 20°	FLEXION 20°→30°	FLEXION 30°
KNEE	FLEXION 60°	FLEXION 60°→30°	FLEXION 30°→0°
ANKLE	P. FLEXION 10°	NEUTRAL	NEUTRAL

Table 13.2.
Normal Locomotion Stance Phase (6)

	INITIAL CONTACT	LOADING RESPONSE	MID-STANCE	TERMINAL STANCE	PRE-SWING
PELVIS ROTATION	FORWARD 5°	FORWARD 5°	NEUTRAL	BACKWARD 5°	BACKWARD 5°
HIP	FLEXION 30°	FLEXION 30°	FLEXION 30°→0°	APPARENT HYPEREXT. 10°	NEUTRAL
KNEE	FULL EXTENSION	FLEXION 15°	FLEXION 15°→0°	FULL EXTENSION	FLEXION 35°
ANKLE	NEUTRAL HEEL FIRST	P. FLEXION 15°	D. FLEXION →10°	NEUTRAL	P. FLEXION 20°

any deviations from the normal patterns of movement. *Second*, the clinician interprets the underlying mechanisms for the gait deviations, taking into account the particular features of the deviations and the patient's musculoskeletal status (muscle strength, range or motion, etc.). There are many ways in which the motions of the body and limbs may deviate from normal during gait, and a comprehensive list is outside the scope of this book. A few important deviations will be described to illustrate clinical gait analysis through the strategy of careful observation followed by analysis.

Gait Deviations at the Ankle

Excessive plantar flexion may be due to a contracture, weakness of tibialis anterior, or overactivity (spasticity) of the calf muscles. During midswing it could produce foot drag, and during stance it reflects inadequate forward rotation of the tibia over the talus. Initial contact with the floor at the beginning of stance may be with the toes or forefoot rather than with the heel. The heel may not be in contact with the floor during midstance, usually because of calf spasticity or ankle contracture. On the other hand, the heel may remain on the floor in terminal stance (absence of roll off) because of calf weakness.

Gait Deviations at the Knee

Inadequate knee flexion may be due to contracture or increased tone in the quadriceps during initial and midswing, or to hamstring weakness or impaired proprioception during loading response. Inadequate extension may be due to contracture of the knee or hip, or weakness of quadriceps or calf muscles. If present during terminal swing, inadequate extension shortens the length of the step, and during stance it increases energy expenditure and may contribute to dragging of the opposite foot.

Gait Deviations at the Hip

Limited flexion may be due to contracture or weak flexor muscles. It may cause toe drag at initial swing and could result in decreased step length and slower velocity. Inadequate extension may be due to flexion contracture at the hip, weakness of the hip extensors, or decreased sensation. It decreases tibial advancement and roll-off and shortens step length. Energy cost is increased. Weakness of the hip abductors produces a Trendelenburg gait with an excessive drop of the pelvis on the side opposite to the stance limb. This may be partially compensated for by a trunk lurch to the involved side or the use of a cane on the opposite side. Arthritis of the hip joint usually produces a similar trunk lurch, and it too can be reduced by a cane in the opposite hand. Ipsilateral dropping of the pelvis during late stance may be due to calf muscle weakness.

It can be seen from the few gait deviations described here that there are often several possible reasons for an altered pattern of movement observed during gait. Careful examination of the patient's musculoskeletal status usually reveals the most likely explanation. The assessment of muscle tone and functional joint ROM in patients with lesions of the central nervous system should be made with the patient standing upright because of the influence of posture on muscle tone.

Gait Aids

Gait aids include a wide variety of walkers, crutches, and canes (Figs. 13.5–13.7). They are extensions of the upper limbs to transmit weight bearing and to provide support in the erect posture. This provides a patient who has severe lower-limb difficulties with 3-point or 4-point supports for walking. It requires sufficient upper limb strength, which may have to be acquired by supervised exercise and usually requires gait training by rehabilitation specialists.

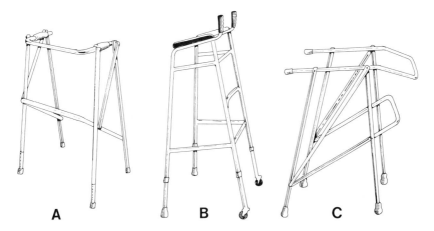

Figure 13.5. Walkers. (A) Standard walker. (B) Forearm support walker. (C) Stairclimbing walker. (Reproduced with permission from: JB Redford, *Orthotics Etcetera*. Baltimore, Williams & Wilkins.)

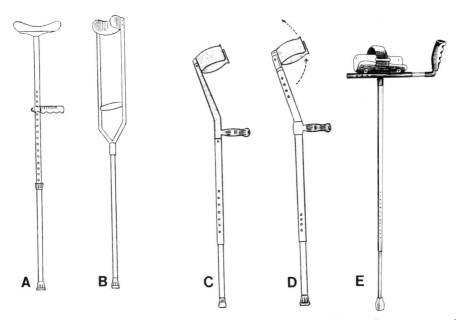

Figure 13.6. Crutches. (A) Telescopic underarm aluminum crutch. (B) Aluminum crutch with U-shaped cuff. (C) Forearm aluminum crutch with stationary forearm piece. (D) Forearm aluminum crutch with adjustable forearm piece. (E) Platform crutch. (Reproduced with permission from: JV Basmajian. *Therapeutic Exercise*. Baltimore, Williams & Wilkins; JB Redford. *Orthotics Etcetera*. Baltimore, Williams & Wilkins.)

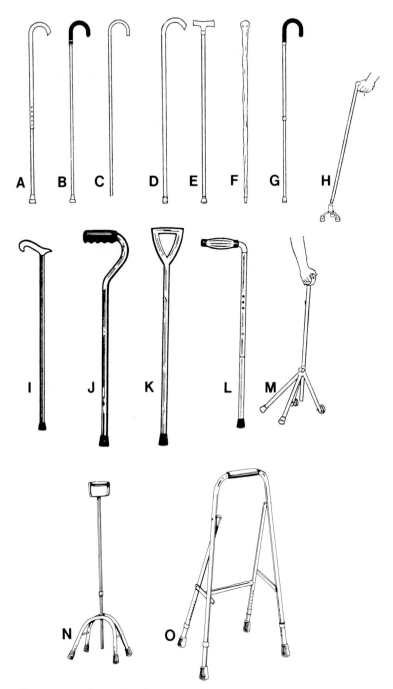

Figure 13.7. Canes. (A) Adjustable aluminum cane. (B) Aluminum cane with rubber-covered handle. (C) Nonadjustable aluminum cane. (D) Crook-top wooden cane. (E) T-top cane. (F) Straight or ball-top cane. (G) Adjustable aluminum cane with rubber-covered handle. (H) Crook-top cane with crab foot attachment. (I) Slant-handled cane. (J) Curved-top cane. (K) Shovel-handled cane. (L) Straight-handled cane. (M) Cane glider with wheels. (N) Quad cane. (O) Walk cane. (Reproduced with permission from: JB Redford. *Orthotics Etcetera*. Baltimore, Williams & Wilkins.)

References

1. Corcoran PJ, Peszczynski M: Gait and gait retraining. In JV Basmajian: *Therapeutic Exericse*, ed 3. Baltimore, Williams & Wilkins Co., 1978.
2. Ellwood PM: Transfers—method, equipment and preparation. In FJ Kottke, GK Stillwell, JF Lehmann: *Krusen's Handbook of Physical Medicine and Rehabilitation*, ed 3. Philadelphia, WB Saunders, 1982.
3. Inman VT, Ralston HJ, Todd F: *Human Walking*. Baltimore, Williams & Wilkins, 1971.
4. Lawton EB: *Activities of Daily Living for Physical Rehabilitation*. New York, McGraw-Hill, 1963.
5. McDonald ET: *Teaching and Using Blissymbolics*. Toronto, The Blissymbolics Communication Institute, 1980.
6. Pathokinesiology Service and Physical Therapy Department, Rancho Los Amigos Hospital: *Normal and Pathological Gait Syllabus*. Downey, Calif., Professional Staff Association of Rancho Los Amigos Hospital, 1981.
7. Schoening H, Iversen IA: Numerical scoring of self-care status: a study of the Kenny self-care evaluation. *Arch Phys Med Rehabil* 49:221–229, 1968.
8. Trombley CA, Scott AD: *Occupational Therapy for Physical Dysfunction*. Baltimore, Williams & Wilkins, 1977.

Vocational Problems

B. POSNER

Some handicapped men and women always have found some jobs with some employers, even though there were no laws requiring it. Those who wanted to hire handicapped people did so; those who didn't want to, didn't. Statistics were vague until recently, but it does seem clear that most handicapped people were out of the mainstream; they simply were not in the public's mind. Then in the 1960s and 1970s, a series of political and sociological explosions rocked the United States. There was the civil rights movement and affirmative action and a breaking down of segregated living patterns throughout the Western world. All of those spilled over, but in delayed reaction, into the ranks of handicapped men and women. They became the last minority to take up the struggle for equality.

We are just now beginning to sort out the impact on the employment of people with disabilities. Below are some of the implications.

SELF-PERCEPTIONS AND PERCEPTIONS OF OTHERS

In the 1960s, handicapped people began asking one another: if other minorities could stand up and demand their full rights as citizens, why not the handicapped minority, with its 12,000,000 adults? They began to organize, form coalitions, and make their demands known at all levels of government—Federal, state, and local. Lawmakers began to take notice. State civil rights statutes were amended to include the handicapped; curb cuts for wheelchairs began to appear in all cities; legislators sought out the views of disabled leaders in planning legislation. Handicapped people became visible for the first time.

Something else happened. They began to gain a new sense of self-worth; they started to perceive themselves not as "damaged people" but as fully capable people who happen to have handicaps. This positive self-perception has carried over into society in general; we (employers included) began to see them in a new light, not as inherent inferiors but as equals. This new positivism has been a major factor in expanding job opportunities for them.

AFFIRMATIVE ACTION

The Rehabilitation Act of 1973 marked a major turning point in the employment of handicapped people in the United States. Two of its provisions, Sections 503 and 504 (brought about by the urging of disabled leaders themselves), prohibited discrimination against handicapped people qualified to hold jobs. No longer could employers blithely turn them down. These sections did more. They required employers to make "reasonable accommodations" for disabled people, to enhance their opportunities to work. We began to see ramps and elevators, special devices for deaf and blind workers, readjustment of duties so disabled people could work, and even more.

More than half the employers of the United States are covered—those with government contracts and those with government grants of all kinds. These have been the pacesetters; their new practices are being emulated by employers not covered by the law—not all, of course, but a growing number. An unexpected result of Sections 503 and 504 has been the building of greater awareness among employers of handicapped people as a source of manpower. They now are being actively recruited by many businesses.

Some Emerging Problems

Affirmative action programs have aggravated a number of problems which always have existed but which have been on America's back burners until now. Among them are the following.

MISMATCHES

Some employers—largely in electronics, computers, and engineering—have been attempting to recruit handicapped workers with little success. Apparently, not too many disabled people are being prepared for careers in these and other fast-growing fields. The reasons include the lack of occupational outlook information by rehabilitation counselors, the lack of the proper kind of early schooling for technical jobs, and some stereotyped thinking which is responsible for keeping disabled people in limited fields.

UPWARD MOBILITY

Handicapped people have not moved up the ranks with the speed of other workers, although conditions show signs of improving in the future. At present, less than 2% of college students are disabled; too many are not getting the proper foundation to move upward. Change is coming, thanks to laws insisting on equal education for all handicapped children, but the pipelines must first be filled.

DISINCENTIVES

The U.S. Census Bureau reveals that 19% more handicapped than nonhandicapped people are out of the labor force—not working, not looking for work, or not counted as unemployed. Why the differential? Among the reasons: inability to handle architectural and transportation barriers (although these are lessening), settling for welfare and other payments, lack of skills to offer employers, and others.

KINDS OF DISABILITIES

Some kinds of disabilities pose more problems with employers than others—epilepsy, history of mental illness, total blindness, and total deafness. Affirmative action has eased the problem somewhat, but many public attitudes remain to be changed.

ADAPTING TO WORK

The past two decades have seen remarkable changes in work place adaptations to disabled people. The cost usually has been lower then expected. Kaiser Corporation in California, for example, decided to remodel its office buildings and was prepared to spend hundreds of thousands of dollars for accessibility. Actual cost was $8500. Lockheed's experience has been similar. Said one executive: "Thus far we have had no unreasonable requirements for major changes . . . every situation is handled separately." Most corporations are finding that the change most often needed is special parking for the handicapped.

Many devices have been created for disabled people. Special amplifiers are in wide use, enabling deaf people to converse on the telephone. Reading machines are available for the blind worker converting the printed word into sound. Special wheelchairs exist to bring mobility to those almost completely paralyzed.

Another kind of adaptation has come into its own: redesigning jobs to meet the capabilities and strengths of disabled workers. This has required more ingenuity than money.

THE RESULTS

Companies which have studied work records of their handicapped employees are virtually unanimous on these points. Performance, safety records, and attendance of disabled workers are as good as and, in many cases, better than, those of all other workers. Insurance rates do not go up when handicapped people are hired. There is surprisingly little prejudice by fellow employees against those with disabilities. The cost of making a building barrier-free is negligible if plans are incorporated in a new building. It does cost more to remodel an existing building, but even then, the price is not prohibitive. Employers generally would be willing to hire more handicapped workers, if rehabilitation and placement agencies could refer more to hiring offices. However, they would have to meet qualifications for jobs.

THE FUTURE

Employment of handicapped people is not at all like it was a mere 2 decades ago. Change is still occurring, and the future will not be at all like the present. A few indicators of the future are as follows:

More research will be devoted to bringing down the price of some of the technological breakthroughs for handicapped people, such as reading machines for the blind and automated wheelchairs for the paralyzed.

More companies will add rehabilitation specialists to their staffs to work with handicapped employees.

There will be much more upward mobility because of better education of handicapped people.

Handicapped people themselves will be called upon to advise employers about hiring practices.

No Utopia—there never is—but a time of expanding opportunities; in short, the future is bright.

Further Reading

1. American National Standards Institute: *ANSI Specifications for Making Buildings and Facilities Accessible to the Physically Handicapped*, New York, ANSI, 1980.
2. Ellner JR, Bender HE: *Hiring the Handicapped*. New York, American Management Association, 1981.
3. Pati GC, Adkins JI Jr: Hire the handicapped—compliance is good business. *Harvard Bus Rev* January-February, 1980.
4. Levitan SA, Taggart R: *Jobs for the Disabled*. Baltimore, Johns Hopkins University Press, 1977.
5. Sugarman JM: *A Citizen's Guide to Changes in Human Services Programs*, Washington, D.C., 1981.
6. White House Conference on Handicapped Individuals: *Final Report, Parts A, B, and C.* Washington, D.C., Government Printing Office, 1977.

Homemaking

M. S. WEISS

Homemaking, in rehabilitation, may be divided into two problem areas. The first is the rehabilitation of the disabled homemaker. This is really a vocational problem in the case of a person for whom the role of homemaker for a family is a major life's work. Moreover, the impairment of a homemaker is detrimental to the economic productivity and well-being of the entire family unit. It is estimated that handicapped homemakers constitute the largest occupational group among the disabled (4).

The second concern is the problem of independent living for the person who must choose between self-reliance and institutional living. This is the case of a disabled person attempting to assume or resume, by choice or necessity, an autonomous life-style away from the family. Until recently, few alternatives existed other than nursing homes or state hospitals.

The approach to the physical rehabilitation of these two groups is similar, although social, psychologic, and economic considerations may differ considerably.

Initially, the basic work skills required by household tasks are assessed. This is accomplished both by history and by observation. These tasks may be categorized as food preparation and serving; light and heavy cleaning tasks; laundry; clothing care; sewing; marketing; financial management; and child care. Simple checklists are available which cover these and

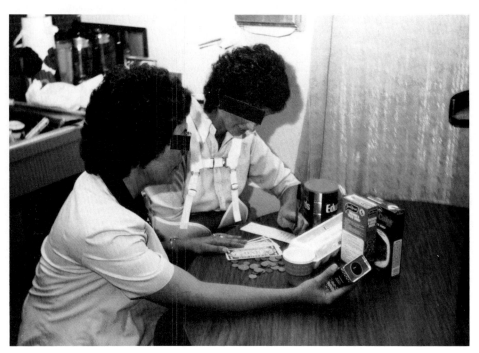

Figure 13.8. Home management skills allow independence in planning, even if physical disability precludes independent execution.

other elements. More elaborate evaluations are often done by occupational therapists or special educators in home economics (Fig. 13.8). Therapy is aimed at achievement of independence in the areas of greatest potential and functional significance.

Approaches to problem areas include training in work simplification (Table 13.3), energy conservation, and adaptive equipment (Fig. 13.9). When physical independence is not possible, the goal becomes managerial independence. The supportive role of the homemaker in parenting roles, maintenance of the emotional health of the family, and other psychosocial tasks may also be impaired and may require rehabilitative efforts. Often, training in homemaking tasks is tied to the other rehabilitation goals in exercise and therapy for recreational and psychological as well as functional gains.

Dynamic factors such as progression or remission of disease and permanence or transience of the living situation (i.e., rental or owned, with family or alone)

should be considered before committing resources to a plan. Frequently, a home visit is required to identify problems of accessibility and space limitations.

In many areas, community-based independent living programs provide services or coordinate community resources to as-

Table 13.3.
Work Simplification Techniques (4)

1. Use both hands to work
2. Lay out work areas within normal reach
3. Slide, don't lift and carry
4. Fixed work station
5. Select equipment that may be used for multiple steps of a task
6. Avoid lifting, use self-supporting tools
7. Use gravity as an assist
8. Pre-position tools
9. Locate controls and switches within easy reach
10. Sit to work whenever possible
11. Select workplace height appropriate for the worker and job
12. Maintain good working condition (light, ventilation, etc)
13. Continue tasks whenever possible

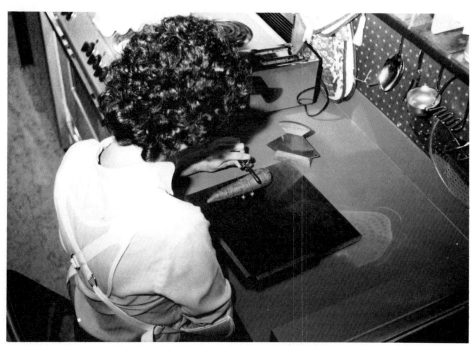

Figure 13.9. Kitchen adaptations may allow a disabled person to be independent in meal preparation.

sist severely disabled individuals in increasing self-determination and minimizing dependency. These programs require substantial consumer involvement. They provide many services, including independent living skills, training, housing, attendant care needs, peer counseling, and advocacy.

In addition to all of the above, individuals vary in "gadget tolerance" and acceptance of intervention in their life. The patient and the family must play an integral role in planning. Such factors often make the difference between effective and ineffective programs.

References

1. Anderson H: *The Disabled Homemaker.* Springfield, Ill., Charles C Thomas, 1981.
2. Erickson G: The accessible home, remodeling concerns for the disabled. *Better Homes and Gardens Remodeling Ideas* Fall: 65–79, 1981.
3. Malick MH, Sherry B: Life work tasks. In *Occupational Therapy*, Hopkins HL, Smith HD: Philadelphia, Lippincott, 1978.
4. Rusk HA: *A Manual for Training the Disabled Homemaker.* Rehabilitation Monograph VII. New York, Institute of Rehabilitation Medicine, 1970.

Recreation and Avocations

M. S. WEISS

That recreation is an important part of life is attested to by the considerable requirements in planning, training, and expense of many popular recreational activities (e.g., skiing, sailing, or scuba diving). Recreation is important to the disabled as well, although the selection and method of participation may be altered. In addition, recreation can be used as a therapeutic tool to help achieve rehabilitation goals.

THE USE OF RECREATION IN REHABILITATION

In the acute rehabilitation setting, the disabled individual and his family may find much idle time. Recreation can provide diversionary stimulation and can be directed to help relieve fear and anxiety, to facilitate self-awareness and acceptance, and to encourage social reintegration of the disabled individual into the family (2).

Later in the course of rehabilitation, recreation can provide a vehicle for social

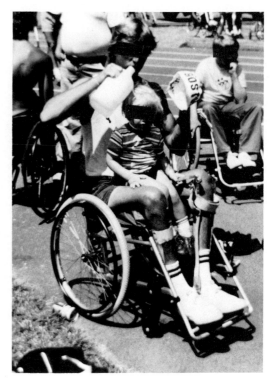

Figure 13.10. Parenting remains an important task for the disabled adult.

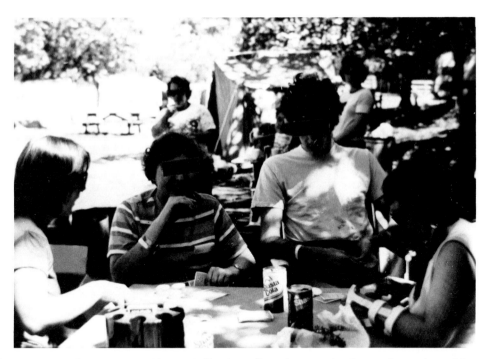

Figure 13.11. Camping provides socialization, diversion, motivation and practice with community skills.

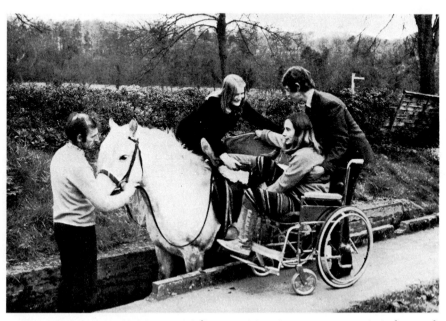

Figure 13.12. For some activities, specialist provision is necessary, as it is here where the special "pit" for the pony assists mounting and the special saddle is necessary. (Reproduced with permission from: JGP Williams and PN Sperry. *Sports Medicine*. Baltimore, Williams & Wilkins.)

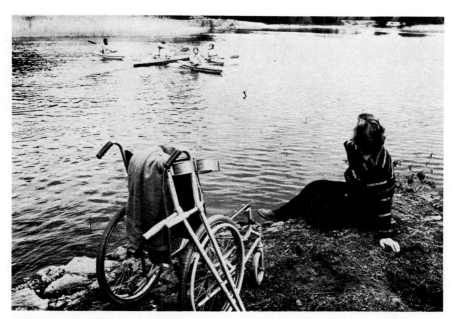

Figure 13.13. Canoeing is an excellent recreation for the disabled person with full upper limb control. (Reproduced with permission from: JGP Williams and PN Sperry. *Sports Medicine.* Baltimore, Williams & Wilkins.)

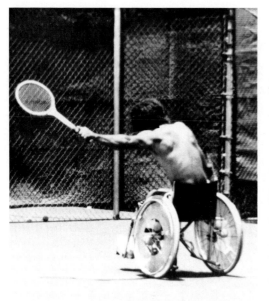

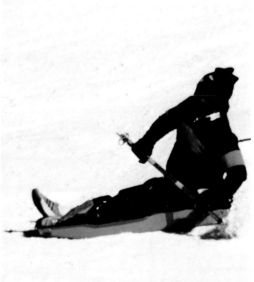

Figure 13.14. Wheelchair tennis is played on a standard court and may be played against an able-bodied opponent.

Figure 13.15. Many ski areas have been made accessible for disabled skiers.

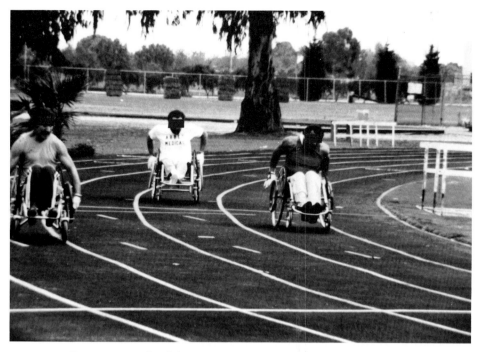

Figure 13.16.   Competitive wheelchair sports are exciting. Serious athletes train rigorously for regional, national, and international games.

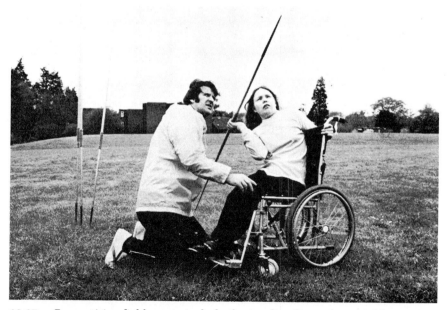

Figure 13.17.   Competitive field sports include the javelin. (Reproduced with permission from: JGP Williams and PN Sperry. *Sports Medicine*. Baltimore, Williams & Wilkins.)

Table 13.4.
A Partial List of Recreation Resources in the USA and Canada

Archery	The National Archery Association Ranks, Pa. 17572
Backpacking	See Wilderness (below)
Basketball	National Wheelchair Basketball Assn. 110 Seaton Building University of Kentucky Lexington, Ky. 40506
Bicycling	Janssen USA 2885 South Santa Fe Englewood, Colo. 80110
Bowling	American Wheelchair Bowling Assn. 2635 N.E. 19th Street Pompano Beach, Fla. 33062
Canoeing	See Wilderness—Minnesota Outward Bound
Flying	American Wheelchair Pilots Assn. 2512 West White Spur Road New River, Ariz.
Golf	John Klein Santa Barbara Comm. Golf Course 3500 McCaw Avenue Santa Barbara, Calif. 93105
Horseshoes	Daniel L. Dagle 4805 Towers Ct., N.E. Salem, Ore. 97301
Hunting & Fishing	Disabled Sportsmen of America P.O. Box 26 Vinton, Va. 24179
Marathon Running	National Spinal Cord Injury Foundation 369 Elliot Street Newton Upper Falls, Mass. 02164
Meets Track & field, soccer, bocca ball, riflery, horseback riding, swimming, weight lifting	National Association of Sports for Cerebral Palsy 66 East 34th Street New York, N.Y. 10016
Meets Track & field, weight lifting, table tennis, swimming, archery (For physically disabled. Stresses competition.)	National Wheelchair Athletic Assn. 2107 Templeton Gap Rd. Suite C Colorado Springs, Colo. 80907
Track & field, soccer, swimming, gymnastics, ice skating, bowling, floor hockey. (For mentally retarded with or without physical disability. Stresses participation.)	Special Olympics, Inc. 1701 K Street, N.W., Suite 203 Washington, D.C. 20006
Motorcycles	Wheelchair Motorcycle Association 101 Torrey Street Brockton, Mass. 02401
Recreation therapy	National Therapeutic Recreation Society 3101 Park Center Dr Alexandria, Va. 22302
Skiing	Arroya P.O. Box 5249 Stanford, Calif. 94305 National Inconvenienced Skiers Assn. Capital Hill Station PO Box 18664 Denver, Colo. 80203 Northern Handicapped Sports and Recreation Association Penn Material Bldg, 3rd Floor Denver, Colo. 80222

Table 13.4—*Continued*

Softball	National Wheelchair Softball Assn Box 737 Sioux Falls, S.D. 57101
Tennis	National Foundation for Wheelchair Tennis 3855 Birch Street Newport Beach, Calif. 92660
Travel	Air Travel Consumer Information Center Department 619F Pueblo, Colo. 81009
Travel	International Directory of Access Guides Rehabilitation International USA 20 W. 40th Street New York, N.Y. 10018
Volleyball	Wheelchair Volleyball Dennis Cherenko 1200 Hornby Street Vancouver, B.C., Canada
Water Skiing	Easy Righter 3N Company Box 24500 Los Angeles, Calif. 90024
Wilderness	Access National Parks Superintendent of Documents Washington, D.C. 20402 Berkeley Outreach Recreation Program 605 Eshleman Hall, Disabled Students Union Berkeley, Calif. 94720 Environmental Traveling Companies 2739 Taravel Street San Francisco, Calif. 94116 Minnesota Outward Bound 1055 East Wayzata Blvd. Wayzata, Minn. 55391 Vinland National Center 3675 Ihduhapi Road P.O. Box 308 Loretto, Minn. 55357

interaction through group activity, allowing for assumption of responsibility and social roles (1). Recreation should allow greater self-assertion in selection of activities than other therapies do. Group planning creates peer pressure and expectations for participation and success. Activities out of the hospital setting give valuable experience in areas of function and adaptation. Physical activities can be selected for medical goals (e.g., strengthening, gait, balance), providing practice, improving speed, motivating patient compliance with therapy, and ensuring carryover out of the rehabilitation setting (4). Outdoor activities encourage one to think of oneself as being well and useful rather than sick and dependent (Figs. 13.10–13.17).

Therapeutic recreation can also provide a safe area for experimentation in physical, social, functional, and avocational pursuits. The process of problem solving, formulating specific goals and methods to attain these goals is something the successfully rehabilitated person does dozens of times each day in dealing with an environment designed for the able-bodied.

Leisure Counseling and Avocational Goals

When first confronted with a disability, one often asks "What can I do?" Sometimes, this is answered in functional terms, such as "you'll be able to walk with braces and crutches," or in vocational terms, such as "you can take up computer programming." Perhaps what is unsaid is the question "What can I do that is fun?" Leisure counseling by a recreation therapist can address this, with therapy programmed to reach avocational goals (3). Previous leisure interests and physical and cognitive capabilities and resources are considered in planning the recreational aspects of a life-style the newly disabled will find satisfactory.

Adaptive Community Recreation Program

Many communities provide recreation programs for the disabled (5). Some of these may be tied to rehabilitation or educational goals through the public school system or community college. Others are administered by departments of parks and recreation. Still others may be adminis-

tered through special interest groups such as the summer camp program of the Muscular Dystrophy Association or recreational program of local chapters of other groups, such as a Stroke Club, Arthritis Club, or Multiple Sclerosis Society. Many disabled athletes have formed organizations for competition and promotion of adapted sports. For a list of groups and resources, see Table 13.4.

References

1. Avedon EM: *Therapeutic Recreation Service.* Englewood Cliffs, N.J., Prentice-Hall, 1974.
2. Haun P: *Recreation, A Medical Viewpoint.* New York, Columbia University Press, 1965.
3. Shank JW, Kennedy DW: Recreation and leisure counseling: a review. *Rehabil Lit* 37:258–262, 1976.
4. Weiss MS, Brown M, *et al*: Recreation therapy program for spinal cord injured patients: Measuring its effect. *Arch Phys Med Rehabil* 61:494, 1980.
5. Whitehouse J (ed): Recreation for disabled people. Physiotherapy, 64:289–301, 324, 329, 1978.

Sexual Issues and Concerns

S. S. COLE and T. M. COLE

There are many issues to consider regarding the sexual health of individuals with physical disabilities. Sexual health is a concept which combines the physiologic aspects of sex functioning and sex acts with personal morals, ethics, and values. In assessing the total impact which physical disability may have on an individual, it is essential to include sexuality in the evaluation. Issues or problems may relate to one's individual identity, the relationships one forms, or to explicit sexual behavior. The extent to which of these aspects of sexuality may be problematic can be assessed through a careful history

and physical examination. This customary medical approach may lead to an understanding of the concrete and symbolic meaning of loss or change on the individual's life (1, 2).

Sex information is acquired throughout the life span, the language of sexuality is developed, and individual values, beliefs, and attitudes are established. When a child is born with a disability or acquires one early in life, it is important for the family to take steps to provide or arrange for the provision of information about sexuality and sex development in a rather direct way, particularly if the child's access to peers and age-appropriate interactions are limited. However, when treating an individual who acquires a disability later in life, perhaps in adulthood after values and sexual experiences have been established, it is important to learn about the pre-existing beliefs, information, and experiences of the disabled person. This information will assist the physician in making realistic assessments and recommendations about continued sexual activity and sexual health for the disabled individual.

The physician should avoid viewing issues around sexual health or sex functioning as "problems." Rather, the professional is encouraged to anticipate situations and events resulting from the disability which would predictably be potential areas of concern. However, focusing only on the lost sexual functions may cause one to overlook a host of issues which may be of more immediate concern to the disabled person, particularly body image, self-esteem, and interpersonal relationships.

BODY IMAGE

A major concern for a physically handicapped person is altered body image. All of us recognize the "body beautiful" ethic prevalent in our culture. Two important concerns might be: "How does my body appear to me?" and "What do I believe others think of my body?" The body is a central part of grooming, style, and mobility in our culture, and its importance becomes even greater when it becomes physically altered. The physician should be sensitive to possible feelings of mutilation, grotesqueness, inadequacy, shame, anger, and self-pity. Many people with physical disabilities frankly admit that they deliberately avoid sexual situations for fear of humiliation or rejection (3).

SELF-ESTEEM

The many ways in which a physical disability influences self-esteem can be anticipated by noting changes and limitations on one's ability to relate to the environment, attractiveness, communicative-cognitive skills, and social status. When an individual is vulnerable to being misunderstood by the public because of grimacing, nonfluent speech, altered gait, drooling, or special equipment needs such as catheters, braces, ostomy bags, or wheelchairs, the costs to one's dignity can be enormous.

The physician must anticipate these vulnerabilities and provide the disabled person with an opportunity for the necessary training and skills to participate again in daily living with a sense of integrity and belonging (4). "For too long, people with a physical or mental handicap have been further handicapped by societal attitudes that said they should not expect and could not have a satisfactory sex life (5)."

There is indeed a two-pronged vulnerability in the fact that society places negative values on being physically disabled and is judgmental about aspects of sexuality which are perceived to be "abnormal." Frustration and decreased self-esteem can be experienced as overwhelming emotions by the disabled individual and perhaps by the family. If the health professional does not address these issues with concern and sensitivity, it will contribute to the development of an emotional disability in addition to the existing physical one.

RELATIONSHIPS

For many people, long separations from a partner or family during hospitalization constitute additional stress on top of the physicial disability. This may disrupt the intimacy of the relationship, whether it be between sexual partners or between parents and children. Feelings of isolation and loneliness can reduce a person's feeling of security. When one member of an intimate relationship is separated from the partner, the fear of abandonment can become a serious concern. The person may become quite vulnerable and dependent on the partner and jealously guard and make demands on the relationship which can have damaging effects. Our society encourages people to seek partners and establish meaningful intimate relationships. When a person experiences a physical disability, one's feelings of physical and emotional competency can be compromised. The caregiver must be careful not to foster the idea that there is no sex life after disability. Instead, the importance and validity of sex should be promoted within the moral and ethical values of the patient.

CATEGORIES OF CONCERNS

Physical disabilities can be grouped into four different categories to prepare the health professional to anticipate the likely areas of concerns and problems (6).

In *Category I* are the disabilities which occur at birth or in early childhood and are of a stable nature. Club foot is an example. Children with nonprogressive disabilities may be limited by the disability and may progress through their psychosexual developmental stages within the limitations. They may be prevented from having the same opportunity as peers in acquiring knowledge and language of sex, and the very practical opportunities of experimentation with their own bodies and with peers. Some children may never experience nudity before another person, including family members, during these important years.

In *Category II* are disabilities which are also acquired in early childhood or before puberty but are progressive and therefore unstable in nature. Juvenile rheumatoid arthritis might be an example. Young people with these types of disabilities may be constantly imposed upon by progressive limitations in their natural development. It is difficult to plan one's life and develop the necessary social skills in preparation for adulthood in the face of progressive

and unpredictable vulnerability. Family support and age-appropriate maturational opportunities in both of these categories of childhood disabilities will play major roles in influencing how much the child is able to grow and mature with peers.

In *Category III* are disabilities which occur in adulthood and are nonprogressive. Many types of traumatic physical disabilities are included in this group. In such situations an adult's sex role patterning may be abruptly altered. Relationships may also be interrupted. Life's work or career plans may be diverted, leading to major changes in the life-style.

In *Category IV* are physical disabilities which are acquired in adulthood but are progressive in nature. Progressive forms of arthritis or the natural aging processes are examples. Persons with progressive adult disabilities will frequently experience increasing limitations which control activities and events in their lives. Increased dependence on medical or outside assistance can interfere with intimacy in relationships. Physical disabilities which probably will lead to death can greatly influence an individual's feelings of stability, wholeness, and sense of control.

Not all rehabilitation professionals are adequately prepared to deal directly with the sexual concerns of the disabled patient or client. Not only may they feel uncomfortable with the topic, but they may also lack institutional or administrative support for this aspect of health care. Training opportunities to increase skills are not commonly available. When sexual issues arise, including sexually inappropriate behavior, it is easy to understand the professional's desire to avoid the situation. Anxiety, lack of information, and the "conspiracy of silence" (1) can contribute to unnecessary suffering by the disabled person. Conversely, not every member of the rehabilitation team should get involved in the details, nor should an overzealous approach be used. Sensitivity, assessment, and communication by the physician regarding sexual concerns of the patient will decrease difficult situations and sexually inappropriate behavior.

SEX ROLE BEHAVIOR

Sex role development and behavior are those aspects of gender identity which we call "maleness-femaleness." Almost always they will be influenced, perhaps even changed, by a physical disability. Attitudes and experiences in masculine and feminine sex development must be understood and integrated by the disabled person and the family. One should attempt to understand pre-existing sex role preferences. The patient's sexual orientation, i.e., heterosexuality or homosexuality, should be determined and not assumed.

Likewise, incidences of sexual assault or trauma which would directly influence attitudes about sexuality should be identified if pertinent to the patient's current sexual history. Helping with sexual behavior problems can best be facilitated by first establishing connections between the problems and the person's background, current environment, and support network. The support network, including family, must be guided and educated into appropriate roles which will help the patient experience affirmation. Denial of sexuality by the family is as inappropriate as is explicit, exploitive, or acting-out behavior by the family.

FAMILIES

Families of patients with head trauma, stroke, or other conditions producing cognitive impairment should be guided in the management of sexually inappropriate or acting-out behavior. Families of children with disabilities should be assisted to provide meaningful sex education for the child and to help the child gain the skills which will lead to responsible sexual decision making.

Perhaps the greatest inconvenience of all will be the impact which the disability produces in the individual's life-style. The position the patient occupied in the family, the relationship the patient had with the family and other close friends, the career which was being pursued, the established role in the community, and concerns related to the duration of the disability will assuredly create anxiety.

PHYSICAL DYSFUNCTION

Negative attitudes toward physical disability may already exist in the individual who has suddenly acquired a disability. Information about sexual health and sex functioning may be limited. Likewise, rigid or restrictive attitudes toward sexual behavior may be part of the individual's personality and values.

Physical functioning may be affected by paralysis, contractures, pain, loss of control of bowel and bladder functioning, medication side effects, spasticity, incoordination, or other neurologic changes. The presence of these conditions may affect one's physical ability to function in sexually intimate activities. If mobility is affected, the potential for sexual activity might be influenced simply by the isolation from social or private experiences which inability imposes on the person.

Limitation of motion may also influence sexual positioning, particularly if the ability to utilize preferred positions has been compromised. For example, if a man who prefers male-on-top positioning for sexual intercourse sustains bilateral above-knee amputations of his legs, he may no longer be able to maintain balance or perform vigorous pelvic thrusting. His sexual self-image may be threatened or destroyed. Without a serious discussion and problem-solving assistance, these situations can further frustrate, influence, and seriously impair relationships. Sexual activity may cease unnecessarily.

The presence of medically necessary equipment such as external urinary drainage systems, urethral catheters, stoma collections bags and braces may be permanent components of the disabled person's life, and therefore will need to be integrated into issues about body image and intimacy. Careful preparation in hygiene should be encouraged for the individual or couple in order to reduce predictable events which would increase feelings of vulnerability and rejection during sexually intimate times.

SEX FUNCTIONING

When assessing the impact a disability has on sex functioning, it is necessary for the professional to identify the knowledge and experiences which existed before the onset of the disability. This will be helpful in identifying what the patient might consider to be a loss or compromise. For men, sexual function can be impaired by loss of sensation or loss of ability to have erection, orgasm, or ejaculation. Fertility is an appropriate concern and must be sensitively discussed. A woman who has experienced a physical disability may notice changes in her usual pattern of sexual arousal during intimacy and may experience a diminished ability to orgasm. Fertility and birth control information must be included in assessment and treatment for all women of childbearing age.

Information about side effects of medications will be helpful to the disabled person. It will also be necessary to conduct a genital examination to assess neurologic impairments. As mentioned earlier, taking a history to include identification of pre-existing concerns or dysfunctions will be helpful. It may be necessary to sort out how much of the current concern around sexual issues is directly influenced by the presence of a disability and how much was pre-existing within the individual or the relationship. Where appropriate, fertility, pregnancy, and delivery information relating to the disability must be discussed with a disabled woman so that she will at all times have the necessary information with which to make responsible sexual decisions and maintain sexual health.

Previous sexual activity and attitudes about sexual behavior can best be assessed by taking a brief sex history. However, as many patients regard the sexual domain as a private rather than a medical concern, questions should be open-ended and supportive rather than overly directive. The interview should be conducted out of hearing of the patient's roommates. Discussion about concepts and preferences of sexual expression should include masturbation, coitus, positioning techniques, breadth of sexual expressions, and past experience.

Assessment, discussion, and intervention with the issues suggested here will positively contribute to increased understanding of sexual health for the patient and will diminish or avoid the development of unnecessary problems. The respect, sensitivity, integrity, professional preparation, and training of the health provider will help to create a sex-positive environment. In a health care setting, such an environment will increase the possibility for people with physical disabilities to feel good about themselves as sexual, adult, responsible, and whole human beings.

References

1. Crewe N: Sexually inappropriate behavior. In Bishop D: Behavioral Problems and the Disabled. Baltimore, Williams & Wilkins, 1980.
2. Cole T: Sexuality and the Spinal Cord Injured. In Green R: Human Sexuality: A Health Practitioner's Text. Baltimore, Williams & Wilkins, 1975.
3. Schiller P: The Sex Profession: What Sex Therapy Can Do, chap 7. Washington, D.C., Chilmark House, 1981.
4. Blum G, Blum B: Feeling Good About Yourself. Mill Valley, Calf., Feeling Good Associates, 1981.
5. Carrera M: Sex: The Fact, the Acts, and Your Feelings. New York, Crown Publishers, 1981.
6. Cole T, Cole S: Sexual Health and Physical Disability. In: Lief H: Sexual Problems in Medical Practice. Monroe, Wisc., American Medical Association, 1981.

Impact of Disability on Family and Society

M. D. Romano

The onset of disability may be likened to the sudden visit of an unwelcome neighbor who appears at the door uninvited and stays forever. Just as a neighbor's imposition in this way is first met with superficial equanimity, if not cordiality, initial responses give way to disruption, and if the neighbor stays long enough, eventually the host family typically reestablishes a homeostasis despite the neighbor's presence, acknowledging it but not capitulating to it. For some families the sudden presence of an uninvited and unwelcome guest will be more disruptive than for others. For them more time is needed for the restoration of homeostasis. So it is when a disability enters a family. There is a period of disruption, or crisis (a breakdown in the usual means of coping (12)), through which the family moves to return to living, with or despite the disability.

If there is anything that can be said with conviction about the impact of disability on families, it is that one cannot generalize about it. Yet the psychological literature is full of dire prognostications (1–3, 8, 9, 14). Among the *assumptions* about what disability does to families are that role reversal invariably occurs when a parent becomes disabled; disabled people are socially isolated and there is social stigma attached to being disabled; family relations are disrupted by disability and social, leisure, and recreational activities change; and families coping with disability are pitiable, or courageous, or chronically depressed.

In actuality, however, there has been relatively little documentation of these predictions. Able-bodied professionals, with good intentions, may be projecting their imagined feelings onto families facing disability. What little research does exist suggests that disability is not, in the long run, the causative factor in family problems, although it may often be blamed (4, 10, 11, 13). Families living with disability are usually socialized to the same beliefs about disability that the rest of the society holds and, consequently, when they face difficulties with rebellious adolescents or financial shortages, they will blame the disability, not realizing that other families without disability may be coping with identical problems.

In considering the impact of disability on families, one must separate early responses related to the onset crisis from the ultimate impact. Homeostasis is restored through the accomplishment of "crisis-specific tasks," each of which is integral to the process (2). Family life is a process rather than a static state, and families are constantly engaged in balancing themselves with other family members and the outside world.

The initial response to a disability in a family may be grounded in a matrix of variables: stage of life at which a family member becomes disabled, the nature of the disabling condition, the ethnocultural identity of the family, and the feelings of the family members.

TIME OF ONSET

When a person is congenitally disabled, his family knows no other way of his being, that is, the disability is at least part of the person from the very beginning. Disabilities acquired after birth (whether acquired in childhood, adulthood, or in old age) introduce the possibility of dissonance between what was and what is. This is not to suggest that dissonance may not also exist for the congenitally disabled person and the family; in that situation, dissonance may reflect what was anticipated and what is.

Resolution involves incorporating the reality of disability as part of the person, not all of him, with a recognition that the disabled person must continue to master life tasks with and despite disability (when, for example, a child born without arms strives to master the environment with feet, mouth, and so forth, if given the opportunity and the encouragement to do so).

If, however, an adult loses his arms, substitution of feet as tools for mastery may be perceived as psychologically difficult (not to mention physically) because the adult has been socialized to see that feet as means of walking rather than as means of grasping objects. The person who loses arms will miss them whereas the person who has never had them cannot miss them in the same way. The experience may be comparable for the family of the disabled person in that it, too, must come to terms with the needs for new ways of doing and for additional ways of being.

NATURE OF THE DISABLING CONDITION

The nature of the disabling condition refers to the disability itself: chronic progressive, chronic remitting, static, or ambiguous, as well as to whether the disabling condition is visible or invisible to others.

The nature of the disabling condition itself imposes certain constraints on the person with the disability and the family. A static disability, such as limb absence, may raise questions of individual potential, but it also presents an unambiguous situation with which the family knows it must permanently live and cope. Such disabilities will not worsen, nor will they remit; they simply are. Chronic progressive and remitting conditions, on the other hand, present ambiguity to families.

Ambiguous situations cause anxiety and raise unanswered questions: "When?" or "How long?" or "Will?" Whether the condition be multiple sclerosis, cancer, diabetes, or any other chronic condition, the family must come to terms with predictable unpredictability.

The visibility of a given condition is also an issue. Visible disabilities demand acknowledgment; invisible disabilities enable the disabled person and his family to "pass for normal" in the world (7). Invisible disabilities present families with the necessity to decide when, how, and who to "tell."

ETHNOCULTURAL IDENTITY

The ethnocultural identity of a family refers to those attitudes and beliefs which have been incorporated unconsciously into a family's belief system and which are grounded in a family's ethnic and religious background and in the larger society in which a family lives. The degree to which families have internalized cultural and/or religious beliefs and pre- and proscriptions about the meaning of disability and about family roles, rights, and rituals may have a significant effect upon a given family's reaction to the onset of a disability. Sex role stereotyping, which is typically culturally defined, has been described as a positive correlate to family alienation with disability (13).

The Judeo-Christian ethic, upon which much of Western culture is founded, defines physical defect as just compensation for sin, i.e., physical stigmata as the visual manifestation of moral impairment (7, 15). Thus, the onset of disability may be perceived by a family as punishment. In some families, where there is a fatalistic acceptance of divine will, onset of disability may be accepted as a test of belief—consider Job who, upon the news of his first losses, ". . .arose, and rent his mantle, and shaved his head, and fell down upon the ground, and worshipped. And said, "Naked came I out of my mother's womb, and naked shall I return thither: the Lord gave, and the Lord hath taken away; blessed be the name of the Lord" (*Job* 1:20–21).

FEELINGS

Associated with the crisis are feelings, for instance, *anxiety.* This may result from the ambiguity of the nature of the disabling condition, from an accepted belief in disability as punishment, or as a result of the recognition that we humans are frail and mortal, confronting the family with a reminder of ephemerality. Anxiety may also arise when disability requires a family to relinquish its fantasy about what family life will be: that idealized version of Mother-Father-Dick-Jane-Baby Sally-Puff-and-Spot who live in a little house with a picket fence in a place where the sun always shines, where Father goes to work each day, and where Mother bakes pies while the children run and play. In actuality, of course, the presence of disability does not preclude work or play or the maintenance of an intact, interdependent, and loving family unit, but in the idealized fantasy of the family, disability is generally not part of the vision.

In addition to anxiety, a family struggling with the onset of disability may feel *anger,* and this anger may be directed either outward toward an abstract or concrete other, or inward. When the anger is turned outward, it may be toward Providence, toward innocent others who become the objects of anger because they are whole and envied or, if appropriate, toward the causative person of the disability, e.g., the driver of the auto in which a family member was injured. When the anger is turned inward, it may take the form of *guilt*—"I should never have let him have that motorcycle"—or anger toward the disabled family member for "breach-of-contract," that is, for breaking the tacit contract upon which the family's life together is predicated. Such tacit contracts exist despite explicit contracts such as marriage vows; we may promise, "For

better or worse, for richer or poorer, in sickness and in health . . .," but the promise is made in the assumption of better, richer, and healthy, not their converse, and when the contract is perceived as broken by the advent of a disability, the disabled person may be perceived as a betrayer. Often, such anger is further complicated by guilt because society places a negative value on mean and angry feelings toward the sick.

Shame is another feeling that some families experience when a family member becomes disabled. Shame is directly related to the imagined social consequences of disability. It is the anticipation of social disgrace for deviance, and its presence in the families of newly disabled persons may reflect family acceptance of disability as the manifestation of moral imperfection, an anticipation of family discreditation by becoming the object of pity or discomfort in others, or of representing the vulnerability of the human condition to others. It might be noted here that not all disabilities are perceived as shameful, or perhaps that some are more shameful than others. War injuries incurred before the Vietnam era have been described as badges of honor while Vietnam veterans with injuries describe being treated as pariahs. Here one can see that culturally accepted righteousness exonerates physical deviance while collective guilt punishes it.

This component of disability is an area of larger, societal ambivalence. Medical and technological advances in this century have made it possible for people with disabilities to survive with potential beyond mere existence. Whereas, in the past, disabled family members could be institutionalized or hidden away at home, scientific progress and broad social change potentially enable disabled people to be full participatory members of society. While justifiably proud of its progress, however, society still simultaneously maintains many of its discrediting attitudes toward disability and has yet to resolve its priorities toward disabled per-

sons. Opportunities for vocational and avocational productivity, for social and educational integration, and even for such
basic rights as enfranchisement and public access through the removal of architectural barriers have become political issues as well as ethical ones (6). The impact
of disability on society is economic, political and social as the larger society struggles to "place" disabled people conso-
nantly within itself. These struggles are
mirrored in the family, with parallels in
the process of restoring family homeostasis and societal homeostasis in response
to the onset of disability.

ROLE OF THE HEALTH CARE SYSTEM

Physicians and other health care personnel are potent resources for families
coping with disability and for the larger
society (5, 16); health providers can edu-
cate about the specific nature and implications of disability, can provide positive
models of acceptance and comfort in dealing with disability, and can encourage the
establishment and maintenance of support systems within extended families,
communities, self-help groups, and consumer organizations. The resolution of
any crisis is potentially a growth process
for those experiencing the crisis, and
planful collaboration, education, and advocacy are the skills that enable mastery
of the tasks necessary to resolve crises
and restore adaptive homeostasis. Moreover, it is health care professionals who
must do further research into the long-
term effects of disabilities on families and
the societal environment in which they
live.

References

1. Anthony E: The mutative impact of serious mental and physical illness in a parent on family life. In Anthony E, Koupernik C: *The Child in His Family*, vol 1, New York, John Wiley & Sons, 1970.
2. Beard M: Changing family relationships. *Dialysis Transplant* 4:36–41, 1975.
3. Bene A: The influence of deaf and dumb parents on a child's development. Psychoanal Study Child 32:175–194, 1977.
4. Buck FM, Hohmann GW: Personality and behavior of children of disabled and nondisabled fathers. Presented at the 87th Annual Meeting of the American Psychological Association, New York, 1979.
5. Dobrof R, Litwak E: *Maintenance of Family Ties of Long-Term Patients: Theory and Guide to Practice*. Washington, D.C., DHEW, 1979.
6. Eisenberg MG, Griggins C, Duval RJ: *Disabled People as Second-Class Citizens*. New York, Springer, 1982.
7. Goffman E: *Stigma: Notes on the Management of Spoiled Identity*. Englewood Cliffs, N.J., Prentice-Hall, 1963.
8. Heslinga K, Schellen A, Verkuyl A: *Not Made of Stone: The Sexual Problems of Handicapped People*. Springfield, Ill., Charles C Thomas, 1974.
9. Hilbourne J: On disabling the normal: the implications of physical disability for other people. Br J Soc Work 3:497–504, 1973.
10. Hohmann GW, Buck FM: Influence of parental disability characteristics on children's personality and behavior. Presented at the 87th Annual Meeting of the American Psychological Association, New York, 1979.
11. Power PW, Dell Orto AE: *Role of the Family in the Rehabilitation of the Physically Disabled*. Baltimore, University Park Press, 1980.
12. Rapoport L: Crisis intervention as a mode of brief treatment. In Roberts RW, Nee RH: *Theories of Social Casework*. Chicago, University of Chicago Press, 1970.
13. Rosenstock FW: *Disabling Illness and Family Alienation*. Washington, D.C., DHEW, 1968.
14. Thomason B, Clifford K: The disabled person and family dynamics. Accent on Living 17:20–35, 1972.
15. Thurer S: Disability and monstrosity: a look at literary distortions of handicapping conditions. Rehabil Lit 41:12–15, 1980.
16. Ziebell B: *As Normal As Possible*. Tucson, Ariz., The Arthritis Foundation, Southern Arizona Chapter, 1976.

CHAPTER FOURTEEN

Special Considerations in Rehabilitation

The Athlete

J. DARRACOTT

This chapter presents a series of short sections, starting with *The Athlete*, which outline situations or patient populations requiring a somewhat modified approach for successful rehabilitation.

PRINCIPLES OF MANAGEMENT OF INJURIES

Although the athlete is considered to have special needs in the management of athletic injuries, the principles involved are identical to those required in the management of the nonathletic soft tissue injury. It is strange to reflect that while the need for early intensive management is generally recognized in athletes indulging in essentially recreational activity, the same is not generally true for injuries affecting work. What is special or different about most athletes is their strong desire for a complete and rapid recovery, and in their special area they function at the limits of their capacity without significant reserve.

Management of soft tissue injuries requires early consultation, accurate diagnosis, intensive treatment, and functional tests of recovery.

Basic Principles

EARLY CONSULTATION

Any soft tissue injury results in loss of function, the degree of which tends to be proportional to the severity of the injury; the aim of treatment is to restore full function as quickly as possible. The earlier the patient is seen, the sooner appropriate treatment can be initiated. The physician providing that consultation must be accessible and prepared to see injuries the same day.

ACCURATE DIAGNOSIS

Accurate diagnosis requires an accurate history; the mechanism of injury and subsequent course usually provide signposts for a diagnosis and identification of the structure injured. The diagnosis must then be confirmed by examination. Without causing unnecessary pain, an effort must be made to identify the injured structure by some form of stress, and

277

other possible causes must be excluded. It is imperative that lesions requiring early surgical intervention (e.g., a complete tear of the medial collateral ligament of the knee) are identified at this stage when direct repair with enhanced results is possible. Rational specific treatment and reasonably accurate prognosis depend on the physician's ability to make an accurate diagnosis.

INTENSIVE TREATMENT

In the same way that few physicians are well trained to assess sports injuries, many therapists lack the particular skills required to treat them. Physicians treating such injuries should develop rapport with a therapist or group of therapists interested in developing the particular skills needed to treat athletes and their injuries. The therapist should be prepared to treat the patient at least daily starting on the day of referral and must ensure that even on weekends appropriate exercises etc. are continued by the patient. As a general rule a little exercise 2–5 minutes hourly is preferable to one 30-minute session. The physician himself should be prepared to instruct the athlete in simple modes of palliation and early exercise routines. As a general rule, rest alone is never adequate treatment.

FUNCTIONAL TESTS OF RECOVERY

The physician should consider the stresses involved before returning the athlete to his sport. The athlete must regain full range of joint movement, full stretch in muscles and ligaments, and full power. Anything less will result in reinjury. If the athlete has a trainer, he should be involved and, particularly in the case of professional athletes, the pressures that are applied to and by coaches should not be allowed to influence the medical decisions on fitness to perform. The physician must ensure that the injured part has been fully stressed under controlled conditions before the athlete returns to full combat.

TREATMENT—GENERAL

The effect of trauma is tissue damage resulting in an inflammatory response. Platelets and macrophages release factors which are mitogenic for fibroplasts and smooth muscle cells which synthesize new collagen to repair the defect (1). As a general rule, treatment should attempt to reduce the swelling and pain of the inflammatory response without propagating the injury, and while not delaying repair should prevent the contractures that occur with collagen maturation.

In the absence of clear evidence that any electrical modality has an effect on inflammation, any form of superficial heat generally provides the palliation required. Traditionally, ice is used early after injury, and some form of heat is used later. Elevation and effleurage (a form of massage) may assist in clearance of the metabolites of tissue damage as will early mobilization in the form of exercise within the limits of pain. Every effort should be made to ensure that muscle power is maintained as near normal as possible.

The use of non-steroidal anti-inflammatory drugs is ill-advised, as the serious side effects (though infrequent) make it impossible to justify their use for injuries which respond so well to appropriate local management. In addition the analgesic effect's masking of pain may result in extension of the injury. For the same reason the superficially attractive injection of local anesthetic and corticosteroids to enable an athlete to perform is culpable if further injury results.

ACUTE INJURIES

Joint

Faced with a painful, swollen joint, the physician must by history and examination exclude fracture or complete ligamentous rupture—which should be referred to a surgeon. In the knee it may be difficult to exclude a meniscal tear for the first few days, but nothing is lost by delaying invasive investigation while treating the attendant features.

(a) Comparative rest by splinting and in the case of weight-bearing joints the use of crutches for the first few days is usually indicated.

(b) Increased fluid within the knee results in a marked increase in intra-articular pressure and pain (2); attempted quadriceps contractions increases this yet further (3). If the fluid is blood, a synovitis will result. If the joint is accessible and particularly if the effusion is tense and causing pain, it should be aspirated, and a Robert-Jones type compression bandage should be applied. Occasionally, the aspiration must be repeated due to reaccumulation of synovial fluid or blood over the first few days, this reaccumulation can usually be prevented by the consistent use of a backslab and crutches.

(c) Palliation of pain traditionally in the form of ice (early) or heat (late).

(d) Exercise—initially isometric contractions progressing to isotonic with full range of movement providing the joint remains "dry."

(e) If meniscal damage is suspected in the knee, the patient should be reviewed every few days until this factor can be excluded; or if firm signs are elicited, until appropriate investigation in the form of double-contrast arthrography or arthroscopy can be carried out.

Ligament

Complete rupture must be demonstrated early, and in the case of lateral ligaments, must be confirmed by stress x-ray (Fig. 14.1). The stress should be applied without either local or general anesthetic because of the risk of turning an incomplete into a complete tear. A complete tear should be referred for early direct repair; there is evidence that the results of surgical repair of complete rupture of the anterior cruciate and medial collateral ligaments of the knee within 1 week are significantly better than those

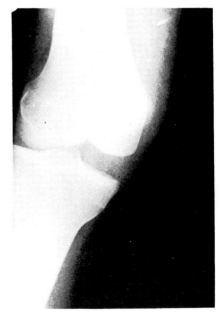

Figure 14.1. X-ray photograph during stress-abduction of a knee in which the medial collateral ligament is torn. (Reproduced with permission from: JGP Williams and PN Sperry: *Sports Medicine.* Baltimore, Williams & Wilkins)

in whom the repair was delayed (4). In general, early direct repair produces better functional results than late ligamentous reconstruction.

Partial tear or Sprain. The management otherwise should follow the basic principles—palliation, relative rest, and mobilization within pain for partial tears of the lateral ligament of the ankle; active mobilization with or without physiotherapy has been shown to achieve significantly better results than immobilization in a POP cast or no treatment (5). A simple sprain should be fully functional in 7–14 days.

Recurrent Sprain. In the case of the ankle, the associated loss of balance due to loss of proprioceptive information from the damaged ligament may increase the likelihood of recurrent sprain. Also there may be loss of full range of movement due to residual ligamentous contracture. A simple balance exercise and stabilizing routine should remedy the situation in 7–

14 days. The temptation to obtain a quick "cure" by injection of corticosteroids should be resisted; the risk is a complete rupture.

Muscle

Strain, "pull," or partial tear, usually at the musculotendinous junction, are treated by simple local palliation of pain, stretching, and graduated exercise from isometric to full range isotonic over the course of 7–10 days. Having suffered a tear, the site of injury will tend to develop a localized contracture with maturation of the new collagen. Careful stretching before and after sports activities may help to prevent further injury.

Muscular hematoma following direct trauma may result in an intramuscular (within the muscle belly) or intermuscular hematoma (at the margin of or between muscle bellies). Clinically, the distinction can be made after 3–4 days when the hematoma of the intermuscular lesion tracks beneath the deep fascia to appear subcutaneously at distant sites. Intramuscular hematoma may cause such muscle necrosis, that overzealous stretching ruptures the muscle. Treatment of the intramuscular lesion therefore is palliation, elevation, effleurage, crutches if necessary, and graduated exercise within pain from isometric to full range isotonic, requiring 4–6 weeks to full recovery. The intermuscular hematoma, once the hematoma has appeared at distant sites, can be worked as hard as possible to full function in 7–10 days.

Myositis ossificans traumatica usually follows muscle hematoma and should be treated similarly to an intramuscular hematoma (6). Rarely is surgical excision required; if so, every effort must be made to maintain the range regained at surgery.

CHRONIC INJURIES

With the advent of middle-aged fitness addiction, failure of bone or tendon to absorb repeated stress, which was formerly infrequent, is now commonplace.

Bone

Stress Fractures. With advancing age there is a gradual loss of bone mass. With normal use, little evidence is seen of bone failure, as exemplified by the number of trabecular microfractures, until the early 40s, after which age the loss of bone is such that there is an exponential increase (7). During running, weight-bearing joints are subjected to large impact loads, up to 15 times body weight. Traditionally, it has been assumed that most of this impact load is absorbed by articular cartilage; however, Radin and his colleagues (8) demonstrated that the major part is absorbed by subchondral bone.

The remodeling of bone required to accommodate to increased load takes many months. New joggers who increase distance and pace in excess of the ability of their bone to accommodate develop failure microfractures in the subchondral area, particularly around the knee, which can be demonstrated by "hot spots" on bone scan. The increased load imposed by running may result in failure. If the localized subarticular bone pain is treated by rest, the scan will eventually become negative, but in response to rest or lack of impact, the bone will become more osteoporotic. Management should be to maintain distance and pace within pain with regular increments to reach maximum over 9–12 months, i.e., to retain the stimulus without causing acute damage.

Chondromalacia patellae, while occurring in the young, has many similarities. Confusion has resulted from the use of a pathological cartilage change as the name of a complex of signs and symptoms. It has been shown that the lesion lies in the bone with osteoporosis, trabecular microfracture, and fragmentation of the subchondral plate; bone scan shows that the process involves not just the patella, but also the tibia and femur (9). While many surgical procedures have been advocated for its management, Bentley (10) has shown that satisfactory results (return to full activities) were obtained in only 25%

in whom the patellar cartilage was shaved and in 35% after cartilage excision and drilling of the subchondral bone; with major rearrangement of the stresses acting on the knee, e.g., after medial transfer of the patellar tendon, the results are improved to 60%, and to 77% after patellectomy. However, at least equivalent results can be obtained by a graduated increase in stress loading within pain over 6–9 months, provided that the patient, trainer, therapist, and physician understand the lesion and its management rationale.

"Shin Splints," with pain at the junction of the lower and middle third of the medial border of the tibia, may result from a chronic strain or tear of the origin of the posterior tibial muscle or from microscopic failure of bone to repeated stress. The symptoms may result from a cortical fracture visible on x-ray and bone scan, or from trabecular failure seen only as a hot spot on bone scan. The muscular lesion can be treated with a heel raise, local palliation, stretching, and graduated exercise. The bone lesion should be recognized as a failure to absorb impact and should be treated as above.

Tendon

Failure of tendon to repeated stress, particularly in the 30+ age group, is seen as localized pain usually near the insertion. The lesion is similar to a tennis elbow—a small tear in a largely collagenous tissue. Treatment should be similar: palliation, friction, massage, and a stretching-exercise routine. Continued stress loading (within pain) is necessary if collagen synthesis is to accommodate to the extra loading required; rest or removal of stress will have the opposite effect. Many months of consistent slow buildup may be required.

WARM UP—WARM DOWN

Most of those involved in sports believe in the benefit of a warmup routine. There is no clear evidence that such routines protect athletes from injury. However, once an injury has occurred, a good warmup and stretching routine may stretch out potential contractures.

References

1. Goldber B, and Rabinovitch M: Connective tissues. In Weiss L and Greep O: ed 4, chap 4. Histology, New York, McGraw-Hill 1977.
2. Caughey DE, Bywaters EGL: Joint fluid pressure in chronic knee effusions. Ann Rheumat Dis 22:106–109, 1963.
3. Jayson MIV, Dixon A St J: Intra-articular pressure in rheumatoid arthritis of the knee, III. pressure changes during joint use. Ann Rheumat Dis 29:401–408, 1970.
4. Warren RF, Marshall JL: Injuries of the anterior cruciate and medial collateral ligament of the knee. Clin Orthop 136:198–291, 1978.
5. Brooks SC, Potter BT, Rainey JB: Treatment for partial tears of the lateral ligament of the ankle. Br Med J 282:606–607, 1981.
6. Lipscomb AB, Thomas ED, Johnston RK: Treatment of myositis ossificans traumatica in athletes. Sports Med 4:111–120, 1976.
7. Darracott J, Vernon-Roberts B, Fazzalari N: Bone changes in osteoarthritis of the hip. Ann R Coll Phys Surg Can 14:225, 1981.
8. Radin EL, Paul IL, Lowy M: A comparison of the dynamic force transmitting properties of subchondral bone and articular cartilage. J Bone Joint Surg 52A: 444–456, 1970.
9. Darracott J, Vernon-Roberts B: The bony changes in "chondromalacia patellae." Rheumat Phys Med 11: 175–179, 1971.
10. Bentley G: The surgical treatment of chondromalacia patellae. J Bone Joint Surg 60B: 74–81, 1978.

Rehabilitation of Children

M. A. ALEXANDER

DEVELOPMENTAL STAGES

The rehabilitation program involves an understanding of the natural history of the disease, the developmental stage of the child, and the interaction of modalities with the child and family. The accomplishment of these steps is predicated on the ability to perform an adequate history and physical. For a child who is not functioning at an appropriate age level, a differential diagnosis must be developed.

In a young child whose motor performance is delayed, this differential must consider the entire central nervous system. Children can be slow in their motor performance because of a global delay secondary to static encephalopathy, may be delayed because of a primary insult to neuromotor control at the cerebral or basal ganglion level, or they may have "motor unit" disease.

EARLY DIAGNOSES

Cerebral palsy represents a neuromuscular disorder which may be taken as a model that makes the concept of evaluation and rehabilitation of many childhood disabilities easier to understand. The history usually gives the diagnosis. Detailed questioning should probe whether the pregnancy, from conception through delivery, had any problems, e.g., excessive weight gain or amniotic fluid, decreased fetal movements, high or low maternal age, problems with fetal heart tones, or difficulties with labor itself. With the advent of natural childbirth, mothers and fathers see more and can remember whether the mother was allowed to hold the child and breastfeed the child immediately or if the child was whisked off to another room to be worked over. Often, the father is more aware of difficulties in the delivery room when questioned closely. The 1- and 5-minute Apgars, as well as birthweight, should be obtained. The history should continue with whether the infant was fed soon after birth or was not fed until the second day of life and how the infant took the bottle when it was offered. Newborn infants have no difficulties in taking from a bottle and do very well with 3 or 4 ounces in a very short period of time (under 15 minutes). Excessive gagging or spitting up may represent a hyperactive gag or discoordinated pharyngeal muscle use.

Many disabled children present with delayed milestones. However, parents of children with cerebral palsy instead may describe their child as "motorically precocious"; their child rolled over from the first few days of life, stood well, and had excellent head control when placed prone. In fact, these children had been accomplishing these motor endeavors through a persistent opisthotonic position or abnormally pronounced standing reflex.

Spina bifida will present an obvious anomaly of the back and spine. Spina bifida is specifically a defect in the vertebral lamina, and the disorder is more appropriately called *myelomeningocele* (MMC). The child with MMC will have extrusion of the spinal cord through the defect in the lamina and into a sack located on the back. As there is both nerve and segmental cord injury and/or dysraphism, any combination of upper and lower motor lesion may exist. Depending on the level of involvement, bladder, bowel, and sexual function, as well as motor control, may be affected. Early in life signs of increased intracranial pressure will alert the neurosurgeon to intervene.

There are a number of excellent catalogues of normal motor milestones (see Table 14.1). Disabilities with limited impact (as in congenital amputations) will show delays in selected milestones. Children with inflammatory disorders may show lags and plateaus which coincide with active disease.

PRIMITIVE REFLEXES

Tonic Neck Reflex

The asymmetric tonic neck reflex is one of the tonic neck reflexes that can be easily elicited and for which there is meaningful standardization. This reflex is present in almost all infants by the third week of life (Fig. 14.2). It normally consists of an extension of the arm and the leg on the side towards which the child's face is rotated. There is a concomitant flexion of the contralateral arm and leg. This change in position of the arms may be more a change in tone and not limb position. This pattern of motor response to head turning is no longer easily detected by 4 months of age. If, as long as the head is rotated to one side, the arms on the chin side of the face are locked in extension and the limbs on the occipital side of the head are locked into flexion, the infant is showing an obligatory asymmetric tonic neck reflex—this is always pathologic.

Other Reflex Responses

In addition to the above reflex, the normal stepping and positive supporting reactions are transitory phenomena in that

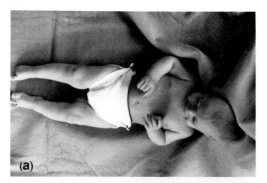
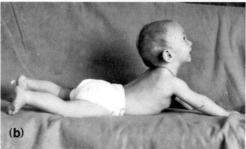
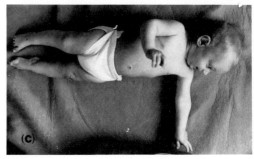

Figure 14.2. Tonic neck reflexes—symmetric (a) flexion and (b) extension; (c) asymmetric. (Reproduced with permission from: B Gowitzke and M Milner: *Understanding the Scientific Basis of Human Movement*, ed 2. Baltimore, Williams & Wilkins.)

Table 14.1
Milestones (Denver Developmental Screening Test) in Months

Milestone	50% Attain (in mos)	100% Attain (in mos)
Smiling	2	5
Sitting	6	8
Speak (dada, mama)	10	13
Standing	11	14
Pincer (index to thumb)	11	15
Walking	12	15
Ride tricycle	24	36

very few newborn infants are capable of supporting their total body weight for more than a few seconds. Children who can consistently bear weight on the lower extremities without any sudden collapsing of the knees and who may also show a tendency to scissor and go into an equinus position are functioning abnormally.

The *Moro* or *startle reflex* should be obtained within the first few weeks of life. It is best elicited by suddenly allowing the head and neck to extend 20—30°. This will cause the arms to open, circumduct, and reach out as if grasping a circular object. To a lesser extent, the lower extremities will assume the same position. It is helpful to note whether the hands open completely and particularly whether there is an asymmetric fisting of the hands. Absence of movement at one shoulder would indicate an upper trunk lesion. This reflex and the asymmetric tonic neck reflex should disappear by 4 months of age.

Another item of precociousness which may actually represent a symptom of CNS insult is the presence of hand dominance under the age of 16 months. A child who is hemiplegic or who has lower motor neuron injury to the brachial plexus will, of necessity, choose the noninvolved arm as his dominant one.

Protective Responses and Socializing

The gradual appearance of protective responses is as important as the disappearance of primitive reflexes. The infant at 6 months of age should be able to prop-sit, and this should include the ability to steady himself with his arms, when slowly displaced from side to side. By 9 months of age an infant is capable of a full-blown *parachute response* which is elicited by bringing the infant rapidly towards the surface onto which the examiner wishes the child to crawl; the arms and legs will extend and be in proper position to assume 4-point contact (Fig. 14.3). Again, noting whether the hands are open and thumbs are out of the palm is a helpful piece of information.

Brazelton (4) has shown that even the newborn infant is capable of snuggling, following an object across 180° of view and responding to its mother's face. Infants who do not interact with adults are suspect of a mental or severe sensory impairment. Newborn infants will make brushing attempts at cloths over their eyes, and by 4 months this is easily accomplished. If the infant at 4 months doesn't react, note whether he is not in-

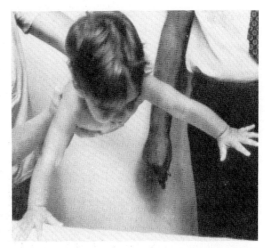

Figure 14.3. Parachute response (in a 10-month-old infant). (Reproduced with permission from: AM Rudolph (ed): *Pediatrics*, ed 16. New York, Appleton-Century-Crofts, 1977.)

terested or disturbed, or whether in fact he cannot bring his hand to his face. At 4 months a child with normal vision will respond to his face in a mirror. A child with severe motor impairment will still react to the examiner, while the mentally retarded child does not react. The motor impairment in a child may then be any combination of upper motor, lower motor, sensory impairment, or intellectual deficit—or even all of the above, as in MMC.

While the onset of ambulation varies from group to group, the absence of ambulation by 18 months is a cause for closer scrutiny. Children initially assume a wide-based stance with the arms in what is called the *high guard position*. With increasing experience the arms come to the side, and the width of the standing base narrows, so that by that time the infant has been walking for 4 to 6 months and the hands are at the sides (2).

The clinician must decide whether there are enough signs to warrant the diagnosis of cerebral palsy. Levine (4) has developed a system based on six categories of motor dysfunction (Table 14.2). If the child is a year old (corrected for prematurity) and meets four of six of his criteria, and is not getting worse, the prob-

Table 14.2
Levine Criteria for Cerebral Palsy[a]

- Postures and movement patterns
- Oral motor patterns
- Strabismus
- Tone of muscles
- Evolution of postural reactions
- Reflexes: deep tendon and plantar

ability is high that he has cerebral palsy. To this should be added a history compatible with a peri- or neonatal problem. If there is any doubt, consultation should be obtained from a pediatric neurologist; otherwise, a treatable cause may be missed.

THE OLDER CHILD AND ACQUIRED CONDITIONS

Rehabilitation problems of children also embrace many conditions described elsewhere in this book, e.g., injuries, burns, musculosketal conditions (e.g., muscular dystrophy, amputees, etc), the need for orthotics and prosthetics, special education and training, psychosocial and sexual maturation, etc. In general, these are best assessed and managed in special facilities by specialists, of whom a growing number are trained in both rehabilitation and pediatrics.

TREATMENTS

Given the appropriate diagnosis, what are the anticipated benefits of therapeutic interventions? The family may already suspect there is a problem, often before the managing physician has been willing to diagnose a problem. This may have led to confusion and hostility on the family's part and behavior which may be counterproductive. The act of intervening with therapy or psychosocial support will lessen the family's anxiety and depression. Parents given a supportive caring clinician are capable of coping with the disability better than if unsupported. As a consequence the act of prescribing any therapy may in and of itself have psycho-

social benefits. It will be up to the physician to decide the degree of intervention and to be scientific about explaining to the family what it is that the intervention may accomplish.

Neurodevelopmental Therapy

A treatment program should follow the development of the child both for gross motor and reflex development. This approach is known as neurodevelopmental therapy (NDT). It is based on the assumption that the child has a static injury to the nervous system. This injury allows for abnormal patterns of motor control to appear, and these in turn force the child to use abnormal compensatory mechanisms to accomplish any volitional motor function. The use of these abnormal motor patterns reinforces tightness and spasticity in certain muscle groups which can go on to fixed deformities and, in turn, can lead to skeletal deformities with growth. The intervention is aimed at helping the child discover normal patterns of motor control. An example is the child who, when placed prone with his arms adducted and elbows extended, is incapable of lifting his head off the surface. However, with his arms rotated and brought above his head and in front of him, there is facilitation of neck extension, and he can raise his head. If the child is worked with in this position and his central nervous system is capable of selecting out the key motor positions and commands to bring about the activity, there is permanent learning of the normal motor response, and the child will continue with that skill. The same neurodevelopmental approach is used for most childhood disorders, as it represents a technique which looks at the entire child and considers motor, sensory, and cognitive disorders. Not only are cerebral palsy and spina bifida motor diseases, but also they are sensory diseases.

Additional Therapy

As the child continues in the neurodevelopmental program the physician may see the child reaching the point at which therapy alone is not controlling the child's motor patterns and subsequent abnormal postures. The tendency to go into equinus, if persistent, will lead to a fixed equinovalgus deformity of the ankle and may necessitate the use of adjunctive interventions if NDT therapy alone is not enough. Early on, inhibitory casting provides a means of positioning the spastic ankle in a neutral position. These are bivalved short leg walking casts. Through poorly understood physiologic reflex loops, the extensor tone in the lower extremities continues to be inhibited, after the discontinuation of the casts or boots. Again it is as if the child has learned the appropriate sensory cues to maintain the necessary motor control to prevent the abnormal pattern from recurring. Should the inhibitory casts initially work and then their effect wear off, rigid plastic ankle-foot orthoses can be incorporated as a long-term adjunctive intervention.

The child with lower motor disease or painful joints will need an orthosis for stability, allowing for the simulation of normal motor patterns. When the ankle can no longer be brought passively to the neutral position with the knee extended, surgery is indicated because there is now a fixed anatomic deformity.

Aids to ADL

As one continues with the child's development and finds that the child is going to be incapable of unassisted gait, crutches and walkers should be added. The child who is not going to be an ambulator but has the intellectual and fine-motor control of some area of the body should have the appropriate electric mobility device prescribed. The child who does not have the experience of independent movement and of cause and effect will find it harder to develop initiative, independence, and self-assertion. Through the use of scooter boards and other mobility devices the child will experience independent movement.

As with adults, the goals of rehabilitation are the provision of function, prevention of tightness, and substitution for dysfunction. Care must anticipate the development of deformities from abnormal muscle action with growth. The child should be seated on a chair with a firm seat and a firm back (shaped to encourage slight lumbar hyperextension) and arm rests (which keep the child from leaning forward). Scoliosis is common in both lower and upper motor neuron diseases. A curve that has progressed beyond 20° needs orthotic intervention. Curves that go beyond 60° usually come to surgical correction. These curves can be prevented or at least retarded with proper positioning and orthotic prescriptions.

Communicative Problems

For the child who is cognitively capable of language but is not showing it, a careful evaluation as to whether the child has a primary expressive and/or receptive disability is most important. With the advent of microcomputers and electronic voices a child who intellectually can master a switching sequence can be understood by peers and have a meaningful life. Careful attention needs to be given to the child who is using gestures or symbols to substitute for inability to produce speech sounds. The physical examination should not be so brusque and threatening that it obscures the childs ability to demonstrate his intellectual skills. A careful history from the family and teachers may turn up potentials that are not obvious on a physical. Certainly the more people from the child's life that corroborate the glimmer of intelligence, the more thoroughly the child's capabilities need to be explored. The rule is look hard, look more than once and, most importantly, listen.

Other Problems

MMC and cerebral palsy account for

most (though not all) pediatric cases that will require rehabilitation, but *muscular diseases* also present important problems. In managing the child with muscular dystrophy, the two cardinal rules are to maintain walking and to avoid deformities. These are accomplished by aggressive therapy, judicious surgery and lightweight polypropylene bracing. At end stage, appropriate respiratory support will improve the handicapped child's quality of life.

Amputees are managed easily by the rehabilitation team with the advent of lightweight terminal devices. Unilateral juvenile amputees should do well if their prostheses are provided at the needed developmental stage, i.e., for upper extremity amputees, 6 months, and for lower extremity, 10 months.

References

1. Holt KS: *Developmental Paediatrics: Perspectives and Practice.* Boston, Butterworths, 1977.
2. Bower TGR: *A Primer of Infant Development.* San Francisco, WH Freeman, 1977.
3. Burnett CN, Johnson EW: Development of gait in childhood. Parts I and II. *Dev Med Child Neurol* 13:196–215, 1971.
4. Brazelton TB, Parker WB, Zuckerman B: Importance of behavioral assessment of the neonate. *Curr Probl Pediatr* 7:4–75, 1976.
5. Levine MS: Cerebral palsy diagnosis in children over age 1 year: standard criteria. *Arch Phys Med Rehabil* 61:385–389, 1980.

Rehabilitation of the Elderly

T. E. STRAX and J. C. LEDEBUR

Growing old is not sudden; we do not wake up one morning to find that we are no longer 25 years old. Physiological and psychological changes take place slowly, and few people, including physicians, are prepared for these changes. Normality in an aging population has never been defined. Until recently, there seemed to be no need to differentiate between aging and illness.

Geriatric medicine has long suffered from lack of enthusiasm and recognition of its importance in the mainstream of contemporary medicine (1–3). Meanwhile, the number of Americans over 65 has been growing at a rate three times faster than the general population. In 1900 one person in 25 was over 65; the ratio is now 1 in 9, and by the year 2000 it will be 1 in 7. By 1990 there will be 27.5 million Americans over the age of 65.

The *evaluation of the geriatric patient* proceeds along many lines: (1) the traditional inventory of medical problems (with traditional therapeutic treatments); (2) dynamic assessment of the patient's psychosocial situation; (3) cognitive and intellectual assessment; (4) functional assessment; and (5) environmental assessment.

The physician must ascertain the patient's functional level within his environment. This is accomplished through ADL checkout and careful questioning of patient and family. If the home environment cannot support the patient's functional status, can it be adapted? Is there an alternate living plan? What are the resources in the community? Could the individual function with a home health aide? Suggestions should be made for alternative housing such as halfway houses and shared houses with common support personnel.

Since all aspects of geriatric rehabilitation cannot be adequately covered in one chapter, we will review some important problems which affect geriatric patients and which have been touched on elsewhere in this book. These include general deconditioning, peripheral vascular disease and amputations, Parkinsonism, fractures, cardiovascular disease, pulmonary disease, pain, depression, organic brain syndrome, sensory impairments, and sexuality.

GENERAL DECONDITIONING

General deconditioning is extremely common because many older people are not active. Muscle bulk, tone, and endurance are diminished. For these people, prolonged hospitalization is often disastrous, and a 10-day stay in the hospital might result in a 20% decrease in muscle strength and bulk. In addition to chronic illnesses, trauma and surgical procedures play havoc. Before an elective surgical procedure is performed, inactive older patients should be taught deep breathing and abdominal splinting techniques, as well as bed mobilization. If the procedure is to be an orthopedic one, it is a good idea to preteach the patient proper gait sequencing and use of adaptive equipment, such as canes or walkers. Postoperatively, training continues, with ADL and bimanual activities added. Before discharge, ADL assessment, and training if necessary, should be performed. Once the individual returns to the community, a continuing program should be set up to increase the strength and endurance of the individual gradually.

PERIPHERAL VASCULAR DISEASE AND AMPUTATIONS

The skin of elderly people is dry, less elastic, and more prone to infection. The loss of fat cells and decreased blood supply lead to an increased incidence of infection and pressure ulcers. Chronic dependency leads to edema which often is nonpitting and not really corrected through long-term use of intermittent positive pressure. One must teach older people to keep their legs elevated when sitting for a prolonged period of time and to wear a support stocking. Skin breakdown should be treated immediately.

Whirlpool

If physical therapy is ordered, whirlpool is usually helpful. The temperature of the bath is extremely important and should be within 10% of the local skin temperature, which means for most patients it should be below 94°F. For every 10% rise of skin temperature there is an almost 100% increase in the metabolic need of the tissues. In normal individuals the tissues have the capacity to dilate vascular beds, giving them about 400% leeway. However, the older patient with severe vascular disease no longer has this reserve; therefore, increases in temperature are extremely dangerous and may lead to tissue damage, necrosis, and possible amputation.

Home Program

The home program for peripheral vascular problems should include bathing the extremity with mild soap every evening, patting it dry, using corn starch in the summer and possibly a mild skin lotion or lubricant in the winter. Nails should be cut by a professional, and shoes should be prescribed to accommodate any foot deformities.

Amputees

Elderly patients may become amputees (see also Chapter 11), and they present two major problems: first, the increased cardiovascular demand of walking and, second, the survival of the remaining extremity in the unilateral amputee. The energy expenditure of a unilateral below knee amputee for ambulation is 10–25% more than normal. The upper limit is much commoner in geriatric patients.

With the bilateral below-knee amputation, this energy expenditure starts to approach 60%. In the case of the unilateral above-knee amputee, energy expenditures for ambulation will approach an increase of 100%, and with the bilateral above-knee amputee, 300–400%. Obviously, with limited cardiovascular reserve, the patient may at some time push beyond the cardiovascular limit. Exercise programs must be tailored to advance the patient accordingly.

Peripheral vascular disease rarely occurs in only one extremity; many unilateral amputees lose the other extremity within 2 or 3 years.

Prostheses are prescribed for patients for functional or cosmetic reasons (see Chapter 7). Patients who want a prosthesis should have one, and those who have sufficient cardiovascular reserve should be taught to walk with or without adaptive devices. All patients should be taught the proper care of the remaining extremity and told to minimize the risk of increased trauma to the remaining extremity or exceeding their cardiovascular limits. Always consider the most stable prosthesis available. In an above knee amputation, this usually means a manual locking knee or a safety knee.

The amputation site is an extremely significant factor affecting the rehabilitation of a geriatric amputee. Only 12–17% of bilateral above knee amputees ever gain the ability to walk even short distances with their prostheses. With one below- and one above-knee amputation, this figure jumps to 25–54%. Some 30–100% of bilateral below-knee amputees learn to walk, and in the case of the unilateral amputee, this figure is about 80%.

MOVEMENT DISORDERS AND PARKINSON'S DISEASE

Tremor, bradykinesia, and akinesia are some of the problems in the elderly. In the case of Parkinson's disease, the major problem is a paucity of movements, flexion of the trunk and head, diminished vital capacity, and a poor dangerous shuffling gait.

Exercises which facilitate righting responses, lateral weight shifting, and kinesthetic proprioceptive awareness improve gait. Reciprocal activities are important. Exercises with distal weights provide a traction response and facilitate phasic movement. Weights placed centrally on the trunk will facilitate postural muscles. Gliders or rollators are useful for Parkinsonian patients, in that the gait sequence is uninterrupted. (A walker, on the other hand, necessitates initiating and ending a movement pattern with each step.) Other aspects of the treatment program should encourage proper breathing techniques, as well as trunk extension and rotation exercises.

With ataxic patients, Frankel's coordination exercises are useful. Central weights are also very useful since they tend to stabilize muscle movements.

FRACTURES

The skeleton of an older person is brittle, and fractures are common. Many have severe osteoporosis, which can be due to many causes, including reduced activity levels, diminished calcium intake, decreased exposure to the sun with diminished vitamin D reserves, and postmenopausal diminished estrogen levels.

Mortality following lower extremity fractures is increased as many elderly people are not able to learn or cannot physically perform nonweightbearing ambulation. To meet this challenge, physicians must consider surgical therapy, including total arthroplasties and multiple pinnings. They enable the patient to bear weight almost immediately.

Programs should emphasize upper extremity strengthening, balance, and gait training with adaptive equipment.

CARDIAC REHABILITATION

The cardiovascular system, like all

other systems, deteriorates as we get older, and many factors determine the rate. Heredity seems to be one of the most important ones, although smoking, obesity, and the presence of stress in one's life, diabetes, and many other factors also come into play. Since many of the people in the geriatric population have some degree of diminished cardiac reserve, all programs must be carefully tailored to the patient.

Exercise Programs

The heart, like any other muscle, deteriorates if it isn't used, and improves with exercise. To design an adequate program one must know the individual's exercise tolerance. Patients are started off at 1.5–3 METs (1 MET is the amount of energy expended—O_2 consumed—while lying at rest)—the level of simple ADL functioning (Table 14.3). A very debilitated cardiac patient might be started off at the lower end of this range. Exercises begin with bed mobility and movements of the upper extremities which have been supported, and then go on to walking followed by riding a more resistive exercise stationary

bicycle. The stationary bicycle is an excellent tool, since most older people feel secure on it, and it can be started without resistance which enables the patient to first range the lower extremities.

PULMONARY DISEASE

Geriatric patients with pulmonary disease have acute and chronic phases, for which specific programs should be initiated whenever possible. In the acute phase, the patient should be placed in a position so that the congested lung can drain easily. This is a sidelying position with the congested lung higher. Percussion and vibration is given to the patient to loosen secretions and aid in this drainage. The patient is instructed to take deep breaths and give short forceful hacking coughs. Patients with weak abdominal muscles or postop surgical patients should have their abdomen splinted to facilitate coughing. When facilitating drainage, the upper segment should be done first and then the lower segment, so as not to spread infection. In general, therapy should be discontinued when the patient

Table 14.3
Cardiac Table

1½–2 mets 4–7 kcal	Desk work, standing, playing cards, and sewing
2.3 mets 7–11 kcal	Auto repairing, typing with a manual typewriter, janitorial work, bowling, golf with an electric cart, fishing, and walking 2 miles/hr.
3–4 mets 11–14 kcal	Wood grain laying and plastering, machine assembly, driving a trailor truck in traffic, welding, cleaning windows, walking 2½ miles/hr, horseshoe pitching, volleyball sixth man noncompetitive, golf (pulling your own bag on a cart), horseback riding at a trot, playing a musical instrument energetically.
4.5 mets 14–18 kcal	Painting, masonry work (like carpentry), walking 3 miles/hr, carrying one's own golf clubs while playing golf, table tennis, tennis doubles, many calisthenics.
5–6 mets 18–21 kcal	Walking 5½ miles/hr, canoeing 4 miles/hr.
6–7 mets 21–25 kcal	Shoveling for 10 minutes, walking 5 miles/hr, playing singles in tennis, hand lawn mowing, skiing in loose snow, and water skiing.
7–8 mets 25–28 kcal	Digging ditches, carrying 8 lb. loads, sawing hard wood, jogging 5 miles/hour, horseback riding at a gallop, basketball, mountain climbing, paddleball.
8–9 mets 28–32 kcal	Shoveling for 10 minutes (lifting at least 14-lb loads), running 5½ miles/hr, squash, social handball.

brings up less than 30 ml of fluid. Patients with congestive heart failure have their fluid usually in the interstitial space, not the bronchi. Therefore, chest physical therapy is not useful, except to facilitate deep breathing.

When an acute event is over, conditioning exercises coupled with deep breathing and relaxation exercises are initiated. This is very important, especially in patients with chronic lung disease. Energy conservation techniques should be taught to all chronic pulmonary patients.

PAIN

Geriatric patients frequently complain of pains, which may be a warning of either a physical or an emotional problem. Occasionally, they are ignored because the physician feels that they are used to obtain attention.

As people get older, patterns of pain change. Headaches become less common; in fact, migraine headaches are rare in the older person. Recurrence of migraine may be a warning of impending stroke. Herpes zoster accounts for 2% of geriatric pain. Foot pain is extremely common, due to tight-fitting shoes, peripheral vascular disease, or arthritis.

Management

After a diagnosis is made and the specific factors have been addressed, one can start with nonspecific conservative treatment for pain relief such as heating modalities, whirlpool baths, icing massage, as well as exercises. By improving muscle tone, posture, and function, pain should be reduced. Occasionally, one may use nerve blocks or transcutaneous electrical stimulators. The latter is useful in patients with herpes, phantom limb, and other neuropathies.

ORGANIC BRAIN DYSFUNCTION AND SENSORY IMPAIRMENTS

Organic brain syndrome (OBS) is a condition in which there is impaired cogni-

tive function due to an irreversible cause such as multiple infarcts or Alzheimer's disease. The term should not be used for sudden reversible changes in cognition such as those caused by metabolic or cardiopulmonary dysfunction. In those cases, the term "acute confusional state" should be used. OBS, confusional states, depression, and sensory impairments share similar symptomatology and may be confused with one another.

Depression

Old age seems to be a time of losses. With advancing age come losses of loved ones through death or infirmity. At retirement, loss of job identity results in further loss of personal identity and self-esteem. Many have not prepared themselves for this time by developing other interests or social contacts. For some, with loss of position comes loss of financial stature, lower standards of living, and loss of control over one's life. Loss of physical capacity compounds the problem. All of these instances and more can cause depression which may be manifested by agitation, withdrawal, insomnia, and inappropriate behavior and may be mistaken for OBS.

Sensory and Cognitive Impairments

Perceptual problems and sensory impairments may also mimic OBS. If one observes a person with figure-ground problems, spatial orientation, right-left discrimination problems, or poor vision, one may see a person who cannot dress, feed, or ambulate independently. Hearing impairments may cause an individual to withdraw, answer inappropriately, and seem confused.

Patients with intact but slowed cognition may also give a more involved picture. It is important when working with such a person to speak slowly, in a nonpressured manner. Allow time for the cognitive processes to take place. Sensory deprivation studies give ample explanation for the results of this older age group whose physical limitations cause the same type of deprivation.

Management. For some patients suffering from organic brain syndrome, therapy can be beneficial. However, programs must be simplified, reduced to their most basic components, and taught in a consistent manner. Often, gestural instructions rather than verbal instruction must be used. "Chaining" a task may also be helpful. This involves structuring down a task to its most basic components; in forward chaining the first step must be achieved and added to step by step. In reverse chaining, the instructor starts with the last step first and works methodically backward in the relearning process. Many of these principles apply when working with visually or hearing-impaired individuals. However, if there is no carryover, chances of successful rehabilitation are not realistic.

SEXUALITY IN THE ELDERLY

Many people feel that sex in old age is improper and impossible. The public views sex in the elderly with humor or derision, and most younger people attribute impotence to older men and loss of physical allure to older women. Children are often shocked to find that their widowed mother or father is involved sexually with a friend. Although there are physiological changes which affect sexual response, older adults are still capable of experiencing and enjoying the full realm of sexuality: fantasy, holding, kissing, the warmth and friendship of a relationship, as well as sexual intercourse and orgasm. The section on *Sexual Issues* in Chapter 13 applies to older people too.

Changes which take place in the older female are decreased vaginal secretion and elasticity. Often, water-soluble lubricants are needed during sexual relations. Some women experience uterine cramps which respond to small doses of estrogen. Many women have slowed onset of orgasm and shortened or reduced intensity of the orgasmic response.

Older men are still capable of penile erection. They may need direct prolonged genital stimulation to achieve erections. The erect penis usually has a decreased girth. It takes a longer time to achieve orgasm, and once orgasm is achieved, the resolution phase is prolonged. Aging men continue to have high levels of interest in having sexual relations. Perhaps, one of every four times that an aging man has sexual intercourse, there may not be specific demand for orgasmic release.

Many men have not been informed of the normal physiological changes in aging. Because of this, males become anxious and sometimes depressed about their temporary inability to have erections. Many withdraw from sexual relations without an explanation to their partners. This imposes celibacy and may lead to depression and anxiety in the partner.

To evaluate if impotence is really psychological, penile nocturnal tumescence studies are helpful. These should be performed, along with counseling and support therapy for both partners. Counseling is also necessary when chronic or acute illness interferes with sexual relations. Often, couples are afraid to resume sexual activity after illnesses such as myocardial infarction. Usually, if an individual is able to climb the stairs to go to the bedroom, he or she is able to have sexual relations.

Our study (4) of institutionalized older people showed that their desires and aspirations are identical to those of older people in the community. Many older people in the community find it difficult to meet and socialize with others. In the case of people who are institutionalized, the institutions usually set the rules and prevent many expressions of sexual intimacy.

SUCCESS RATE OF REHABILITATION

Comprehensive rehabilitation for the geriatric patient works. The Philadelphia Geriatric Center demonstrated this through a 3-year study (4) of 100 patients who had lost sufficient ADL and/or ambulation to warrant their moving to the next lower level of dependent care. Of these patients 76% had significant heart disease, and 24% had organic brain syndrome.

Of the 100 patients, 82 were rehabilitated to the point that they could return to their previous living arrangements. Only nine went on to a more dependent level of care.

Four years after the initial study, all of the patients were reidentified to see if they had maintained their gains. Although 37 had died during the 4-year study period, only 11 had lived less than 1 year after being discharged from the rehabilitation program. This meant that 89% lived long enough to benefit from the program. There were 46 ex-patients who were still living in the community; thirty-seven of them could be found for the follow-up study, and almost all of them were still independent in ambulation, dressing, toileting, and feeding.

SUMMARY

Comprehensive rehabilitation of the older patient does improve the quality of the patient's life by helping to achieve independence in the areas of ambulation and activities of daily living. This enables the older people to live in community settings for longer periods of time. To achieve this type of result one must deal with a comprehensive rehabilitation team, which needs some special training in the handling of geriatric patients. This training should be in the area of developing programs to motivate this particular patient population. Most of the techniques used in therapy are standard techniques that are used in other rehabilitation programs.

References

1. Gryfe CI: Reasonable expectation in geriatric rehabilitation. J Am Geriatr Soc 20:237–238, 1979.
2. Richel WE: The Geriatric Patient. New York, H.P. Publishing, 1978.
3. Rusk HA, Reed MHM: Rehabilitation of the aging. Bull NY Acad Med 49:1383, 1971.
4. Strax T, Ledebur JC: Rehabilitating the geriatric patient: potentials and limitations. Geriatrics 34:99–101, 1979.

Behavior and Rehabilitation

D. S. BISHOP

Helping the disabled and dealing with the psychosocial-behavioral aspects of their situation is a demanding challenge. This chapter highlights the complexity and offers some clinical solutions. Other sources of additional knowledge and approaches are readily and reasonably available (2, 5, 7).

Rehabilitation requires several shifts from the thinking and focus of acute medical care. With disability the deficits are all too clear so that efforts must shift to include a more careful assessment of strengths. Acute medical care usually requires that the patient be "looked after" while in the rehabilitation process they should be collaborators and later assume independent responsibility. The focus also shifts from attempting complete recovery to achieving a level of functional capacity that is appropriate and realistic. The important question about behavior then becomes: "Yes, there are several difficulties, but which ones, if changed right now, will really alter the patient's capacity to function?"

THERE ARE MANY POSSIBLE EXPLANATIONS

It is far too easy to say of a disabled patient's behavior, "OK, but after all, it's just a normal response to the situation." Such simplicity usually represents avoiding the difficulty of careful assessment. Behavior in the context of disability is complex; any number of possible explanations can be invoked, and several may be correct in a given situation.

Example: "Depression"

To illustrate, let us use depression as an example and discuss six possible etiologies. First, depression may be a variant of the normal mood changes we all experience. Second, depression may reflect pessimistic and depressive personality traits. Third, the depression may be a manifestation of a significant psychiatric disorder. Physical disability grants no immunity to psychiatric disease and may even trigger its onset. Both can occur together and yet be unassociated. Fourth, the depression may be part of the psychosocial response to disability. Worry about the future, self-doubt, depression, anxiety; any one of a range of phenomena may occur as people confront their disability. The severity may vary and may be short lived or protracted. Fifth, the depression may represent an intensification of premorbid personality characteristics. A person with a depressive personality may become more depressed when faced with a crisis or with biological changes. Sixth and last, the depression may be due to specific biological changes or deficits. Examples are the lassitude of hypothyroidism, the apathy and irritability associated with frontal lobe disorders, or the depression caused by medications such as cortisone or some antihypertensives.

Many explanations are therefore possible. In reality, a combination is usually the case, and clarifying the role of each possible source is required and demands careful assessment.

USING SEVERAL MODELS AIDS ASSESSMENT AND TREATMENT

The challenge is how to best go about assessing and understanding such a complex set of interacting variables. First, one requires a repertoire of basic interviewing skills (4, 6). Second, you have to be aware of and able to handle your own response to the circumstances you confront, be sensitive, and be able to control the session in a responsive manner. Third, you need an outline of the content areas you need to assess. What do you ask about? Table 14.4 outlines the areas to be explored first and is self-explanatory. The following section will therefore focus on additional areas that, if explored, provide a sound initial understanding of the person and his situation.

This guide incorporates the use of several models of behavior. The basic concepts each incorporates can be described operationally so that a set of questions or probes is obvious for each, the doctor-patient relationship can be understood, and they suggest possible interventions. An overview and outline that can be taken to an interview is presented in Table 14.5.

Learned Behavior

With this model you explore how behavior has been learned through operant conditioning, modeling, and phobias. *Operant conditioning* focuses on rewards—we go where the cookies are. You therefore find out what the person likes and dislikes. This is done in general and also with regard to views about hospitals, doctors, and medical staff. This information is helpful in delineating what leverage you can use with the patient to obtain cooperation and what you should avoid (censures). It is not uncommon for health professionals without such knowledge to reward the very behaviors they dislike.

One patient told of how he would throw

Table 14.4
Outline of Areas to Be Assessed

Stage	Content
1. Orientation	What does patient expect from session.
2. Presenting Problem	Exploration of disability (chronology of events, emotional-personal reactions at stages, experience with disability previously, and expectations). Reaction to medical system and professionals. View of future.
3. Strengths and/or Problems (prior to and arising from disability)	Check the following areas for patients personal perception and reactions to possible difficulties. Family: biological and marital School/work Financial Avocational-leisure activities Friends and socialization network Mobility: (1) General (out or housebound?) 2) Specific (e.g., paralysis) Sexuality: (1) relationships and (2) physical function Activities of daily living (eating, sleeping, dressing, hygiene) Problems in meeting medical care needs Bowel and bladder function Rehabilitation program and components
4. Mental Status	Do first if serious disturbance of thought, memory, orientation
5. Background	Family history (medical and psychiatric) Developmental stages Schooling
6. Develop a problem list	From 3, 4, and 5.
7. Shift and explore behavior via different models (see Table 14.5)	

himself out of his wheelchair at 7:30 p.m. and be put to bed as punishment. In fact, he liked to go to bed about 8 and this mechanism allowed him to get there before the usual 10 o'clock that facilitated the staff. He commented, "Boy, did I ever have them well trained."

Modeling is another way we learn to behave. This is the "monkey-see, monkey-do" concept, and is based on how we all learn by observing others. Ask about people the patient has known that experienced significant illnesses or disability, about how well the patient perceives that they handled their situations, and look for similarities to the patient's own behaviors. A parent who became a chronic and complaining individual following an illness may provide the model for similar behavior in the patient. Positive models

can provide explanations for current adaptive behavior. You, too, are a model, and if you brush aside emotionally laden and uncomfortable topics, you model avoidance.

Phobias are fears of specific situations. Disabling falls or car accidents with serious sequelae can sometimes lead to height or driving phobias. Hospitals, medical procedures, catastrophic first attempts to renew relationships, and sexual experience are other common sources of phobia development. Ask about situations that currently create significant anxiety and discern their origins.

Many new behavioral approaches are being tested in the treatment of neurological deficits which in recent years were unresponsive to therapy. Biofeedback-augmented physical therapy of stroke pa-

Table 14.5
Different Models of Behavior

Model and Component	Questions and Problems	Doctor-Patient Relationship	Possible Interventions
Learning			
1. Operant conditioning (we go where the cookies are)	Who liked and disliked / What patient likes or dislikes / Teachers, friends or enemies, parents, sibs, health professionals	May indicate what doctor can do to reinforce behavior and what will censure it	Operant conditioning program. Use rewards to reinforce compliance and behavior
2. Modeling (monkey see, monkey do!)	Who patient knows that had disability and how they handled it	Physician should model appropriate behavior and responses	Reinforce positive model techniques—if no effective models, expose to successful patients.
3. Phobias	Clarify if patient has phobias and explore those related to disability (e.g., falling, being caught in fire, soiling self)	Check patient is not phobic for hospitals or doctors	Desensitization / Relaxation training (use imagery to avoid physical problems)
Adaptation			
1. Defense mechanisms	Check if some being overly or inappropriately used.	See references for details / Projections (anger at you is about patient) / Watch denial over time—don't confront.	
2. Coping strategies	How has person handled losses and stresses in past? Do these have adaptive capacity in current context?	Reinforce positive past coping strategies.	Help patient use previous adaptive coping / Help patient learn new methods if previous ones are maladaptive
Family			
1. Role in family	How does patient behave in family / Consider need for family assessment	Watch that you may be caught in role of parent, spouse, etc. and patient in negative family role	Assess family for clarification of role
2. Family assets	What particular strengths and supports do family provide	Engage family as collaborators: Don't disenfranchise.	Engage family
Biological			
1. Deficits	Mental status to check organic brain dysfunction (disorientation, memory, cognitive dysfunction) / Consider if behavior is mediated by central nervous system deficit.		Aggressive attention to medical problems / Special rehabilitation techniques for CNS deficits

2. Iatrogenic — Review other systems (e.g., CV, metabolic) for problems — Medication for some deficits

Review potential behavior difficulties secondary to medications or treatment. — Consider alternative medications

Check for alcohol and drug abuse. — Don't addict patient to meds

3. Biologically based psychiatry disease — Mental Status — Treat as indicated

tients and other types of neural loss is now becoming available in many rehabilitation centers (Figs. 14.4 and 14.5)

Adaptive Behavior

Disability often leads to conflicts that create psychodynamic stress for patients. For example, if they have had trouble with dependency, becoming more so as a result of disability can potentiate the problem. This will lead to increased anxiety and may amplify both defense mechanisms and previous coping strategies.

We all use a range of defense mechanisms and some to a greater extent than others. It is important to determine which ones are used most by a given patient. Good psychiatric texts provide a detailed description and discussion of them (4, 6) so that only a few examples will be used here. It must be remembered that most are unconscious mechanisms and that they cannot be altered simply by conscious effort.

Reaction Formation, Displacement, Projection, and Denial. These are often seen in disabled populations. With *reaction formation*, the person responds with an emotion that is opposite to one that creates conflict and anxiety. The overly pleasant and ingratiating patient in a rehabilitation ward may be doing this, and you should be alert to the anger that it hides. With *displacement*, the conflict that resides in one area is transferred to a less threatening one. Expressing anger at a nurse when really mad at the doctor or focusing on a painful limb to avoid painful emotions are examples. Discussion of the apparent topic (nurse or limb pain) will be frustratingly unsuccessful, as the real conflict area needs to be addressed. You can deal with this by asking questions like, "I wonder who else makes you angry?", or "There must be a lot of painful things happening to you. Can you tell me about some of them?"

With *projection*, people accuse others (or objects) of negative attributes they cannot accept in themselves without con-

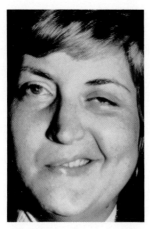

Figure 14.4. Patient 8 years after ablative right facial nerve palsy and "unsuccessful" nerve graft. (Reproduced with permission from: JV Basmajian. *Biofeedback—Principles and Practice for Clinicians.* Baltimore, Williams & Wilkins.)

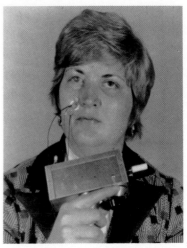

Figure 14.5. EMG feedback training of right facial muscles of patient in Figure 14.4. The returning activity in the muscles activates a buzzer in the battery-operated portable biofeedback device. This patient was "cured" in several weeks of training.

flict and anxiety. Blaming health professionals for not doing their job, or a wheelchair for not working properly, may be projecting one's own sense of not doing one's job or working as one would like!

Denial is an unconscious defense mechanism whereby the person refuses to accept the reality of a situation. The term is much abused in the case of the disabled. At times it is used as a derogatory label for nonconformity or poor compliance rather than to label a defense mechanism. However, the possible positive and negative consequences are poorly understood. Denial is usually seen by helpers as negative, but there are reports of its utility. For example, denial during the acute phase of a myocardial infarction is associated with a good outcome, but its continuing use into the postacute phase is associated with a bad outcome. The use of this mechanism therefore requires further study, and you should take care before assuming it explains the patient's problems. If correctly identified during the acute phases, it should probably be viewed as adaptive, and the expectation should be held that when the person is ready, he will talk.

Coping strategies are another way we all adapt to difficulties. These are the conscious and habitual patterns used to deal with conflicts. Ask the person to identify stresses from the past and then inquire about how they were dealt with. The previously used pattern will often be employed to deal with disability. However, the disability may render the method inadequate or inappropriate. The use of physical activity to relieve frustration is impossible for the quadriplegic and is contraindicated in the arthritic, but it is an aid to the paraplegic in developing compensatory motor functions. Intellectual pursuits will not help a cognitively disabled head injury victim cope, but it may be very useful to a quadriplegic.

Those born with, or developing a disability early in life will develop coping strategies that incorporate the handicap. Problems occur only if the strategy is maladaptive and thereby becomes a longstanding pattern of poor coping.

Risk taking and *social supports* may be major factors in developing positive coping skills. I personally feel that the ability to take risks and do the unexpected may be closely tied to achieving maximum potential. The recent movies "The Other Side of the Mountain" and "Coming Home" offer many examples of adaptive risk taking.

Family Behavior

Understanding the family patterns and considering the family ramification of treatment approaches can also help us to understand behavior. This area is a very large one (3). Ask yourself if the behavior is similar to the patient's pattern in the family because these patterns are often replicated in other settings. As an example, I saw a girl who cowered from her father and clung to her mother in the clinic. At school, she cowered from male teachers and was overly clinging with female teachers. Similar problematic behaviors with authoritarian doctors and maternal nurses might be expected in a hospital setting.

The problem behavior may also result from failure to appropriately involve the family. Sometimes the marital partners have worked out very helpful patterns where one becomes the main source of leadership and aid for the other. Focusing on the individual and not involving the partner can short-circuit this and lead to negative results. Witness the case where the husband had been able to solve problems well, but he would begin by going over it all with his wife. Her reflections on his comments helped him put things in perspective and provided her with a sense of being helpful. When hospital staff worked with him alone, he was less effective, and the wife became picky with them. He had lost an important resource, and she had been alienated—which compounded the problem. When staff identified areas that needed to be dealt with, and left solutions to the two of them, the husband again became an effective problem solver, the wife an effective collaborator.

At times, the family may not have the skills or capacity to address the tasks, and they then require additional help. However, it is always important to involve them.

Biological Behavior

Central nervous system deficits, disruption of other body systems, medications, and some psychiatric diseases all represent biological states that can strongly influence and determine behavior (4, 6). A careful and detailed mental status will elucidate the phenomena suggesting that one of these is the case.

There are a host of behavior side effects from medications, and the possibilities increase with combination and interaction problems. Alcohol and drug abuse or addiction can be associated with the onset of disability and can be part of a poor response pattern. Physicians must be careful not to become part of the addiction process.

Biologically based behavior problems require careful assessment, aggressive treatment of the medical, addictive, and psychiatric problems, and then a reassessment to delineate unremitting difficulties that may be addressed via the other models. In general, biologically mediated behavior should be treated first—obviously, you can't desensitize a delirious patient.

SUMMARY

Disability presents complex behavior responses and demanding challenges. Several models of behavior are usually required for a sound understanding, and good assessment is an integral part of good management.

References

1. Balkany-Butt L, Balkany-Butt N, Armstrong M, Werner G: Crisis intervention techniques and spinal cord injury. In Bishop D: *Behavioral Problems and the Disabled: Assessment and Management.* Baltimore, Williams & Wilkins, 1981.
2. Bishop DS: *Behavioral Problems and the Disabled: Assessment and Management.* Baltimore, Williams & Wilkins, 1981.
3. Bishop DS: Family problems and disability. In Bishop D: *Behavioral Problems and the Disabled:*

Assessment and Management. Baltimore, Williams & Wilkins, 1981.

4. Kaplan HI, Freedman AM, Sadock BJ: *Comprehensive Textbook of Psychiatry/III.* Baltimore, Williams & Wilkins, 1980.

5. McDaniel JW: *Physical Disability and Human Behavior*, Chapter 3. Toronto, Pergamon, 1969.

6. Nicoli AM, Jr: *Harvard Guide to Modern Psychiatry.* Cambridge, Harvard University Press, 1978.

7. Shontz FC: Psychological adjustment to physical disability: Trends in theories. *Arch Phys Med Rehabil* 59:251–254, 1978.

Progressive Disorders

C. M. GODFREY

Despite the advances in modern medicine and the improvement of therapeutic regimens, many disorders continue to show a progression of disease and attendant disability. Even though the major active elements of rheumatoid arthritis are suppressed, the demyelination of multiple sclerosis is halted, or the spasticity of hemiplegia is controlled, the usual course is that things will be worse.

This deterioration applies to the diseased tissues and also to other organs. The long-term diabetic on insulin frequently progresses to a neuropathy, with changes in muscles. The suppression of carcinoma by chemotherapy may mean damage to the neuromusculoskeletal system. The reduction of general activities because of any disease process may lead to unwanted secondary results, and even in cerebral palsy a "nonprogressive disease," there are undesirable sequelae resulting from a chronically low level of activity.

PLANNING

The physician's responsibility, in concert with the patient and the family, is to anticipate and meet these problems. To do this effectively, there must be a plan.

There are four target areas upon which all efforts should focus in the care of progressive disorders: the maintenance and enhancement of the ability of the patient to do physical activities, the intactness of the family unit, the assertion of the patient's identity, and the education of the patient and family about the disease.

In the planning process it is necessary to realize that there is a different rate of progression in many disorders. The patient with multiple sclerosis may be stable or may suddenly regress to a lower level. The rheumatoid arthritic may have a slow downhill course. Parkinsonism is progressive and continuous with a gradual decrease of all physical activities. The patient with cancer may have progressive complaints of tiring, inability to match last year's performance and, eventually, to perform at an acceptable rate. These variations require that the physician play a major planning role in an individual strategy for the patient.

Team Burnout

A large factor in such a plan is physician fatigue. Burnout of the medical team is a common complication in the treatment of progressive disorders. Frequently, members of the health team fail to pursue aggressively the most recent developments in medical science which can affect the patient and are unaware of new techniques which may enhance the victim's ability to achieve a more satisfying life. Once a label is affixed, medical thinking tends to work in stereotypes, e.g., "… and it is common knowledge that it is difficult to change the natural history of amyotrophic lateral sclerosis."

Exercise

This need to up-to-date knowledge applies particularly in the field of physical restoration, where loss of muscle power prevents patient mobility. For example, the exercise training of diabetics demands a grasp of newer biochemistry findings.

In other disorders, such as rheumatoid arthritis, recent work suggests that speed-specific exercises can selectively lead to power improvements while, with tuning of the velocity, they minimize the high intra-articular pressures (1, 2), described by Jayson et al. (3).

In the hemiplegic patient, the use of electromyographic biofeedback training has opened new areas (4). Using kinematic data (5), Perry et al. (6) have shown that the patient with multiple sclerosis can benefit from the fitting of a rocker-sole. These are but a few examples.

Family Support

One of the major threats to the patient is a breakup of the family unit. Chronic sickness, particularly when associated with significant disability, places a great strain on the husband-wife relationship. With older families there is a reasonable tendency to remain together, with the spouse of the hemiplegic patient accepting the responsibility of caring—although this may come at a time when the spouse's own health is not at its best. Setting up a realistic program which does not absorb the full time of the spouse can forestall problems here if it is accepted that life goes on for the normal person with the pursuit of nonpatient centered activities. Set up a spouse "vacation," just to get away from it all for a few weeks. This break can be timed with a short admission to a rehabilitation center for a "recycling" program for the patient, to look at and upgrade recently lost abilities.

With the younger family and progressive disorders such as multiple sclerosis, planning is more difficult. The disablement, which may frequently involve emotional and sexual disinterest, frequently leads to the spouse seeking pleasure outside the house with ultimate complete removal. The best means of avoiding this is frank discussion regarding the necessity for the disabled person to recognize the needs of the able person.

Such a discussion may be fruitless because of the self-centeredness of many people who have a chronic disability. It is difficult for the healthy person to realize the preoccupation that may seize victims of a disease. All thoughts, words, or actions during a day are shaped by how it affects the body. Will it cause more pain? More disability? Will it mean that I lose more of myself? This egocentricity, especially noticeable with progressive disability, conditions all reactions. It becomes a great struggle to maintain one's identity.

So it is necessary early in the course of a progressive illness to talk about a rearrangement of family responsibilities. Is there a possibility of job sharing? Can the traditional roles be exchanged and the wife become the breadwinner while the husband performs household tasks with some assistance? Can we anticipate a cash shortfall and adjust for it by knowing exactly what can be expected from social assistance programs?

Part of this process entails the preservation of individualism of the diseased person. Each of us is a composite of various activities and thoughts. With a reduction of physical and mental stimuli, our personalities change with a loss of self-identity. This closing in of the perimeters of our activities must be compensated for by an opening of other areas in which we can function with reduced abilities. The arthritic patient who cannot do strenuous physical activities can be encouraged to expand to nonphysical recreation, such as an interest in music or participation in group activities which requires a good deal of telephoning.

This preservation requires a realization of what is to be expected from the disease process. Realistic goals must be set, which means an openness and frankness between physician and family. Part of this can be promoted by a willingness to share the advisory field by consultation or referrals to other areas of expertise. This is important to prevent doctor shopping. Part of this process must involve the maintenance of hope, not by a "Pollyanna approach" but by the promotion of a melange of faith, optimism, and humor.

Contract

One of the best techniques of achieving the desired end is to establish a contract with the patient and the family. What do you expect the patient to be doing a year from now, or 2 years from now? What consultations do you plan on a regular or intermittent basis? What level of physical and mental activity do you anticipate and what level is acceptable to the patient and the family? With this in mind a written contract is helpful to assure yourself and the patient that the accepted end is being reached, and that unrealistic expectations do not persist.

The care of patients with progressive disorders can be rewarding and can be an opportunity for personal growth of the patient, the family, and the physician.

References

1. Moffroid MT, Whipple RH, Hofkosh J et al: A study of isokinetic exercise. *Phys Ther* 49:735–747, 1969.
2. Coyle EF, Feiring DC, Rotkis TC, Cote RW, III, Roby FB, Lee W, Wilmore JH: The specificity of power improvements through slow and fast isokinetic training. Personal communication, 1981.
3. Jayson MIV, Dixon AJ: Intra-articular pressure in rheumatoid arthritis of the knee. II Effect of intra-articular pressure on blood circulation to the synovium. *Ann Rheumat Dis* 29:266, 1970.
4. Basmajian JV, Kukulka CG, Narayan MG et al: Biofeedback treatment of foot-drop after stroke compared with standard rehabilitation technique: effects on voluntary control and strength. *Arch Phys Med Rehabil* 56:231–236, 1975.
5. Godfrey CM: Kinematics—a dimension of collagen disorders. *J Rheumatol* 7:594–595, 1980.
6. Perry J, Gronley JK, Lunsford T: Rocker shoe as walking aid in multiple sclerosis. *Arch Phys Med Rehabil* 62:59–65, 1981.

Intractable Pain

W. E. FORDYCE

Chronic pain is prototypic of the importance of incorporating behavioral science into health care delivery as a complement to medical science. In chronic illness, including chronic pain, neither medical nor behavioral science can do the job without the other.

Pain is thought of as a sensory system. That short-sighted view is based solely on "disease model" concepts. We can know a person has pain *only* by behavior: verbal or nonverbal. Those communications about pain-suffering will hereafter be termed *pain behaviors.*

When observing pain behaviors, in whatever form, the diagnostician must recognize the proper question is: "What causes those pain behaviors to occur?" not "Is the pain 'real'?", or "What body damage factor causes these pain behaviors to occur?" Pain behaviors may occur because of body damage or other factors.

The next important distinction is between acute (recent onset) and chronic pain. Clinically, the proper management methods of acute pain, if applied to chronic pain, likely will make the problem worse. Similarly, proper management for chronic pain, if applied to acute pain, is usually ineffective. Trauma-induced pain has a finite healing time, beyond which the expression of pain behaviors *must* take on a different meaning from those true at onset. Furthermore, pain behaviors, like all other behaviors, are sensitive to learning-conditioning effects.

As a result, the protracted expression of pain behaviors (as occurs in prolonged healing time or in recurring episodes of injury and pain) ensures exposure to potential learning-conditioning effects. If conditioning occurs, pain behaviors will persist past healing time and indefinitely into the future. The proper evaluation of chronic pain, therefore, requires a blending of medical and behavioral science (or learning-conditioning) concepts.

Traditionally, pain behaviors not accounted for on the basis of physical findings have been attributed to emotional or motivational factors and acquire labels such as psychogenic, conversion reaction, or hysteria. This is but another application of a disease model perspective, although now the "disease" is attributed to the psyche. Resort to psychogenic concepts is not the only alternative to an "organic" or "body damage" explanation; nor has it been an effective one.

HOW LEARNING-CONDITIONING MAY COME TO INFLUENCE OR CONTROL PAIN BEHAVIORS

Before proceeding, another important conceptual point needs to be understood: how we label things exerts great influence on how we perceive them. For example, a sensory experience labeled by the sufferer as "pain" is likely to "hurt" more than if labeled as "tension" or "heat." That is so because the label evokes the network of associations attached to the term by past experience, thereby intensifying the effect.

It is commonplace to use the language of pain to express suffering. We may, for example, say that some person "gives me a pain in the neck." We do not mean there is nociception in the neck; nor do we mean that person produces pain. We mean that person causes suffering, though we use the label "pain." Confounding of pain-suffering adds immeasurably to the persistence of pain behaviors. It misdirects patient behavior and misleads diagnosticians. Pain behaviors tend to become associated with a host of prior suffering experiences which, because they have been aversive, contribute to avoidance learning.

Pain behaviors, like all other behaviors, are sensitive to conditioning effects. They may come under control of or be substantially influenced by conditioning in either of two ways.

Direct Reinforcement of Pain Behaviors

Pain behaviors (verbal or nonverbal) tend to elicit reinforcing actions from those around the suffering person. Common examples are special attention and other forms of supportive behaviors from spouse or family members; sanctioned and even prescribed rest; prescribed analgesics delivered on a *prn* (take only as needed) regimen—the traditional way for prescribing analgesics. In each setting, the consequences (i.e., attention, rest, analgesics) are pain behavior contingent. They occur or are delivered only when the patient communicates by word or action that there is pain-suffering. *Contingent* reinforcement has great potency in producing conditioning effects.

Indirect Reinforcement of Pain Behaviors (Avoidance Learning)

Escape behavior is defined as behavior which terminates an aversive stimulus, as in withdrawing the hand from a hot stove. Avoidance behavior is defined as behavior which postpones—perhaps indefinitely—an aversive stimulus. These can be grouped together as avoidance learning. It has long been known that avoidance learning, once established, is very durable. Little ongoing reinforcement is needed to maintain an established avoidance response.

There are two principal ways avoidance learning plays a role in maintaining chronic pain behavior, as well as in contributing to the persistence of pain behaviors associated with recent onset. The first concerns the social or situational consequences which follow when a person takes protective action in response to pain-suffering. A housewife with back pain may recline on the couch to ease the pain of her back after making beds or vacuuming a rug. In doing so, she eases the pain and earns "time out" from what may be an aversive activity in its own right: housework. A man with an unsatisfying job, who spends the day at home easing the pain of his aching back, also earns "time out" from the aversive job. In both cases, pain behaviors may be directly reinforced by the easing of pain by rest but also may be indirectly reinforced by time out from aversive stimuli. When there is wage replacement funding from insurance, the cost of being sick is reduced and perhaps eliminated, making even more potent the avoidance-learning effects of rest.

These forms of reinforcement of pain behaviors approximate what has long been termed "secondary gain." They play significant roles in many problems of chronic pain. Unless examined and understood, the nature of the pain problem will elude the diagnostician, and needless and irrelevant investigations and therapies may be instituted.

There is a second way avoidance learning enters. Stimuli associated with aversive stimuli may themselves take on aversive properties. A recent onset pain patient with a hip or leg injury may experience during healing time that walking more than 100 m leads to a marked increase in pain-suffering. There is the risk that cues internally or in the environment indicative of an approach to the walking distance of 100 m will become capable of eliciting the pain behaviors. It is an antic-ipatory response, as well as an example of avoidance learning. To paraphrase: "Past experience has told me that exceeding 100 meters will lead to significantly greater pain. I must, therefore, stop when I near the 100 meter mark." In some cases the person seems directly to experience the pain. In others, it may only be anticipated. In either case, the result is the same—he or she stops.

A second example: the vast majority of middle-aged women who complain of lower quadrant abdominal or pelvic pain have long been found to find intercourse aversive *antecedent* to the pain problem. The pain behaviors yield time out from the aversive activity of intercourse.

The pattern just described has also been termed *superstitious overguarding*. It is commonly observed in chronic pain patients.

IMPLICATIONS FOR THE PRACTICING PHYSICIAN AND OTHER HEALTH CARE PROFESSIONALS

Evaluation of Chronic Pain

- In trauma-initiated chronic pain there must be exploration of both physical finding and learning-conditioning factors. Either or both in any mix may produce and maintain the pain behaviors. Learning-conditioning factors become more important after healing time has elapsed.
- Behavioral evaluation of chronic pain must examine not only what the person says but also what he or she does. What is the activity level? What activities are limited or avoided because of "pain"? What are the social consequences of pain behaviors?

Treatment or Management of Pain

- Avoid pain behavior contingent regimens: *prn* or take-only-as-needed analgesics, working-to-tolerance exercise-rest regimens (e.g., "Let pain be your guide") *after* healing time.

- Explain to your recent onset pain patients that medications and rest are effective only during healing time. Therefore, set them to expect that those therapies will be discontinued following healing.
- Build into the regimen restoration of activity. Rest or "light duty" should be prescribed only for the interval sufficient to produce healing of soft tissue injury. There should then be a reintroduction of exercise and activity. Spell out the number of repetitions of a prescribed set of exercises each day, with an incrementing rate.
- Involve the spouse or significant others in the explanations of the treatment

plan to optimize prevention of chronicity.

For more details about the methods described here and underlying conceptual and empirical bases, see the following references.

References

Block AR: Multidisciplinary treatment of chronic low back pain: a review. *Rehab Psychol* 27:51–63, 1982.

Fordyce WE: *Behavioral Methods in Chronic Pain and Illness*. St. Louis, CV Mosby, 1976.

Fordyce WE *et al*: Family doctor *vs.* chronic pain. *Patient Care* 12:216–261, 1978.

Roberts A, Reinhardt L: The behavioral management of chronic pain: long-term follow-up with comparison groups. *Pain* 8:151–162, 1980.

Sternback R (ed.): *The Psychology of Pain*. New York, Raven Press, 1978.

Rehabilitation Management of Burns

S. V. FISHER

Over 2 million persons in the United States are burned each year, at least 100,000 are hospitalized (2). Because of increased emphasis on burn care over the last two decades, the survival rate has improved dramatically, and the length of hospitalization has decreased (3). With more severely burned patients surviving, the risk of disability from the sequela of burns increases. Physical medicine and rehabilitation should be involved from the onset of burn injury through long-term follow-up care. The burn rehabilitation team helps to position, splint, and exercise the acutely burned victim. During the hospitalization, the team continues its therapies and contributes to the education of patients and families, and the provision of psychological care; later, the team may provide or arrange vocational counseling.

Burns may be classified by causative agent, depth of burn, the percent of total body surface burned (6), and by the American Burn Association criteria (10). (See Table 14.6 and Fig. 14.6.) Other factors considered to determine the severity of burn are location of burn, age, pre-existing illness, smoke inhalation, and other associated injuries. Electrical energy which is converted to heat in the less conductive tissues causes injury which may seem relatively minor initially but not infrequently causes deep tissue necrosis. Although blood vessels and nerves have a low electrical resistance, they can often sustain significant injury, necessitating amputations and causing central and peripheral nervous system pathology (1).

REHABILITATION GOALS AND CARE

The major rehabilitation goals are: (1) proper wound care and skin healing; (2) preservation of function through main-

Table 14.6
Burn Classification

A. Causative Agent
   (1) Thermal
      (a) Heat
      (b) Cold
   (2) Electrical
   (3) Chemical
   (4) Radiation
B. Depth of Burn (6)
   (1) Older Terminology
      1st degree–epidermis injured
      2nd degree—dermis partially damaged
      3rd degree—all dermis destroyed
      4th degree—muscle, nerve, and bone damaged
   (2) Newer Terminology

Superficial partial thickness	Epidermis and upper part of dermis injured
Deep partial thickness	Epidermis and large upper portion of dermis injured
Full thickness	All skin destroyed

C. Size of Burn—"Rule of Nines" (6)
   Head = 9% body surface area (BSA)
   Each upper extremity = 9% BSA
   Each lower extremity = 18% BSA
   Anterior trunk =   18% BSA
   Posterior trunk =   18% BSA
   Perineum =   1% BSA
D. American Burn Association Classification (10)[a]
   (1) Minor: <15% BSA partial thickness (10% child)
            <2% BSA full thickness (not involving eyes, ears, face, or perineum)
   (2) Moderate: All 15–25% BSA (10–20% in child)
              2–10% BSA full thickness (not involving eyes, ears, face, or perineum)
   (3) Major: All > 25% BSA partial thickness (20% in child)
            ≥10% BSA full thickness
            All burns to face, eyes, ears, feet, perineum
            All electrical
            All inhalation
            All burns with fracture or major tissue trauma
            All with poor risk secondary to age or illness

[a] Most moderate and all major burns should be hospitalized.

taining range of motion and strength; (3) minimizing hypertrophic scarring and maximizing cosmetic outcome; (4) reducing pain behavior; and (5) providing psychological and vocational counseling. These goals are comparable for inpatient and outpatient burn care (See Table 14.7).

OUTPATIENT

For optimal outpatient burn care, the patient and family must be cooperative and willing to be seen for frequent follow-up care. Pain is a major complaint with even the smallest burn, and responds well to cooling initially and later occlusion with a dressing or skin substitute. Patients assume a flexed position for comfort. The prevention of contractures requires early institution of proper positioning and exercise techniques and continued vigilance. Splinting is rarely necessary for the outpatient.

The outpatient's wound must be cleansed once or twice daily by the hospital staff or the patient and family. If a burn extends over a joint, it should be exercised through the full ROM 4 times a day. Elevation for edema control is para-

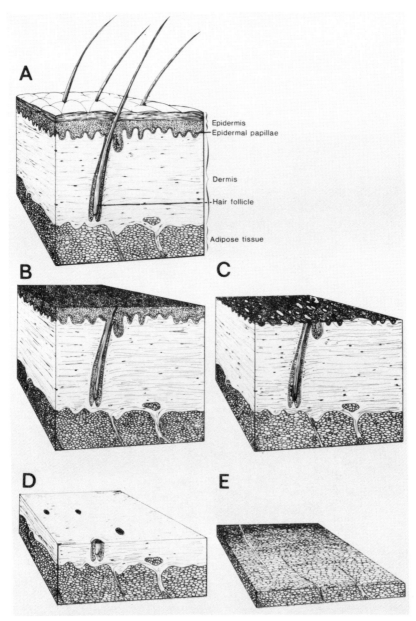

Figure 14.6. Depth of burns: (A) Normal skin. (B) Superficial partial thickness (1st degree). (C) Superficial partial thickness (2nd degree). (D) Deep partial thickness (2nd degree). (E) Full thickness (3rd degree).

mount, especially for foot and hand burns. Close medical supervision must be provided, and hospital admission is indicated if cellulitis, unusual pain, or purulent drainage are noted.

Removal of broken blisters with gentle mechanical debridement of the wound is initially needed, but intact blisters are not disturbed (9). A topical antimicrobial agent helpful in alleviating pain and effective against most common pathogens is used, or a biological dressing may be used instead. With the use of closed wound treatment, the pain is decreased, and the active motion necessary to prevent contractures is less painful.

Table 14.7
Outline of Burn Rehabilitation Problems

Area Affected	Goal	Exercise	Positioning	Appliance and Splinting
Face	Decrease scarring, prevent microstomia and ectropion	Facial exercise	Elevation, no pillows if ears affected	Microstomia appliance, Jobst hood, face mask
Anterior neck	Maintain neck ROM	A & PROM (active & passive range of motion exercises)	Hyperextension mattress	Neck splint
Shoulder	Maintain ROM, strength, minimize anterior/posterior axillary fold webbing	Reciprocal pulleys; A & PROM stressing flexion, abduction, rotation; overhead walker during ambulation	Abduction, flexion, external rotation, elevation	Clavical strap, total contact abduction axillary splint, overhead suspension when supine
Elbow	Maintain ROM and strength	A & PROM stressing flexion, extension, and supination	Usually extension, may need to alternate flexion & extension	Total contact extension splint
Hand & wrist	Maintain ROM & strength, independence in ADLs, edema control	A & PROM, ADL activity, strengthening, coordination exercises	Initial: elevate hand usually 70° flexion MCP, extension of PIP & DIP, 15° wrist extension, thumb opposition	Initial: intrinsic plus resting splint, finger troughs acutely
		(Note: convalescent hand care is beyond chapter scope—see bibliography for information)		
Hips	Maintain ROM, strength	Ambulation, stair climbing, stationary bicycle, A & PROM stressing hip extension and abduction	Hips abducted to 15° prone & supine lying, avoid rotation	Uncommon
Knees	Same	Ambulation, stair climbing, stationary bicycle, A & PROM	Usually extension	Total contact posterior extension splint for popliteal burns
Ankle	Same Edema control	Ambulation, stair climbing, stationary bicycle, A & PROM, heel cord stretching	Neutral	Elastic support ankle-foot orthosis in neutral position
Foot	Same Edema control	Ambulation	Dorsal burn: toes plantar flexed	Elastic support dorsal burn: extra depth shoes with flexion of toes
			Plantar burn: toes neutral position	Plantar burn: padded sandals

Rehabilitation Considerations

Active ROM exercise helps to control edema and preserve joint and muscle function better than passive ROM. Gentle stretching at the end of the active range and sustaining this stretched position are advantageous when there is limitation of motion as well as for the uncooperative patient or child. Exercises should be performed at least four times daily. When not exercising, the patient should be either positioned for gravity-assisted edema control or should be engaged in activities or play designed to maintain strength, ROM, and independence in ADL. Pressure wraps will assist in edema control. Ambulation, stair climbing, and stationary bicycle riding are helpful in maintaining lower extremity ROM, strength, and cardiovascular fitness.

INPATIENT REHABILITATION

If the goals of treatment are not being met as an outpatient, the burn victim should be admitted to the hospital for a more structured treatment approach before the wounds become infected or contractures develop. Severely burned victims are admitted to the hospital where the specialized care of the burned patient is beyond the scope of this chapter (12, 13, 18). The burn rehabilitation team becomes involved sooner or later.

Hydrotherapy

Viable tissues must be treated gently during bathing and exercise. Hydrotherapy, although controversial, has been traditional in burn care—but is by no means universally used. Hydrotherapy may be immersion or spray type (4). Immersion hydrotherapy provides a comfortable method of dressing removal for wound care and provides an excellent time for ROM exercises. Active motion is again preferred to passive.

Exercise

Exposed tendons become dry and frag-ile and so are covered with a biologic dressing. With the exceptions of the PIP and DIP joints of the hand, where no motion is allowed when tendons are damaged, only gentle active ROM is allowed. When ROM is performed, stretching of the tendons is not done. Once granulation tissue covers the tendon area, grafts will adhere, and the tendon strength will improve. At that time, more vigorous ROM exercises may be resumed.

Bed Positioning

The patient should be positioned to help reduce edema and to counteract the usual contracture burn position (Table 14.7). This is an important consideration in the burn victim. In most cases, the best positioning is elevation and extension of the part, with the exception being at the shoulder where the position is elevation, abduction, and flexion. The positioning is designed to counteract the natural wound contracture.

Splinting

Splinting by specialists can play an important role in the management of the burned patient (4, 5, 7, 11). Splints should be custom-made, modified as necessary, and should distribute pressure in such a way as to prevent pressure ulcers. Splints should be as comfortable as possible and yet position the joint opposite the contracted burn position. Splints cannot replace exercise and should be removed frequently to inspect the underlying tissues and to have the patient exercise. Splints are most effective for children or when the patient is unresponsive, sleeping, confused, or uncooperative. They may be applied after skin grafting to immobilize both the graft and the joints proximal and distal to the graft (to maintain the skin at maximum tissue length).

SCARRING

The prevention of hypertrophic scars (Figs. 14.7 and 14.8) is a major goal in

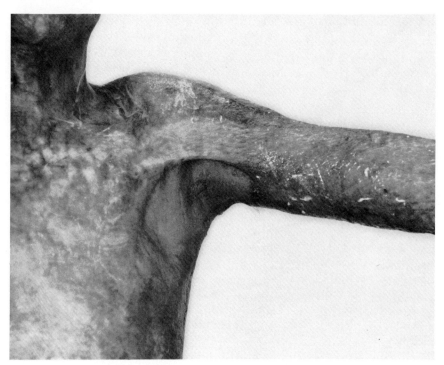

Figure 14.7.   Anterior axillary contracture with webbing. Note blanching of skin across web with attempted abduction of arm. This preventable contracture can be reduced with proper positioning, splinting, and exercise.

rehabilitation of burn patients and may require several years of care after injury (5, 7, 11). Pressure (approximately capillary blood pressure) against the skin has given good success. It is hypothesized that the pressure acts initially by edema control and later by promoting early collagen maturation. Elastic garments, such as the Jobst® pressure garments and elastic bandages, are quite effective on the extremities and trunk but less effective on highly contoured areas. The garments need to be ordered in pairs to allow washing. Pressure must be applied at least 23 hours/day, and garments need to be checked frequently since they become inelastic, and the patient's weight, edema, and healing process fluctuate. In contoured concave areas such as axilla, between the breasts, in the midback, etc., the garment may need to be augmented with the use of foam or silicone elastomer to give total contact and equal pressure to all areas (Fig. 14.9).

A progression of elastic wraps to tubular elastic to commercial garments is suggested since early application and use of the garments causes shearing, blistering, and skin breakdown. If blisters do occur, they are punctured and drained, and pressure is continued whenever possible.

FACE

Scarring of the face is particularly disturbing. The face, because of its many contours and important structures, needs specialized pressure techniques. Jobst face masks are available and used at many burn centers. A silicone elastomer or thermoplastic splint is used with the Jobst to maintain the highly contoured facial structures. Transparent face masks, although time consuming to fabricate, offer the best solution to applying pressure to the face (4, 8). A disadvantage is that the fabrication and modification of this mask takes a very experienced therapist or orthotist who must make frequent modifi-

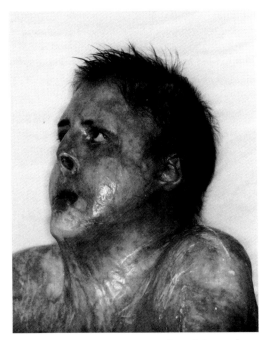

Figure 14.8. Severe face and neck burn demonstrating contractures with loss of neck shelf, rounded shoulders, distortion of mouth, and ectropion. Note blanching of skin over chin with attempted extension of neck. Early application of neck and face splints could have reduced disfigurement by minimizing skin-connective tissue contracture and hypertrophic scarring.

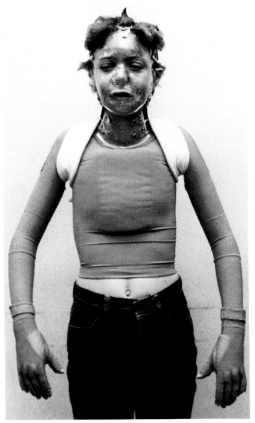

Figure 14.9. Compression orthotics. Transparent face and neck splints, Jobst long-sleeved vest and gloves, elastomeric thumb and finger web spreaders, chest elastomeric conformer, and figure eight axillary compression appliance.

cations as scarring is reduced and edema subsides.

NECK

Foam collars are frequently used for neck burns; however, total contact is difficult to maintain. Foam is well tolerated by fragile tissue. As healing progresses the transparent neck splint is effective in maintaining the neck shelf, minimizing the hypertrophic scarring, and preventing neck flexion contractures. All neck splints need to be individually fabricated.

HAND

Hyperextension at the MCP joints and flexion of the PIP and DIP joints with thumb adduction is the typical contracted burned hand position. The edema in the dorsum of the hand aggravates the con-

tracted position. Initially, the use of splints to flex the MCP joints and maintain the thumb web in addition to elevation and compression to reduce edema is critical. Individual finger gutter splints are used to help prevent boutonniere deformities when the dorsal hood mechanism is in jeopardy. Special attention must be given to the web spaces of the fingers during the convalescence stages to prevent webbing (Figs. 14.9 and 14.10).

PAIN

Burns are obviously painful, and the pain must be dealt with on a 24-hour basis for the patient. Each burn center has its

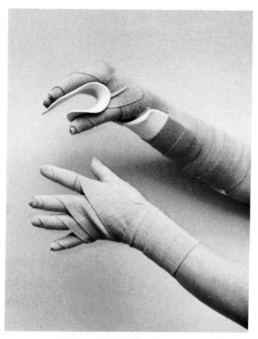

Figure 14.10. A resting hand splint for proper acute burn positioning. A "boxer" figure 8 wrap to reduce edema.

port and family education is important. Early psychological intervention as well as vocational counseling is thought to hasten adjustment and earlier return to work.

FOLLOW-UP CARE

Frequent outpatient follow-up is essential to provide psychological support and to supervise and modify the care plan. The patient should be aware of all common problems such as sensitivity to sunlight, pruritus, blistering of fragile skin, heat or cold intolerance, skin dryness with need for moisturizing, loss of sensation and precaution for skin breakdown.

The follow-up should continue until all scars are matured, all reconstructive surgery is completed, and the patient has returned to society and a satisfactory vocation. This follow-up care may involve the entire rehabilitation team and, because it takes several years, especially in children, it requires planning and commitment.

own pain regimen. When analgesics are to be used, continuous oral long half-life analgesics on a regular scheduled therapeutic regime are superior to short-acting medications on an "as needed" basis. Therapeutic intervention utilizing self-hypnosis relaxation techniques are valuable in reducing anxiety and pain behavior. Behavior modification techniques can enhance compliance with the therapy programs.

NEUROPATHY

Peripheral polyneuropathies are relatively common sequelae of burns from multiple causes and require appropriate rehabilitation therapy. Localized neuropathy, however, due to pressure or stretching of a peripheral nerve are preventable by proper positioning, splinting, and avoidance of inappropriate stretching.

COUNSELING

Counseling for adjustment to disfigurement and disability as well as family sup-

References

1. Artz CP: Electrical injury. In Artz CP, Moncrief J, Pruitt BA Jr (eds): *Burns: A Team Approach.* Philadelphia, WB Saunders, 1979.
2. Artz CP: Epidemiology, causes and prognosis. In Artz CP, Moncrief J, Pruitt BA Jr (eds): *Burns: A Team Approach.* Philadelphia, WB Saunders, 1979.
3. Feller I, Tholen D, Cornell RG: Improvements in burn care, 1965 to 1979. *JAMA* 244:2074–2078, 1980.
4. Johnson CL, O'Shaughnessy EJ, Ostergren G: *Burn Management.* New York, Raven Press, 1981.
5. Larson DL *et al*: Contractures and scar formation in the burn patient. *Clin Plast Surg* 1:653–666, 1974.
6. McDougal WS, Slade CL, Pruitt BA Jr: *Manual of Burns.* New York, Springer-Verlag, 1978.
7. Park DH, Evans BE, Larson DL: Prevention and correction of deformity after severe burns. *Surg Clin North Am* 58:1279–1289, 1978.
8. Rivers E, Strate R, Solem L: The transparent face mask. *Am J Occup Ther* 33:108–113, 1979.
9. Shuck JM: Outpatient management of the burn patient. *Surg Clin North Am* 58:1107–1118, 1978.
10. American Burn Association: *Specific Optimal Criteria for Hospital Resources for Care of Patients with Burn Injury.* New York, American Burn Association, 1976.
11. Yeakel M: Occupational therapy. In Artz CP, Moncrief J, Pruitt BA Jr: *Burns: A Team Approach.* Philadelphia, WB Saunders, 1979.

APPENDIX

I. Myofascial Pain Syndromes and Their Treatment

D. G. SIMONS

In the seven pages that follow, Plates I–VII illustrate special techniques described in Chapter 11. The most common trigger point-referred pain pattern, a stretch technique, and the spray pattern for individual muscles are shown. The most likely placement of the trigger points in each muscle is located by a *short straight flat arrow*. The usual pattern of pain referred by trigger points in a muscle is shown in *solid black*; the extended patterns of more active trigger points are *stippled*. The *large 3-dimensional arrows* emphasize the direction of pressure exerted by the operator to stretch the muscle in the *relaxed* patient. *Dashed lines* indicate the path on the skin followed by the stream of vapocoolant spray; their *arrowheads* point the direction.

HEAD AND NECK PAIN

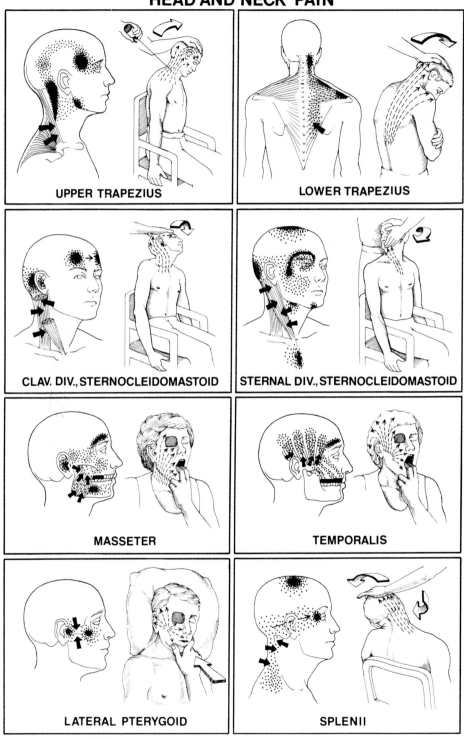

UPPER TRAPEZIUS

LOWER TRAPEZIUS

CLAV. DIV., STERNOCLEIDOMASTOID

STERNAL DIV., STERNOCLEIDOMASTOID

MASSETER

TEMPORALIS

LATERAL PTERYGOID

SPLENII

PAIN PATTERN   TRIGGER POINT

Plate I

HEAD AND NECK PAIN (CONTINUED)

SHOULDER AND UPPER EXTREMITY PAIN

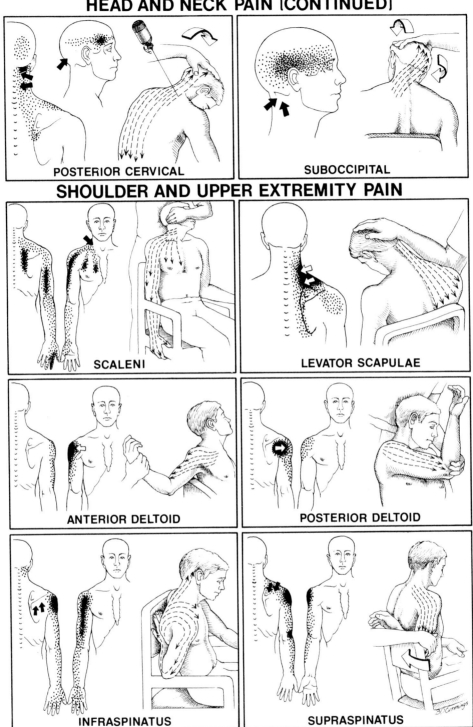

POSTERIOR CERVICAL

SUBOCCIPITAL

SCALENI

LEVATOR SCAPULAE

ANTERIOR DELTOID

POSTERIOR DELTOID

INFRASPINATUS

SUPRASPINATUS

PAIN PATTERN   TRIGGER POINT

Plate II

SHOULDER AND UPPER EXTREMITY PAIN (CONTINUED)

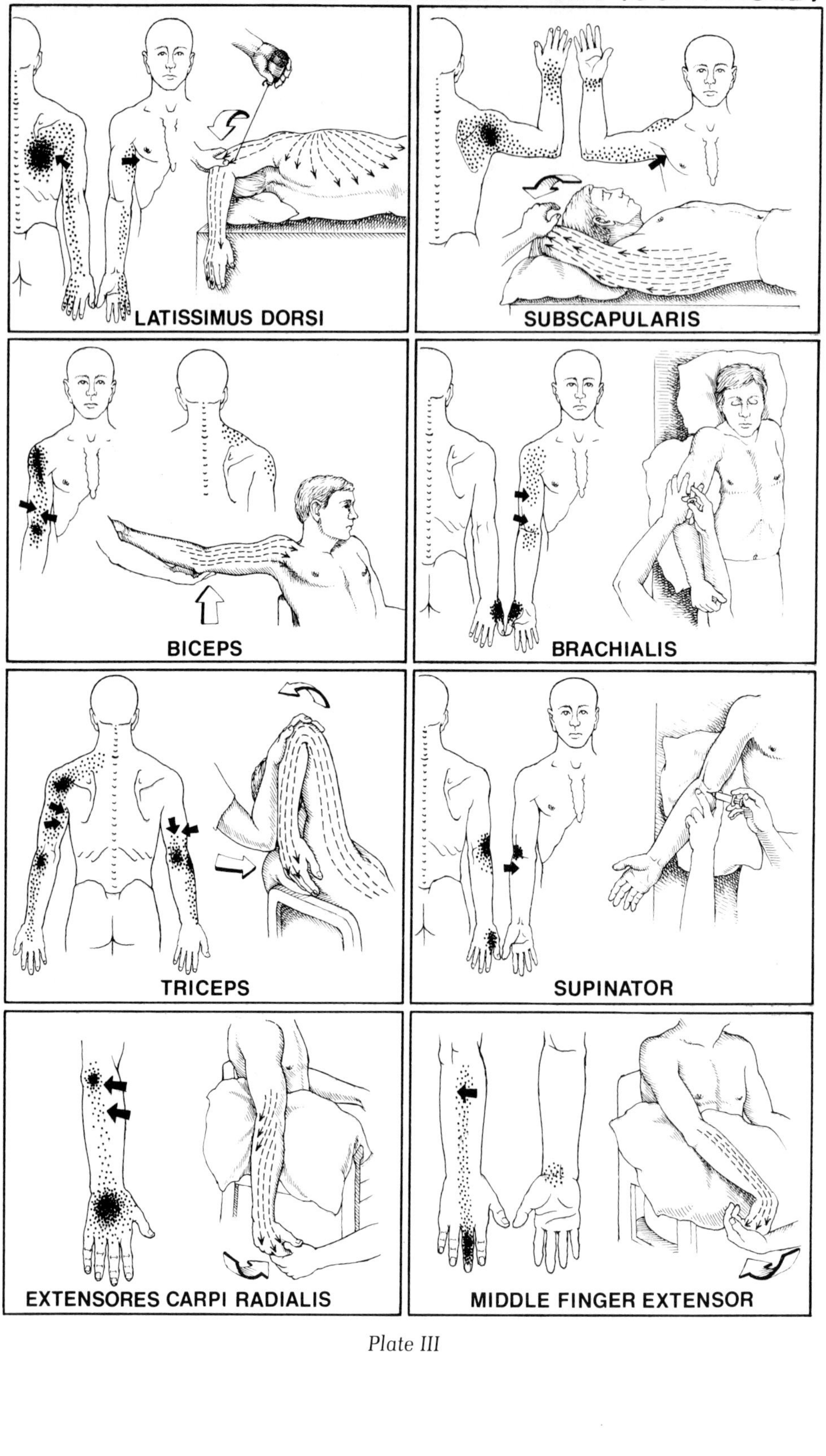

LATISSIMUS DORSI

SUBSCAPULARIS

BICEPS

BRACHIALIS

TRICEPS

SUPINATOR

EXTENSORES CARPI RADIALIS

MIDDLE FINGER EXTENSOR

Plate III

SHOULDER AND UPPER EXTREMITY PAIN (CONT.)

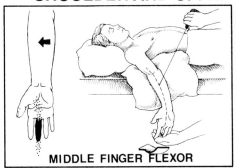

MIDDLE FINGER FLEXOR

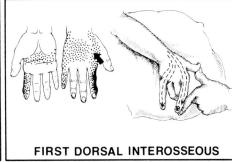

FIRST DORSAL INTEROSSEOUS

TRUNK AND BACK PAIN

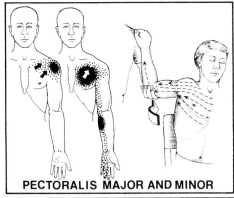

PECTORALIS MAJOR AND MINOR

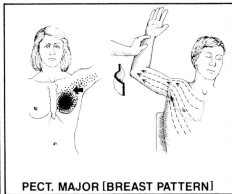

PECT. MAJOR [BREAST PATTERN]

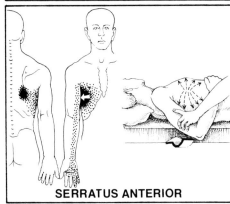

SERRATUS ANTERIOR

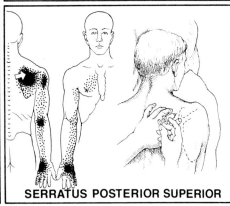

SERRATUS POSTERIOR SUPERIOR

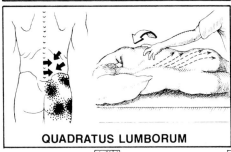

QUADRATUS LUMBORUM

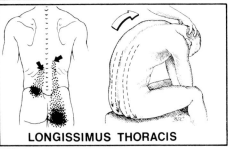

LONGISSIMUS THORACIS

PAIN PATTERN ▨   TRIGGER POINT ➡

Plate IV

TRUNK AND BACK PAIN (CONTINUED)

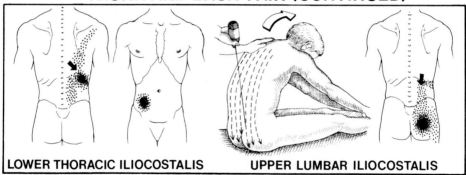

LOWER THORACIC ILIOCOSTALIS   **UPPER LUMBAR ILIOCOSTALIS**

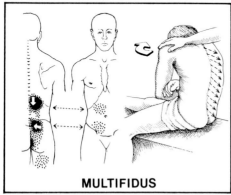

MULTIFIDUS

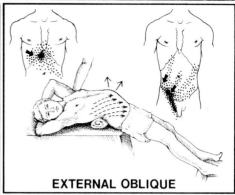

EXTERNAL OBLIQUE

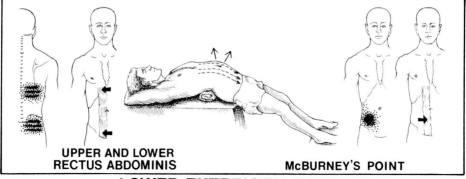

**UPPER AND LOWER
RECTUS ABDOMINIS**   **McBURNEY'S POINT**

LOWER EXTREMITY PAIN

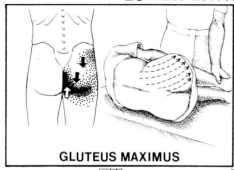

GLUTEUS MAXIMUS

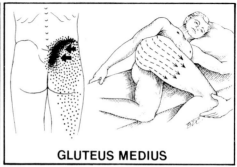

GLUTEUS MEDIUS

PAIN PATTERN ⬚ TRIGGER POINT ➡

Plate V

LOWER EXTREMITY PAIN (CONTINUED)

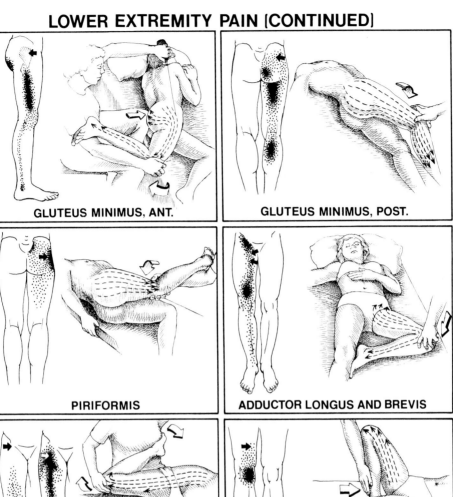

GLUTEUS MINIMUS, ANT.	GLUTEUS MINIMUS, POST.
PIRIFORMIS	ADDUCTOR LONGUS AND BREVIS

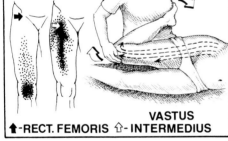

VASTUS
↑-RECT. FEMORIS ⇧-INTERMEDIUS

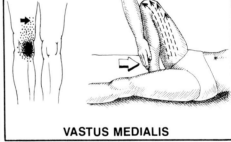

VASTUS MEDIALIS

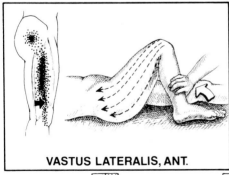

VASTUS LATERALIS, ANT.

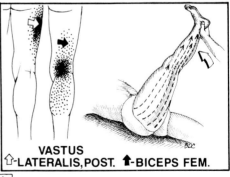

VASTUS
⇧-LATERALIS, POST. ↑-BICEPS FEM.

PAIN PATTERN ▨ TRIGGER POINT ➡

Plate VI

LOWER EXTREMITY PAIN (CONTINUED)

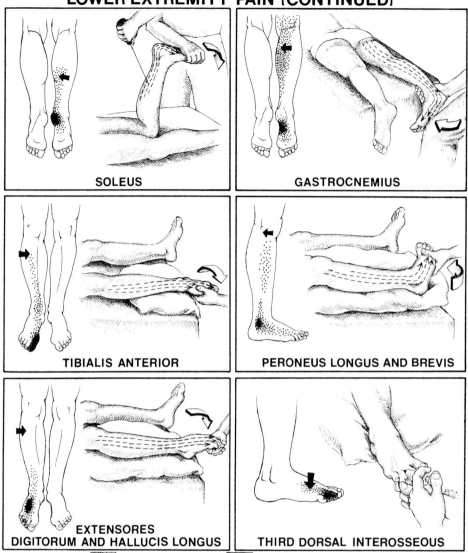

SOLEUS

GASTROCNEMIUS

TIBIALIS ANTERIOR

PERONEUS LONGUS AND BREVIS

EXTENSORES DIGITORUM AND HALLUCIS LONGUS

THIRD DORSAL INTEROSSEOUS

PAIN PATTERN   TRIGGER POINT

Plate VII

APPENDIX

II. Tables and Figures of Major Muscles, Joints, and Peripheral Nervous System

J. V. BASMAJIAN

This section is an aid for students (and their teachers), primarily to reduce the need for searching through other textbooks for applied anatomical information. Of course it is not complete; to make it complete would require assembling material enough to fill a book. Almost all the material is derived from my textbooks published by the Williams & Wilkins Company, our present publisher: *Primary Anatomy; Grant's Method of Anatomy; Therapeutic Exercise*. They should be consulted for greater coverage. Several tables are based on material in Kendall, Kendall, and Wadsworth: *Muscle Testing and Function*, also published by Williams & Wilkins.

Table A1.
Range of Joint Motion

Joint	Action	Degrees of Motion
Shoulder	Flexion	180
	Extension	45
	Adduction	40
	Abduction	180
	Medial rotation	90
	Lateral rotation	90
Elbow	Flexion	145
Forearm	Pronation	80
	Supination	85
Wrist	Flexion	80
	Extension	70
	Abduction	20
	Adduction	45
Hip	Flexion	125
	Extension	10
	Abduction	45
	Adduction	40
	Medial rotation	45
	Lateral rotation	45
Knee	Flexion	140
Ankle	Flexion	45
	Extension	20
Foot	Inversion	40
	Eversion	20

Table A2.
The Spine and Its Motion

	Cervical	Lumbar
Forward flexion	65°	95°
Extension backward	50°	35°
Lateral flexion	40°	40°
Rotation	55°	35°

(ᵃ From: J. V. Basmajian: *Therapeutic Exercise*, ed 3. Baltimore, Williams & Wilkins.)

Table A3.
Derivatives of the Brachial Plexus within the Limits of the Axilla

| Cords | Terminal branches | Collateral branches | |
	Mixed (motor and sensory)	Motor	Cutaneous
Lateral	1. Musculocutaneous 2. Lateral root of median	1. Clavicular head of pectoralis major (and upper part of sternocostal head)	
Medial	1. Medial root of median 2. Ulnar	1. Sternocostal head of pectoralis major 2. Pectoralis minor	1. Med. cutan. n. of arm 2. Med. cutan. n. of forearm
Posterior	1. Axillary 2. Radial	1. Subscapularis 2. Latissimus dorsi 3. Teres major	
From the musculocutaneous From the radial		1. Coracobrachialis 1. Triceps (long head) and	Post. cutan. n. of arm
From the 5, 6, and 7 roots of the plexus		1. Serratus anterior	

Table A4.
Segmental Innervation of Muscles of Shoulder and Upper Arm Supplied by Brachial Plexus[a]

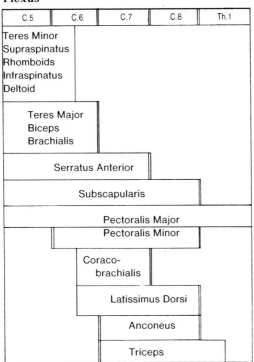

| C.5 | C.6 | C.7 | C.8 | Th.1 |

Teres Minor
Supraspinatus
Rhomboids
Infraspinatus
Deltoid

Teres Major
Biceps
Brachialis

Serratus Anterior

Subscapularis

Pectoralis Major
Pectoralis Minor

Coraco-brachialis

Latissimus Dorsi

Anconeus

Triceps

* Modified after Bing, and Haymaker and Woodhall.
([a] From: J. V. Basmajian. *Grant's Method of Anatomy.* Baltimore, Williams & Wilkins.)

Table A5.
Muscles Acting upon the Shoulder Girdle

Simple elevation	Simple depression	Elevation with upward rotation of glenoid cavity	Depression with downward rotation of glenoid cavity	Protraction or forward movement	Retraction or backward movement
Trapezius (upper) Lev. Scapulae Serratus anterior (upper)	Pect. minor Subclavius Pect. major and Lat. dorsi	Trapezius (upper) Trapezius (lower) Serratus anterior	Lev. scapulae Rhomboids Pect. minor Trapezius (mid.) Pect. major and Lat. dorsi	Pect. minor Lev. scapulae Serratus anterior and Pect. major	Trapezius (mid.) Rhomboids and Lat. dorsi

* *Note:* Pectoralis major and latissimus dorsi act on girdle indirectly, through the humerus.

Table A6.
Muscles Acting on the Shoulder Joint with Their Approximate Spinal Nerve Segments

Flexion		Extension		Abduction	
Deltoid (clav.)	5, 6	Deltoid (postr.)	5, 6	Deltoid (mid.)	5, 6
Supraspinatus	5, 6	Pect. major (st.)	7, 8, 1	Supraspinatus	5, 6
Pect. major (clav.)	5, 6	Teres major	5, 6		
Biceps	5, 6	Lat. dorsi	7, 8		
Coracobrachialis	7	Triceps (long)	7, 8		
5, 6 (7)		5, 6, 7, 8, 1		5, 6	

Adduction		Med. rotate		Lat. rotate	
Deltoid (postr.)	5, 6	Deltoid (clav.)	5, 6	Deltoid (postr.)	5, 6
Pect. major (cl.)	5, 6	Pect. major (clav.)	5, 6	Infraspinatus	5, 6
Pect. major (st.)	7, 8, 1	Pect. major (st.)	7, 8, 1	Teres minor	5, 6
Coracobrachialis	7	Subscapularis	5, 6		
Teres major	5, 6	Teres major	5, 6		
Lat. dorsi	7, 8	Lat. dorsi	7, 8		
Triceps (long)	7, 8				
5, 6, 7, 8, 1		5, 6, 7, 8, 1		5, 6	

Table A7.
Muscles Acting on the Elbow Joint

Subdivisions of the joint	Flexors	Nerve segments	Nerve	Extensors	Nerve segments	Nerve
Humeroulnar	Brachialis	5, 6	Musculocutan.	Triceps Anconeus	7, 8	Radial
Humeroradial	Biceps Brachioradialis Pronator Teres	5, 6 (5), 6 6	Musculocutan. Radial Median			

Table A8.
Segmental Innervation of Muscles of Forearm and Hand[a]

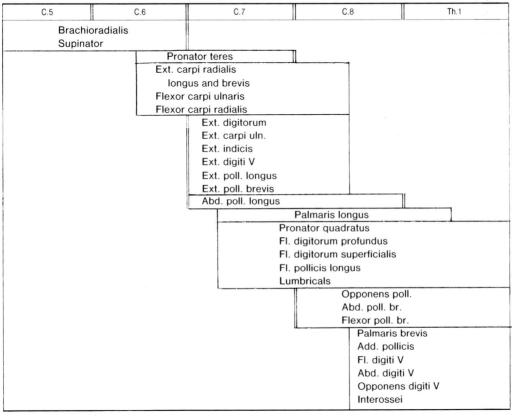

C.5	C.6	C.7	C.8	Th.1

Brachioradialis
Supinator

Pronator teres
Ext. carpi radialis
longus and brevis
Flexor carpi ulnaris
Flexor carpi radialis

Ext. digitorum
Ext. carpi uln.
Ext. indicis
Ext. digiti V
Ext. poll. longus
Ext. poll. brevis
Abd. poll. longus

Palmaris longus
Pronator quadratus
Fl. digitorum profundus
Fl. digitorum superficialis
Fl. pollicis longus
Lumbricals

Opponens poll.
Abd. poll. br.
Flexor poll. br.

Palmaris brevis
Add. pollicis
Fl. digiti V
Abd. digiti V
Opponens digiti V
Interossei

* Modified after Bing, and Haymaker and Woodhall.

([a] From: J. V. Basmajian. *Grant's Method of Anatomy*. Baltimore, Williams & Wilkins.)

Table A9.
Muscles Acting upon the Radioulnar Joints and Their Nerves and Nerve Segments

Pronators	Segment	Nerve	Supinators	Segment	Nerve
Pronator quadratus	(7), 8, 1	Anterior inter-osseous	Supinator	5, 6	Posterior interos-seous
Pronator teres	6	Median	Biceps	5, 6	Musculocuta-neous
Fl. carpi radialis	6	Median	2* dorsal muscles of the thumb	(6), 7, (8)	Posterior interos-seous

* The extensor pollicis brevis arises from the radius and therefore cannot assist in rotation.

Table A10.
Muscles Acting on the Radiocarpal Joint and Their Nerve Segments

Flexion		Extension		Abduction		Adduction	
Fl. c. ulnaris	8, 1	Ex. C. ulnaris	7	Ex. c. radialis longus	6, 7	Ex. c. ulnaris	7
Fl. c. radialis	6	Ex. C. radialis longus	6, 7	Ex. c. radialis brevis	6, 7, 8	Fl. c. ulnaris	8, 1
Palm. longus	7, 8, 1	Ex. C. radialis brevis	7	Fl. c. radialis	6		
Abd. poll. long.	7			Abd. poll. long.	7		

Table A11.
Muscles Acting on Fingers

Metacarpophalangeal Joints				Proximal Interphalangeal Joints		Distal Interphalangeal Joints	
Flexion	Extension	Abduction	Adduction	Flexion	Extension	Flexion	Extension
1. Interossei 2. Lumbricals (3. Long flexors)	Long extensors	Dorsal inteross. Abd. Dig. V	Palmar Inteross.	1. Flex. Dig. Superfic. (2. Flex. Dig. Prof.)	1. Interossei 2. Lumbricals (3. Long extensors)	Flex. Dig. Prof.	1. Interossei 2. Lumbricals

Table A12.
Muscles Acting on Thumb

Carpometacarpal Joint					Metacarpophalangeal Joint		Interphalangeal Joint	
Flexion	Extension	Abduction	Adduction	Opposition	Flexion	Extension	Flexion	Extension
Flexor Poll. Br.	1. Abd. (2. Poll. Ext. Poll. Br.) (3. Ext. Poll. L.)	1. Abd. Poll. L. 2. Abd. Poll. Br.	1. Add. Poll. (2 1st Dorsal Inteross.)	Opponens Poll.	Flex Poll. L. Flex. Poll. Br.	1. Ext. Poll. Br. (2. Ext. Poll. L.)	Fl. Poll. L.	Ext. Poll. L.

Table A13.
Muscle: Root Innervation[a]

[a] (After Kendall, Kendall, and Wadsworth.)

SPINAL SEGMENT	THORACIC T1,2,3,4	THORACIC T5,6	THORACIC T7,8	THORACIC T9,10,11	THORACIC T12	LUMBAR L1	LUMBAR L2	LUMBAR L3	LUMBAR L4	LUMBAR L5	SACRAL S1	SACRAL S2	SACRAL S3
ERECTOR SPINAE	X	X	X	X	X	X	X	X	X	X	X	X	X
SERRATUS POST. SUP.	X												
TRANS. THORACIS	X	X	X										
INT. INTERCOSTALS	X	X	X	X	(X)								
EXT. INTERCOSTALS	X	X	X	X	(X)								
SUBCOSTALES	X	X	X	X									
LEVATOR COSTARUM	X	X	X	X									
OBLIQUUS EXT. ABD.		(X)	X	X	X	x	x						
RECTUS ABDOMINIS		x	X	X	X	x							
OBLIQUUS INT. ABD.			x	X	X	X							
TRANSVERSUS ABD.				X	X	X							
SERRATUS POST. INF.				X	x								
QUAD. LUMBORUM					X	X	X	X					
PSOAS MINOR						X							
PSOAS MAJOR						x	X	X	x				
ILIACUS						(X)	X	X	x				
PECTINEUS							X	X	x				
SARTORIUS							X	X	(X)				
QUADRICEPS							X	X	X				
ADDUCTOR BREVIS							X	X	X				
ADDUCTOR LONGUS							X	X	x				
GRACILIS							X	X	X				
OBTURATOR EXT.								X	X				
ADDUCTOR MAGNUS							x	X	X	x	x		
GLUTEUS MEDIUS									X	X	X		
GLUTEUS MINIMUS									X	X	X		
TENSOR FAS. LAT.									X	X	X		
GLUTEUS MAXIMUS										X	X	X	
PIRIFORMIS										(X)	X	X	
GEMELLUS SUPERIOR										X	X	X	(X)
OBTURATOR INTERNUS										X	X	X	(X)
GEMELLUS INFERIOR									X	X	X	(X)	
QUADRATUS FEMORIS									X	X	X	(X)	
BICEPS (LONG HEAD)										x	X	X	x
SEMITENDINOSUS									x	X	X	x	
SEMIMEMBRANOSUS									x	X	X	x	
BICEPS (SHORT HEAD)										X	X	X	
TIBIALIS ANTERIOR									X	X	x		
EXT. HALL. LONG.									x	X	X		
EXT. DIGIT. LONG.									X	X	X		
PERONEUS TERTIUS									X	X	X		
EXT. DIGIT. BREVIS									x	X	X		
PERONEUS LONGUS									x	X	X		
PERONEUS BREVIS									x	X	X		
PLANTARIS									x	X	X	(X)	
GASTROCNEMIUS											X	X	
POPLITEUS									X	X	X		
SOLEUS										x	X	X	
TIBIALIS POSTERIOR									(X)	X	X		
FLEX. DIGIT. LONG.										X	X	X	(X)
FLEX. HALL. LONG.										X	X	X	
FLEX. DIGIT. BREVIS									x	X	X		
ABDUCTOR HALLUCIS									x	X	X		
FLEX. HALLUCIS BREVIS									x	X	X		
LUMBRICALIS I									x	X	X		
ABD. DIGITI MINIMI											X	X	
QUAD. PLANTAE											X	X	
FLEX. DIGITI MINIMI											X	X	
OPP. DIGITI MINIMI											X	X	
ADUCTORS HALLUCIS											X	X	
PLANT. INTEROSSEL.											X	X	
DORSAL INTEROSSEL.											X	X	
LUMBRICALES II. III. IV									(X)	(X)	X	X	

Table A14.
Muscles: Root Innervation[a]
[a] (After Kendall, Kendall, and Wadsworth.)

SPINAL SEGMENT	C1	C2	C3	C4	C5	C6	C7	C8	T1
HEAD & NECK EXTENSORS	X	X	X	X	X	X	X	X	X
INFRAHYOID MUSCLES	X	X	X						
RECTUS CAP. ANT. & LAT.	X	X							
LONGUS CAPITUS	X	X	X	(x)					
LONGUS COLLI		X	X	X	X	X	(x)		
LEVATOR SCAPULAE			X	X	X				
SCALENI (A.M.P.)			x	X	X	X	X	X	
STERNOCLEIDOMASTOID	(x)	X	x						
TRAPEZIUS (U.M.L.)		x	X	X					
DIAPHRAGM			x	X	x				
SERRATUS ANTERIOR					X	X	X	x	
RHOMBOIDS, MAJ. & MINOR				x	X				
SUBCLAVIUS					X	X			
SUPRASPINATUS				x	X	x			
INFRASPINATUS				(x)	X	X			
SUBSCAPULARIS					X	X	x		
LATISSIMUS DORSI						X	X	X	
TERES MAJOR					x	X	x		
PECTORALIS MAJ. (UPPER)					X	X	X		
PECTORALIS MAJ. (LOWER)						X	X	X	X
PECTORALIS MINOR						(x)	X	X	x
TERES MINOR					X	X			
DELTOID					X	X			
CORACOBRACHIALIS						X	X		
BICEPS					X	X			
BRACHIALIS					X	X			
TRICEPS						x	X	X	x
ANCONEUS							X	X	
BRACHIALIS (SMALL PART)					X	X			
BRACHIORADIALIS					X	X			
EXT. CARPI RAD. L & B.					x	X	X	x	
SUPINATOR					x	X	(x)		
EXT. DIGITORUM						X	X	X	
EXT. DIGITI MINIMI						x	X	X	
EXT. CARPI ULNARIS						x	X	X	
ABD. POLLICIS LONGUS						x	X	X	
EXT. POLLICIS BREVIS						x	X	X	
EXT. POLLICIS LONGUS						x	X	X	
EXT. INDICIS						x	X	X	
PRONATOR TERES						X	X		
FLEX. CARPI RADIALIS						X	X	x	
PALMARIS LONGUS						(x)	X	X	x
FLEX. DIGIT. SUPERFICIALIS							X	X	X
FLEX. DIGIT. PROF. I & II							x	X	X
FLEX. POLLICIS LONGUS						(x)	x	X	X
PRONATOR QUADRATUS							x	X	X
ABD. POLLICIS BREVIS						x	x	x	x
OPPONENS POLLICIS						x	x	x	x
FLEX. POLL. BREV. (SUP. H.)						x	x	x	x
LUMBRICALES I & II						(x)	x	X	X
FLEX. CARPI ULNARIS							x	X	x
FLEX. DIGIT. PROF. III & IV							x	X	X
PALMARIS BREVIS							(x)	X	X
ABD. DIGITI MINIMI							(x)	X	X
OPPONENS DIGITI MINIMI							(x)	X	X
FLEX. DIGITI MINIMI							(x)	X	X
PALMAR INTEROSSEI								X	X
DORSAL INTEROSSEI								X	X
LUMBRICALES III & IV							(x)	X	X
ADDUCTORS POLLICIS								X	X
FLEX. POLL. BREV. (DEEP H.)								X	X

Table A15.
Summary of Upper Limb Muscles[a,b]

Spinal Segment

4	5	6	7	8	1	MUSCLE	Abduction	Lat. Rotat.	Flexion	Med. Rotat.	Extension	Adduction	Flexion	Extension	Supination	Pronation
							SHOULDER						ELBOW		FOREARM	
4	5	6				Supraspinatus	Supraspin.									
(4)	5	6				Infraspinatus		Infraspin.								
	5	6				Teres minor		Teres mi.								
	5	6				Deltoid	Deltoid	Delt., post.	Delt., ant.	Delt., ant.	Delt., post.					
	5	6				Biceps	Biceps, l.h.		Biceps			Biceps, s.h.	Biceps		Biceps	
	5	6				Brachialis							Brachialis			
	5	6				Brachioradialis							Brachiorad.		Brachiorad.	Brachiorad.
	5	6	7			Pectoralis maj., Upp.			Pect. mj., u.	Pect. mj., u.		Pect. mj., u.				
	5	6	7			Subscapularis				Subscap.						
	5	6	(7)			Supinator									Supinator	
	5	6	7			Teres major				Teres mj.	Teres mj.	Teres mj.				
	5	6	7	8		Ext. carpi rad. l. & b.							Ext. c. r. l.			
		6	7			Coracobrachialis			Coracobr.			Coracobr.				
		6	7			Pronator teres							Pron. teres			Pron. teres
		6	7	8		Flex. carpi rad.							Fl. c. rad.			Fl. c. rad.
		6	7	8		Latissimus dorsi				Lat. dorsi	Lat. dorsi	Lat. dorsi				
		6	7	8		Ext. digitorum										
		6	7	8		Ext. digit. min.										
		6	7	8		Ext. carpi ulnaris										
		6	7	8		Abd. poll. long.										
		6	7	8		Ext. poll. brev.										
		6	7	8		Ext. poll. long.										
		6	7	8		Ext. indicis										
		6	7	8	1	Pect. maj., lower				Pect. mj., l.		Pect. mj., l.				
		6	7	8	1	Triceps					Tri., l.h.	Tri., l.h.		Triceps		
		(6)	7	8	1	Palmaris long.							Palm. l.			Palm. l.
		(6)	7	8	1	Flex. poll. long.										
		(6)	7	8	1	Lumb. I & II										
		6	7	8	1	Abd. poll. brev.										
		6	7	8	1	Opponens poll.										
		6	7	8	1	Flex. poll br. (s. h.)										
			7	8		Anconeus								Anconeus		
			7	8	1	Flex. carpi ulnaris							Fl. c. ul.			
			7	8	1	Flex. digit. super.										
			7	8	1	Flex. digit. prof.										
			7	8	1	Pronator quad.										Pron. quad.
			(7)	8	1	Abd. digiti min.										
			(7)	8	1	Opp. digiti min.										
			(7)	8	1	Flex. digiti min.										
			(7)	8	1	Lumb. III & IV										
				8	1	Dor. interossei										
				8	1	Palm. interossei										
				8	1	Flex. poll. br. (d.h.)										
				8	1	Add. pollicis										

[a] (After Kendall, Kendall, and Wadsworth.)
[b] Listed according to spinal segment innervation and grouped according to joint action.

WRIST				CARPOMETACARPAL OF THUMB & LITTLE FINGER AND METACARPOPHALANGEAL JOINTS					PROX. INTERPHAL.		DISTAL INTERPHAL.	
Extension	Flexion	Abduction	Adduction	Extension	Abduction	Flexion	Opposition	Adduction	Extension	Flexion	Extension	Flexion
Ext. c. r. l & b		Ext. c. r. l & b										
	Fl. c. rad.											
Ext. dig.				Ext. dig.					Ext. dig.		Ext. dig.	
				Ext. dig. min.					Ext. dig. min.		Ext. dig. min.	
Ext. c. ul.			Ext. c. ul.									
	Abd. poll. l.	Abd. poll. l.			Abd. poll. l.							
	Ext. poll. b.			Ext. poll. b.					Ext. poll. b.			
Ext. poll. l.		Ext. poll. l		Ext. poll. l.					Ext. poll. l.		Ext. poll. l.	
				Ext. ind.					Ext. ind.		Ext. ind.	
	Palm. l.											
	Fl. poll. l.					Fl. poll. l.						Fl. poll. l.
						Lumb. I, II			Lumb. I, II		Lumb. I, II	
					Abd. poll. b.							
							Opp. poll.					
						Fl. poll. b. (s)						
	Fl. c. ul.		Fl. c. ul.									
	Fl. dig. sup.					Fl. dig. sup.				Fl. dig. sup.		
	Fl. dig. pro.					Fl. dig. pro.				Fl. dig. pro.		Fl. dig. pro.
					Abd. d. min.							
							Opp. d. min.					
						Fl. d. min.						
						Lumb. II, III			Lumb. III, IV		Lumb. III, IV	
				Dor. int.	Dor. int.				Dor. int.		Dor. int.	
					Palm. int.			Palm. int.	Palm. int.		Palm. int.	
						Fl. poll. b. (d)				Fl. poll. b. (d)		
								Add. poll.				

Table A16.
Summary of Lower Limb Muscles[a, b]

Spinal Segment

Lumb. 1	2	3	4	5	Sac. 1	2	3	Muscle	HIP Flexion	HIP Adduction	HIP Med. Rotat.	HIP Abduction	HIP Lat. Rotat.	HIP Extension	KNEE Extension	KNEE in flexion Lat. Rotat.	KNEE in flexion Med. Rotat.
1	2	3	4					Psoas major	Psoas maj.			Psoas maj.	Psoas maj.				
(1)	2	3	4					Iliacus	Iliacus			Iliacus	Iliacus				
	2	3	(4)					Sartorius	Sartorius			Sartorius	Sartorius				Sartorius
	2	3	4					Pectineus	Pectineus	Pectineus							
	2	3	4					Adductor long.	Add. long.	Add. long.							
	2	3	4					Adductor brev.	Add. brev.	Add. brev.							
	2	3	4					Gracilis		Gracilis							Gracilis
	2	3	4					Quadriceps	Rect. fem.						Quadriceps		
	2	3	4					Adductor mag.	Add. m. (ant.)	Add. mag.							
		3	4					Obturator ext.		Obt. ext.			Obt. ext.				
			4	5	1			Adductor mag.		Add. mag.				Ad. m. post.			
			4	5	1			Tibialis ant.									
			4	5	1			Ten. fas. lat.	Tensor f.l.		Tensor f.l.	Tensor f.l.			Tensor f.l.		
			4	5	1			Gluteus minimus	Glut. min.		Glut. min.	Glut. min.					
			4	5	1			Gluteus medius	G. med., ant.		G. med., ant.	Glut. med.	G. med., post.	G. med., post.			
			4	5	1			Popliteus									Popliteus
			4	5	1			Ext. dig. long.									
			4	5	1			Peroneus tertius									
			4	5	1			Ext. hall. long.									
			4	5	1			Ext. dig. brev.									
			4	5	1			Flex. dig. brev.									
			4	5	1			Flex. hall. brev.									
			4	5	1			Lumbricalis I									
			4	5	1			Abductor hall.									
			4	5	1			Peroneus longus									
			4	5	1			Peroneus brevis									
		(4)	5	1				Tibialis post.									
			4	5	1	(2)		Gemelli inferior				Gem. inf.	Gem. inf.				
			4	5	1	(2)		Quadratus fem.		Quadratus f.			Quadratus f.				
			4	5	1	(2)		Plantaris									
			4	5	1	2		Semimembranosus						Semimemb.			Semimem
			4	5	1	2		Semitendinosus						Semitend.			Semitend
			4	5	1	(2)		Flex. dig. long.									
				5	1	2		Gluteus maximus	G. max., low.			G. max., upp.	Glut. max.	Glut. max.			
				5	1	2		Biceps, short h.								Bic., s.h.	
				5	1	2		Flex. hall. long.									
				5	1	2		Soleus									
				(5)	1	2		Piriformis				Piriformis	Piriformis	Piriformis			
				5	1	2	(3)	Gemelli superior				Gem. sup.	Gem. sup.				
				5	1	2	(3)	Obturator int.				Obt. int.	Obt. int.				
				5	1	2	3	Biceps, long h.						Biceps l.h.		Bic., l.h.	
			(4)	(5)	1	2		Lumb. II, III, IV									
					1	2		Gastrocnemius									
					1	2		Dorsal inteross.									
					1	2		Plantar inteross.									
					1	2		Abd. dig. min.									
					1	2		Adductor hall.									

[a] (After Kendall, Kendall, and Wadsworth.)
[b] Listed according to spinal segment innervation and grouped according to joint action.

ANKLE			FOOT		METATARSOPHALANGEAL JOINT				Proximal Interphalangeal joints		Distal Interphalangeal joints	
Flexion	Dorsiflex.	Plant flex.	Eversion	Inversion	Extension	Flexion	Abduction	Adduction	Extension	Flexion	Extension	Flexion
Sartorius												
Gracilis												
	Tib. ant.			Tib. ant.								
Popliteus												
	Ext. d. long.		Ext. d. long.		(2-5 dig.) Ext. d. long				(2-5 dig.) Ext. d. long		(2-5 dig.) Ext. d. long	
	Peroneus t.		Peroneus t.									
	Ext. hall. l.			Ext. hall. l.	Ext. hall. l.				Ext. hall. l.		Ext. hall. l.	
					(1-4 dig.) Ext. dig. br				(1-4 dig.) Ext. dig. br		(1-4 dig.) Ext. dig. br	
						(2-5 dig.) Flex. dig. br				(2-5 dig.) Flex. dig. br		
						Flex. hall. br.						
						2nd dig. Lumb. I			(2nd dig.) Lumb. I		(2nd dig.) Lumb. I	
							Abd. hall.					
		Peroneus l.	Peroneus l.									
		Peroneus b.	Peroneus b.									
		Tib. post.		Tib. post.								
Plantaris		Plantaris										
Semimemb.												
Semitend.												
		Flex. dig. l.		Flex. dig. l.		(2-5 dig.) Flex. dig. l				(2-5 dig.) Flex. dig. l		(2-5 dig.) Flex. dig. l
Bic., s.h.												
		Flex. hall. l.		Flex. hall. l.		Flex. hall. l.				Flex. hall. l.		Flex. hall. l.
		Soleus										
Bic., l.h.												
						(3-5 dig.) Lumb II-IV			(3-5 dig.) Lumb II-IV		(3-5 dig.) Lumb II-IV	
Gastroc.		Gastroc.										
						(2-4 dig.) Dor. int			(2-4 dig.) Dor. int		(2-4 dig.) Dor. int	
						(3-5 dig.) Plant. int			(3-5 dig.) Plant. int		(3-5 dig.) Plant. int	
							Abd. d. min.					
								Add. hall.				

Table A17.
Muscles Acting on the Hip Joint

Circumductors			
Flexors	Extensors	Abductors	Adductors
Iliopsoas	Gluteus maximus	Gluteus medius	Adductor magnus
Tensor fasciae latae	The three hams	Gluteus minimus	Adductor brevis
Sartorius	Adductor magnus	(Tensor fasciae latae)	Adductor longus
Pectineus	(ham part)		
		Piriformis	Pectineus
Rectus femoris		Sartorius	
Adductor longus			Gluteus maximus
Adductor brevis			
Adductor magnus			Short muscles
(Obt. part)			Obturator internus
			Gemelli
			Obturator externus
			Quadratus femoris

	Rotators	
	Medial	Lateral
	Gluteus medius	Gluteus maximus
	Gluteus minimus	Short muscles
	(Tensor fasciae latae)	Piriformis
		Obturator internus
		Gemelli
	Adductor magnus	Obturator externus
	(ham part)	Quadratus femoris
	Pectineus	Iliopsoas
	Upper adductor mass	

Table A18.
Muscles Acting upon the Knee Joint (All the Muscles That Cross It)

Nerve supply	Muscles	Accessory actions	Main actions
Sup. gluteal Inf. gluteal	Iliotibial tract T. fasciae latae Gluteus max. (part)	Retain knee in the extended position	
			Extensors
Femoral	Quadriceps femoris Rectus femoris V. intermedius V. lateralis V. medialis		
	Sartorius		Flexors
Obturator	Add. gracilis	Rotate leg medially	
Tibial division of sciatic	Semitendinosus Semimembranosus Popliteus		
	Gastrocnemius Plantaris		
	Biceps (long)		
Peroneal division of sciatic	Biceps (short)	Rotate leg laterally	

Table A19.
Segmental Innervation of Muscles of Hip and Thigh

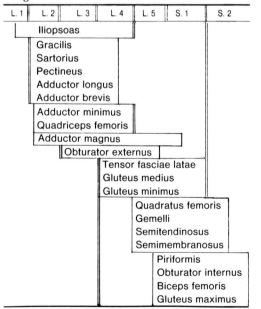

| L. 1 | L. 2 | L. 3 | L. 4 | L. 5 | S. 1 | S. 2 |

Iliopsoas
Gracilis
Sartorius
Pectineus
Adductor longus
Adductor brevis
Adductor minimus
Quadriceps femoris
Adductor magnus
Obturator externus
Tensor fasciae latae
Gluteus medius
Gluteus minimus
Quadratus femoris
Gemelli
Semitendinosus
Semimembranosus
Piriformis
Obturator internus
Biceps femoris
Gluteus maximus

* Modified after Bing, and Haymaker and Woodhall
[a] (From: J. V. Basmajian: *Grant's Method of Anatomy*. Baltimore, Williams & Wilkins.)

Table A20.
Muscles Acting on Ankle Joint

Plantarflexion	Dorsiflexion
1. Soleus	1. Tibialis anterior
2. Gastrocnemius	2. Extensor hallucis longus
3. Peroneus longus	
(4. Plantaris)	(3. Extensor digitorum longus and peroneus tertius)
(5. Peroneus brevis)	
(6. Tibialis posterior)	

Table A21.
Muscles Acting on Intertarsal Joints

Inversion	Eversion	Plantarflexion
1. Tibialis anterior	1. Peroneus longus	1. Peroneus longus
2. Tibialis posterior	2. Peroneus brevis	2. Tibialis posterior
	3. Peroneus tertius	3. Abductor hallucis
		4. Abductor digiti minimi
		5. Flexor digitorum brevis
		(6. Peroneus brevis)
		(7. Long flexor tendons to toes)
		(8. Lumbricals and quadratus plantae)

Table A22.
Segmental Innervation of Muscles of Leg and Foot[a]

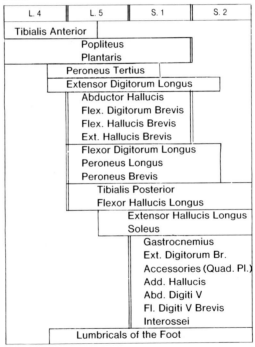

* Modified after Bing, and Haymaker and Woodhall

[a] (From: J. V. Basmajian: *Grant's Method of Anatomy.* Baltimore, Williams & Wilkins.)

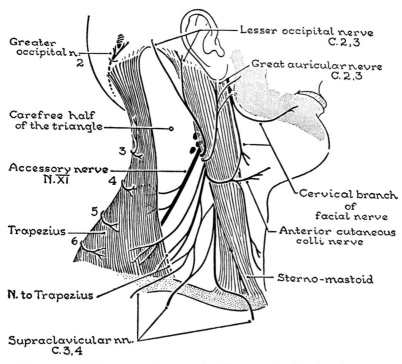

Figure A1. The superficial nerves of the neck. Of these, the facial and accessory are motor. (*Nerves of neck: anterior cutaneous = transverse.*) (From: J. V. Basmajian. *Grant's Method of Anatomy.* Baltimore, Williams & Wilkins.)

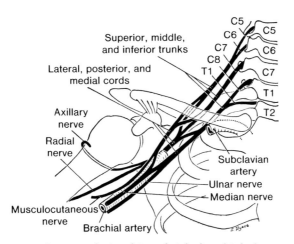

Figure A2. Course and main relationships of right brachial plexus (semischematic).

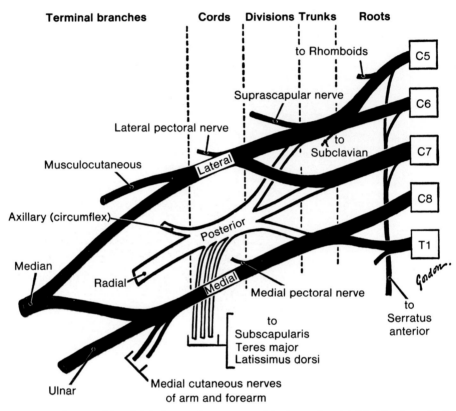

Figure A3. Scheme of brachial plexus, its parts, and its branches (right side, from in front).

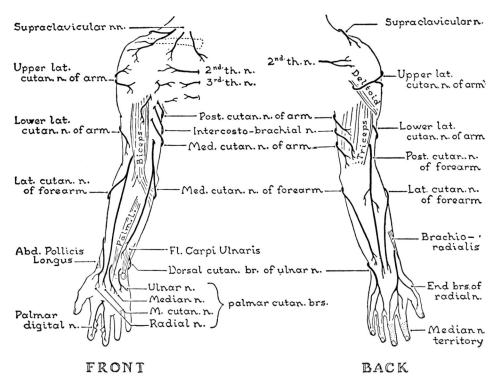

Supraclavicular nn.
Supraclavicular n.
Upper lat. cutan. n. of arm
2nd. th. n.
3rd. th. n.
2nd. th. n.
Deltoid
Upper lat. cutan. n. of arm
Lower lat. cutan. n. of arm
Post. cutan. n. of arm
Intercosto-brachial n.
Med. cutan. n. of arm
Biceps
Triceps
Lower lat. cutan. n. of arm
Post. cutan. n. of forearm
Lat. cutan. n. of forearm
Med. cutan. n. of forearm
Lat. cutan. n. of forearm
Palmaris
Brachio-radialis
Abd. Pollicis Longus
Fl. Carpi Ulnaris
Dorsal cutan. br. of ulnar n.
End brs. of radial n.
Ulnar n.
Median n.
M. cutan. n.
Radial n.
palmar cutan. brs.
Palmar digital n.
Median n. territory

FRONT   BACK

Figure A4.   The cutaneous nerves of the upper limb. (From: J. V. Basmajian: *Grant's Method of Anatomy.* Baltimore, Williams & Wilkins.)

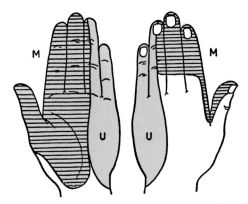

M   M
U   U

Figure A5.   Distribution of median and ulnar nerves in the hand. (From: J. V. Basmajian. *Grant's Method of Anatomy.* Baltimore, Williams & Wilkins.)

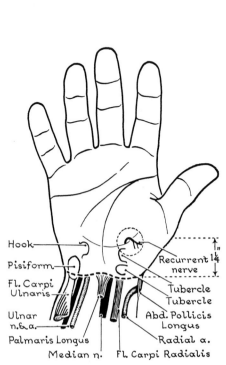

Hook

Pisiform

Fl. Carpi Ulnaris

Ulnar n. & a.

Palmaris Longus

Median n.

Recurrent 1¼" nerve

Tubercle

Tubercle

Abd. Pollicis Longus

Radial a.

Fl. Carpi Radialis

Figure A6.   Surface anatomy of the front of the wrist: a key position. (From: J. V. Basmajian: *Grant's Method of Anatomy.* Baltimore, Williams & Wilkins.)

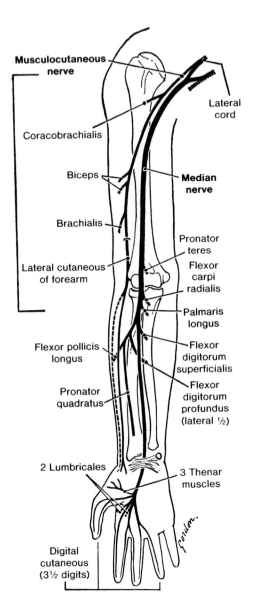

Musculocutaneous nerve

Coracobrachialis

Biceps

Brachialis

Lateral cutaneous of forearm

Flexor pollicis longus

Pronator quadratus

2 Lumbricales

Digital cutaneous (3½ digits)

Lateral cord

Median nerve

Pronator teres

Flexor carpi radialis

Palmaris longus

Flexor digitorum superficialis

Flexor digitorum profundus (lateral ½)

3 Thenar muscles

Figure A7.   Distribution of right musculocutaneous and median nerves (semischematic). (From: J. V. Basmajian: *Primary Anatomy.* Baltimore, Williams & Wilkins)

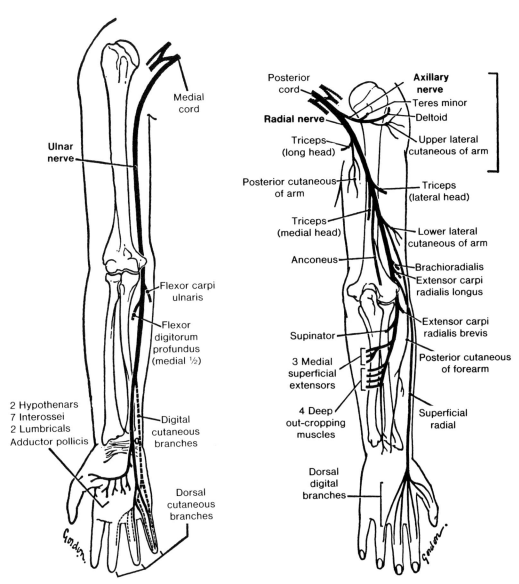

Figure A8.   Distribution of right ulnar nerve (semischematic). (From: J. V. Basmajian: *Primary Anatomy*. Baltimore, Williams & Wilkins).

Figure A9.   Distribution of right radial and circumflex (axillary) nerves (semischematic, from behind). (From: J. V. Basmajian: *Primary Anatomy*. Baltimore, Williams & Wilkins.)

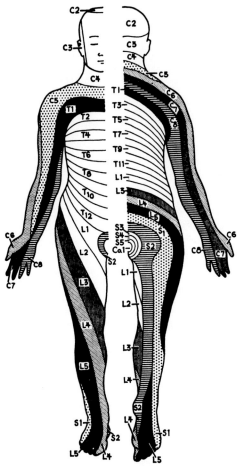

Figure A10.   Dermatomes: the strips of skin supplied by the various levels or segments of the spinal cord. (From: J. V. Basmajian: *Grant's Method of Anatomy*. Baltimore, Williams & Wilkins.)

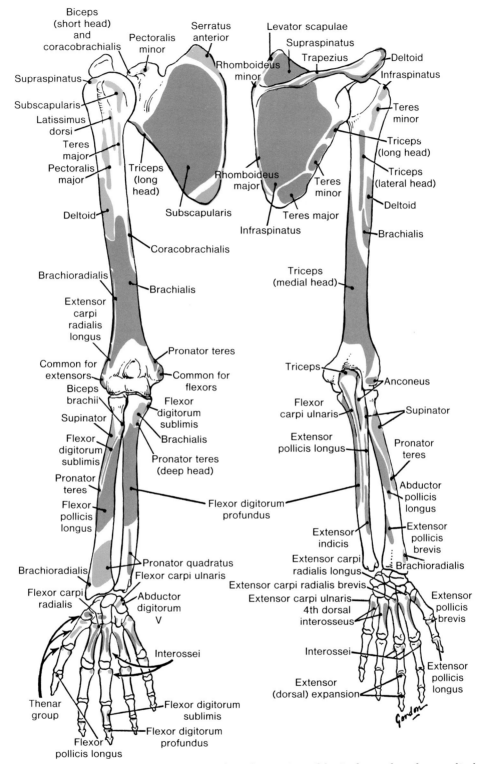

Figure A11.   Anterior view of origins (red) and insertions (blue) of muscles of upper limb.
Figure A12.   Posterior view of origins (red) and insertions (blue) of muscles of upper limb.

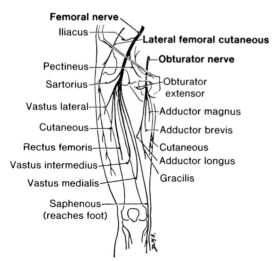

Figure A13. Nerves of front of thigh (From: J. V. Basmajian: *Primary Anatomy*. Baltimore, Williams & Wilkins.)

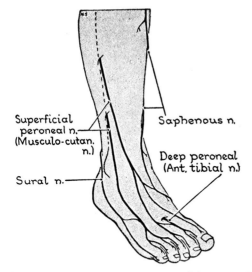

Figure A14. Cutaneous nerves of dorsum of foot. (From: J. V. Basmajian: *Grant's Method of Anatomy*. Baltimore, Williams & Wilkins)

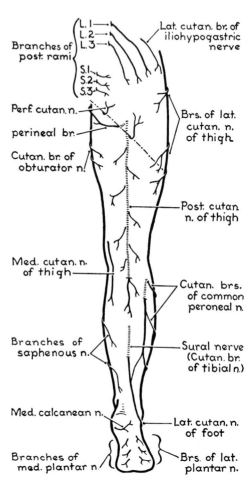

Figure A15. Cutaneous nerves of back of lower limb. (From: J. V. Basmajian: *Grant's Method of Anatomy*. Baltimore, Williams & Wilkins.)

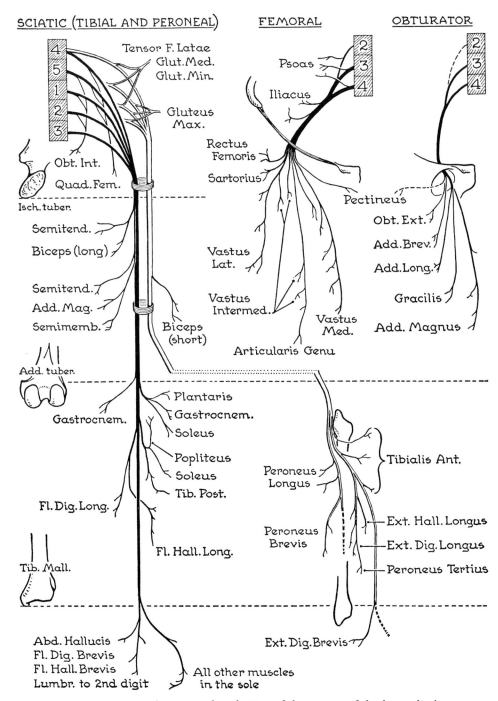

Figure A16.   The motor distribution of the nerves of the lower limb.

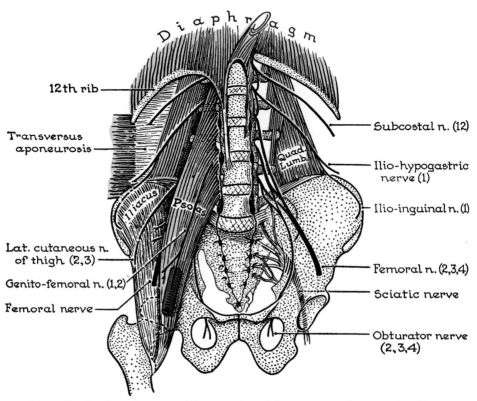

Figure A17.   The lumbar plexus and the muscles of the posterior abdominal wall. (From: J. V. Basmajian: *Grant's Method of Anatomy.* Baltimore, Williams & Wilkins.)

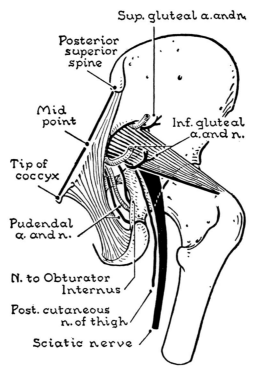

Sup. gluteal a. and n.

Posterior
superior
spine

Mid
point

Tip of
coccyx

Pudendal
a. and n.

Inf. gluteal
a. and n.

N. to Obturator
Internus

Post. cutaneous
n. of thigh

Sciatic nerve

Figure A18. Structures passing through the "door" to the gluteal region. (From: J. V. Basmajian: *Grant's Method of Anatomy*. Baltimore, Wilkins & Wilkins.)

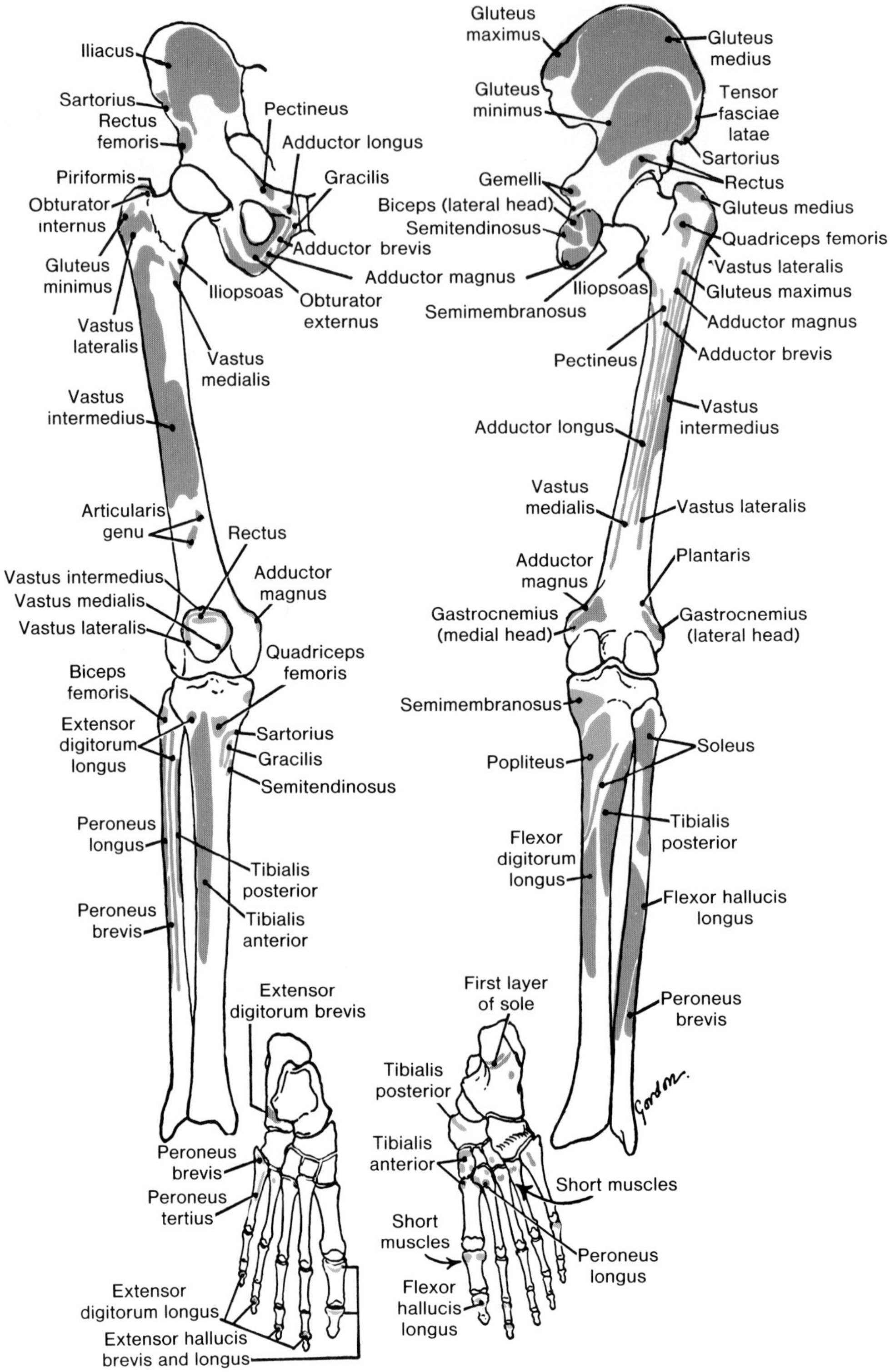

Figure A19. Anterior view of origins (red) and insertions (blue) of muscles of lower limb.
Figure A20. Posterior view of origins (red) and insertions (blue) of muscles of lower limb.

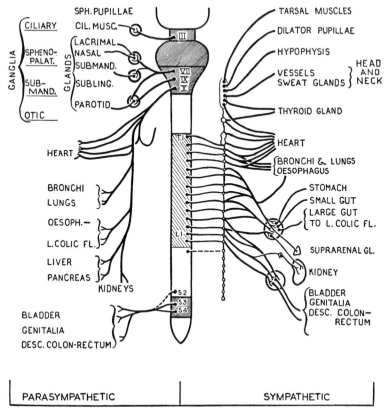

Figure A21.   General plan of the autonomic nervous system. (From: J. V. Basmajian: *Grant's Method of Anatomy.* Baltimore, Williams & Wilkins.)

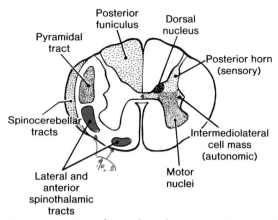

Figure A22.   Schematic cross-section of spinal cord. (From: J. V. Basmajian: *Grant's Method of Anatomy.* Baltimore, Williams & Wilkins.)

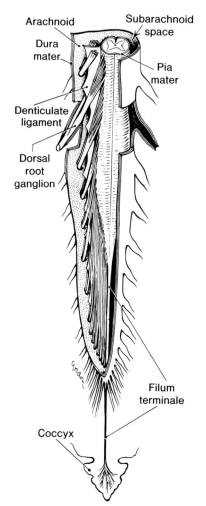

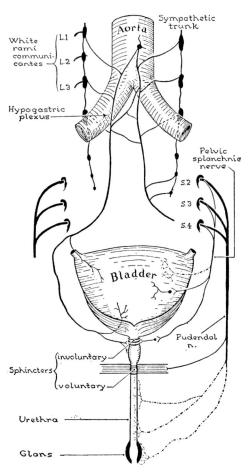

Figure A23. Cauda equina and spinal cord exposed from behind. On right side structures in subarachnoid space have been removed. (From: J. V. Basmajian: *Primary Anatomy.* Baltimore, Williams & Wilkins.)

Figure A24. Diagram of the nerve supply of the bladder and urethra. (From: J. V. Basmajian: *Grant's Method of Anatomy.* Baltimore, Williams & Wilkins)

Index

Page numbers in *italics* indicate figures. A t after the page number indicates a table.